Other monographs in the series, Major Problems in Clinical Surgery:

SOLID
LIVER
TUMORS

by

James H. Foster, M.D.

Director, Department of Surgery
Hartford Hospital
Hartford, Connecticut

and

Martin M. Berman, M.D.

Department of Pathology
Hartford Hospital
Hartford, Connecticut
Assistant Professor of Pathology
University of Connecticut Health Center
Farmington, Connecticut

Volume XXII in the Series
**MAJOR PROBLEMS IN
CLINICAL SURGERY**
PAUL A. EBERT, M.D.
Consulting Editor

W. B. Saunders Company, Philadelphia, London, Toronto, 1977

W. B. Saunders Company: West Washington Square
Philadelphia, Pa.   19105

1 St. Anne's Road
Eastbourne, East Sussex BN21 3UN, England

1 Goldthorne Avenue
Toronto, Ontario M8Z 5T9, Canada

Solid Liver Tumors   ISBN   0-7216-3824-4

Last digit is the print number: 9   8   7   6   5   4   3   2   1

To

J. ENGLEBERT DUNPHY, M.D.

and

IVAN L. BENNETT, JR., M.D.

Who taught so well the virtues of
hard work, hard facts, and a light touch.

Foreword

In the practice of surgery there are areas in which individuals have infrequent experience, and for this reason it is practically impossible to present a reasonable state of the art. This monograph concerning solid liver tumors represents almost a year's research and travel by the authors to obtain data from enough patients to derive conclusions which would have statistical significance. In certain instances the lesions are so rare that only case histories can offer any indication of outcome. This monograph represents the most extensive and detailed information on lesions of the liver that are rarely encountered, but when found, a source document such as this monograph will be of utmost importance.

PAUL A. EBERT, M.D.

Preface

An attempt has been made to draw together what is known about solid liver tumors and their treatment. Enough experience has accumulated during the first two decades since the anatomic basis of safe liver resection was established to allow conclusions and cautious optimism. Liver cancer in the adult and the child is often curable, and it is hoped that this book will encourage an aggressive approach to the diagnosis and management of patients with these rare lesions. The place of liver resection for metastatic cancer has been clarified, and the rapidly expanding field of study of benign liver tumors has been reviewed. By the time this monograph is published, I suspect that the information included about hepatocellular adenomas may be obsolete, but a start has been made. The book is largely based on data collected by visiting 98 hospitals across the United States of America to study the clinical histories, pathology, and postoperative course of patients undergoing resection of solid tumors of the liver.

The 1974 Liver Tumor Survey suffers from the inadequacies of any retrospective chart review, and it would have provided more useful information if all patients with liver tumors from each institution could have been studied. However, a large amount of data has been accumulated, and it is hoped that the advantages of a uniform look at this experience by two students of these diseases will in part offset the obvious deficiencies.

Whatever the scientific merit of this monograph may prove to be, it can certainly stand as an outstanding example of the willingness of the medical profession to share information openly and freely. This review would not have been possible without the cooperation of many hundreds of surgeons, pathologists, hospital administrators, medical record librarians, and tumor registrars across the country. Our debt to each of these is enormous, and I hope that they will derive some small satisfaction from seeing the work completed.

I would also like to express my thanks to the Directors of the Hartford Hospital for their financial support of the travel costs of this study and to the administration and staff of the Hospital for their patience and support during its completion.

Finally, gratitude beyond the power of words to convey must be paid: (1) to Cathy White, Clinical Librarian, for assistance in collecting the reported experience of others; (2) to Margaret Foster, Research Assistant for help in organizing and analyzing the data; and (3) to Joan Lively, Tama Zimmerman, and, most particularly Mary Beth O'Brien for making those many phone calls, typing hundreds of letters, and preparing the drafts and final manuscript.

JAMES H. FOSTER, M.D.
MARTIN M. BERMAN, M.D.

Contents

Chapter One

INTRODUCTION AND GENERAL CONSIDERATIONS

INTRODUCTION AND GENERAL CONSIDERATIONS

Three decades after the giant steps forward taken in surgical care as a result of the experiences of World War II, and two decades after the pioneering contributions of Pack,[7] Lortat-Jacob,[5] and Quattlebaum,[8] liver resection now seems firmly established as an operation that can be undertaken on an emergency or elective basis with a reasonable expectation that the patient will survive the operation and postoperative course. Yet experience with liver resection for solid tumors is very limited in the U.S. — largely because of the rarity of primary solid tumors and the reluctance of surgeons to resect deposits of metastatic cancer. Ong,[6] Lin,[4] Tung,[9] Honjo,[3] Balasegaram,[1] and other Asian surgeons have reported large series of liver resections for primary liver cancer in adults, but their experience is limited to malignant tumors of childhood, benign tumors, and metastatic disease.

Most of the critical questions about liver tumors still remain unanswered. What causes neoplastic change in a noncirrhotic liver? Do the primary tumors that occur in the noncirrhotic livers of "western" patients behave differently from the more common tumors that occur in parts of Asia and Africa? Are birth control pills and other drugs carcinogenic, or is it just that certain liver tumors occur in the same population as the one that takes contraceptive medication? What is the best way to find and diagnose the various types of liver tumors? Is primary liver cancer ever curable by resection? What are the criteria that determine resectability and/or curability? Should metastatic cancer in the liver be excised? Can relief of symptoms from hormone-producing endocrine tumors be achieved by palliative resection of liver metastasis? Are there methods short of resection that can be used to slow the growth of either primary or secondary liver tumors? What are the techniques by which a mass lesion can be resected safely from this very vascular organ? And so on.

No Western surgeon or physician has a sufficiently wide experience with liver tumors and their resection to provide reliable answers to these and other questions. Published reports tend to emphasize only one or, at best, a few limited aspects of the subject—such as operative technique, pathologic classification, or specific etiologic or geographic factors—and there is a paucity of long-term survival information.

What was needed was a way to draw together the experience of several centers—to pool information, to form a "critical mass." National cooperative surveys for several diseases have been made by mailed questionnaire, but the classification, and even the nomenclature, of liver tumors and liver operations varied a great deal from institution to institution. A decision was reached, therefore, to study first-hand patient records and the gross and microscopic appearance of patients' liver tumors by a series of personal visits.

The Directors, Administrators, and Surgical Staff of Hartford Hospital were generous enough to grant time and funds sufficient to allow me to visit a number of hospitals around the U.S. during 1974. Thanks to the extraordinary cooperation of many old and new friends, a large amount of information was gathered. This monograph is written to explore what was learned from that survey and from a study of the reported experience of others. The lessons of that analysis have been tempered by a modest personal experience with liver tumors and liver resection, and refined by the association of a skilled pathologist.

The resulting format may be confusing to the reader in that new information is intermingled freely with reported experiences. Certain conventions have been chosen to simplify the reader's task, and much of the patient data has been relegated to appendices at the end of the book. There remain in the chapters that follow, however, more tables and more numbers than are usually acceptable to a reader looking for straightforward information to help him care for a particular patient. This surfeit of statistical data perhaps is justified on the grounds that much confusion still exists about the nomenclature of diseases and operations for solid tumors of the liver. By assembling a wide base of factual data, we hope to build a solid platform upon which a clinical decision can be made today and upon which others can rest new information in the future.

To limit our task, we have excluded from further consideration simple cysts, hemangiomas, tumors of the major extrahepatic bile ducts and their bifurcation, and bile duct adenomas (hamartomas).

Perhaps the most exciting new development in the care of patients with liver tumor is total hepatectomy with transplantation. Patients with carcinoma who received liver transplants were purposely excluded from the 1974 Liver Tumor Survey in order to limit the scope of our project. The current status of patients transplanted for tumor is briefly summarized in Chapter Twelve.

In general, the pathologic classification of primary tumors that we have chosen follows that recommended by Edmondson in his 1958 Armed Forces Institute of Pathology Fascicle 25.[2] Chapters Four through Seven discuss the major groups of primary solid tumors—i.e., primary epithelial carcinoma in adults, primary epithelial carcinoma in children, primary benign tumors, and a miscellaneous group into which were placed the cystadenomas, cystadenocarcinomas, primary sarcomas, hamartomas, and malignant vascular tumors. Separate chapters are devoted to secondary liver tumors that have involved the liver by embolic metastasis (Chapter 8) or by direct invasion (Chapter 10). The chapters on specific types of tumor are preceded by a brief summary of the historical aspects of liver resection for solid tumor (Chapter 2) and by a discussion of the current status of diagnostic techniques (Chapter 3). The final chapters of the monograph are devoted to the techniques of liver resection, and to a review of the literature on the results achieved by transplantation and by nonresectional therapy of primary and secondary liver tumors.

METHODS

TERMINOLOGY

of Pathology

Specific discussions of the nomenclature of various primary tumors of the liver will be included in the several chapters that follow, but certain general guidelines have been chosen. The more cumbersome prefixes "hepatocellular" and "cholangiocellular" have been used, rather than the simpler "liver cell" and "bile duct" proposed by Edmondson,[2] for two reasons. First, the phrase "bile duct carcinoma" brings to the mind of most surgeons a tumor of the major extrahepatic biliary ducts, whereas "cholangiocellular carcinoma" or the shorter (and interchangeable) "cholangiocarcinoma" means a solid intrahepatic mass lesion originating in smaller ducts. Second, we have chosen the longer adjectives because past and present usage and proposed national and international classification systems seem to favor the Latin-rooted terms. The word "hepatoma" is ambiguous and confusing and is not used. The two major categories of epithelial tumors of childhood are called "hepatoblastoma" and "hepatocellular carcinoma" corresponding with the most prevalent current usage.

The adjective "mixed" has been used in various ways by different pathologists. For tumors of adults, "mixed" is used hereafter to mean a combination of hepatocellular and cholangiocellular elements in the same lesion, a rare circumstance, but one that will be considered in Chapter Four. "Mixed" has been used when referring to tumors of childhood to describe tumors made up of mixed epithelial and mesenchymal elements. We have placed all these lesions under the heading of "hepatoblastoma" and, to avoid confusion, we have not used the adjective "mixed" when discussing pediatric tumors.

of Operation

Right and left "lobectomy" refers to the removal of approximately one-half of the mass of the liver by division through the central plane, defined by the distribution of the portal venous branches and major bile ducts. "Extended" lobectomy refers to the inclusion of any significant part of the contralateral lobe together with a regular lobectomy. With the exception of left lateral segmentectomy, all other partial lobectomies, however large, are referred to in this book as "wedge" resections. The term "hemihepatectomy" is not used, and removal of the liver to the left of the umbilical fissure is called "left lateral segmentectomy."

of Survival

An "operative death" is defined as any death within 30 days of liver resection, or at any time prior to hospital discharge if directly related to the operation. Long-term survival is listed in the many tables that follow, using four abbreviations. "AFD" means that the patient was alive and free of any evidence of disease at the time of the last follow-up; "AWD" means alive with disease evident; "DWD" means dead with disease. In a few instances patients with known residual tumor died of other causes, but they have all been included under the category "DWD." "DOD" means dead without evidence of disease. Not all of these patients were autopsied, but there was no evidence of tumor when the patient died of some other obvious cause, usually long after liver resection.

Survival figures are actual rather than actuarial. For example: if

100 patients were operated upon and 90 survived the operation, two-year survival figures are calculated by constructing a fraction, the numerator of which is the number of patients living 24 months or longer, and the denominator of which is 90, minus the number of patients alive at less than 24 months and minus the number of patients lost to follow-up.

1974 LIVER TUMOR SURVEY – METHODS

Personal visits were made to 98 hospitals in 48 cities in 28 states and the District of Columbia to collect information about patients undergoing liver resection for solid tumors. Figure 1–1 notes the location of these cities, and Appendix I lists the hospitals visited and the names of the primary sponsors in each hospital who coordinated the visit. The hospitals were selected by the surgeon-author for the following reasons: (1) proximity to Hartford, Connecticut; (2) proximity to professional meetings attended during 1974; (3) the presence of friends of the surgeon-author or of reporters of significant experience with liver tumors; and (4) the willingness of the institution to allow a visit.

Letters were written to each of the primary sponsors requesting permission to review the records of patients who had undergone resection for solid tumors in their institution since the year of 1960. Refusals were rare and usually were based either on an inability of busy Record Room personnel to promise the required extra effort or on the intention of the institution to publish its own study of this subject. Assurances were made to each institution that their contribution would be recognized and that the confidentiality of surgeon, patient, and the institution would be respected. The administrative requirements necessary to effect permission varied a great deal from institution to institution. In some cases this was done quite informally with the Chief of Surgery, and in others it required the action of multiple decision-making bodies within the hospital.

After receiving initial approval, the surgeon-author wrote to the Medical Record Librarian, the Chief of Pathology, and the Tumor Registrar in each institution, and phone calls were made to confirm the final details of the proposed visit.

When record selection was based upon coded pathologic diagnosis, the review process proved to be inefficient because of the large number of pathologic categories, the confusion in terminology of primary tumors, and the fact that most patients with biopsy-proof of primary and secondary liver carcinoma never came to resection. A selection process based on the coded diagnosis of "liver resection" proved to be

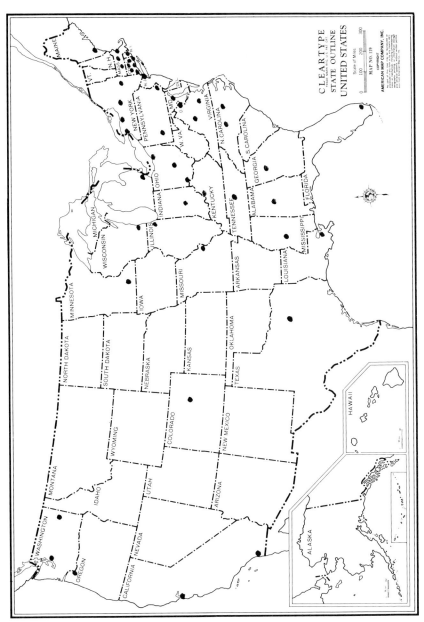

Figure 1–1. Cities visited during the 1974 Liver Tumor Survey.

more efficient. Patients who had undergone resection for liver cyst, hemangioma, bile duct adenoma (hamartoma), abscess, hydatid disease, trauma, and other non-neoplastic diseases were excluded. However, patients with mesenchymal hamartomas, cystadenomas, and cystadeno-carcinomas were included. From the hospital records for each patient with a resected tumor, a flow sheet was prepared that contained information on age, sex, preoperative symptoms, physical examination, laboratory and other diagnostic tests, the details of operation, surgical pathology, the postoperative course, and the post-hospitalization follow-up. The histologic sections and any available gross photographs of the tumor were reviewed in the Pathology Department of the involved hospital, and, finally, the Tumor Registry was visited to obtain the most current follow-up information.

In many cases further follow-up information was obtained by letter or phone call to the involved physician, and in several instances a Tumor Registrar has kept the surgeon-author informed about the later course of a patient since the end of the survey.

Often there were several hundred charts waiting for review from which only a few cases were found to be suitable for inclusion in the survey. In other hospitals most of the available records were usable. There was no guarantee given by any institution or by the author that all cases of liver resection for solid tumor would be included in the survey. The selection was entirely random, depending on whatever the Record Room could make available on the day of the surgeon-author's visit. Therefore, the study may suffer both from the inadequacies of an incomplete sample, and from our policy of including only *resected* liver tumors rather than the whole experience with resected and nonre-sected neoplasms.

In this fashion more than 650 abstracts were prepared, from which a subsequent review process selected 621 for final inclusion. Twelve hospitals or group clinics contributed more than ten cases, and 36 other institutions contributed between five and ten cases. The records of three large private clinics (Lahey, Cleveland, and Mayo) were analyzed in the Clinic offices, and then subsequent visits were made to the associated hospitals to study the pathology. Through the great kindness of Dr. Irving Ariel, permission was obtained to review the files of the George Pack Foundation in New York City where the operative, pathology, and office-visit records of many patients were made available for analysis. However, the complete hospital record and histologic slides were not available for this one group of patients, and most of these cases were not included in the survey unless the available record provided a clear and unequivocal picture of the problem and its outcome.

After the visits were completed, each participating hospital was asked to send to the pathologist-author the histologic material on all primary liver tumors. Great cooperation was received, and Dr. Berman has had a chance to review the vast majority of primary liver tumors. Although skilled in the diagnosis of liver tumors before the survey began, Dr. Berman found that the unusual privilege of reviewing a large number of cases brought together at one time allowed him to achieve a perspective that matured as his experience grew. Review and re-review resulted in the final categorization that formed the solid basis on which the remainder of this monograph rests.

An initial pathologic classification was made of all the primary liver tumors, and then clinical correlations were made that will be discussed in the following chapters. Dr. Berman has organized and written most of the pathology information included in Chapters Four through Seven.

Several cases previously reported in the literature have been reviewed and included in the 1974 LTS. Whenever this is known to be so, the cases have been cross-referenced in the text of this monograph. Those cases not previously reported will remain anonymous. Their inclusion in this book should not compromise their availability for study and reporting by others.

As the voluminous literature on liver tumors and their resection, which dated back as far as 1879, was reviewed and abstracted, certain liberties were taken. Using modern criteria for pathologic classification and the knowledge gained from the 1974 LTS, we have retrospectively reinterpreted data and reclassified names given to specific tumors and operations in several instances. Whether this somewhat presumptuous activity can be justified by the privilege of hindsight will have to be decided by the reader. The following chapters will identify original references that can be rechecked by the doubtful.

REFERENCES

1. Balasegaram, M.: Hepatic surgery: a review of a personal series of 95 major resections. Aust. N. Z. J. Surg. *42*:1, 1972.
2. Edmondson, H. A.: Tumors of the Liver and Intrahepatic Bile Ducts. Section VII — Fascicle 25, Atlas of Tumor Pathology. Armed Forces Institute of Pathology, 1958.
3. Honjo, I., and Mizumoto, R.: Primary carcinoma of the liver. Am. J. Surg. *128*:31, 1974.
4. Lin, T. Y.: Primary cancer of the liver, quadrennial review. Scand. J. Gastroenterol. (Suppl.) *6*:223, 1970.
5. Lortat-Jacob, J. L., and Robert, H. G.: Hepatectomie droite régleé. Presse Med. *60*:549, 1952.
6. Ong, G. B., and Leong, C. H.: Surgical treatment of primary liver cancer. J. R. Coll. Surg. *14*:42, 1969.
7. Pack, G. T., and Baker, H. W.: Total right hepatic lobectomy; report of a case. Ann. Surg. *138*:253, 1953.
8. Quattlebaum, J. K.: Massive resection of the liver. Ann. Surg. *137*:787, 1952.
9. Tung, T. T.: Chirurgié d'exérèe du foie. Hanoi, 1962.

Chapter Two

HIGHLIGHTS IN THE HISTORY OF LIVER TUMORS AND THEIR RESECTION

INTRODUCTION

The history of our knowledge of liver tumors and the surgeon's role in their therapy can be separated into three major eras. The first dates from ancient times to about 1880. Information was anecdotal, and operation was only done on an emergency basis when a traumatic wound or an unexpected finding forced the surgeon's hand. The second or middle era began with that great burst of activity that occurred in all types of abdominal surgery in the 1880s and continued until World War II. Operations on the liver were done electively for the first time. However, cases were rare, follow-up information was incomplete, techniques were not based on anatomy, and, in the absence of a sound pathologic classification, the consolidation of knowledge was difficult. Although little progress was made in the surgery of the liver between World Wars I and II, it was a productive period for consolidation of earlier experiences, and this chapter owes a great debt to those English-language encyclopedists of a more leisurely era who searched and documented what had gone before.

The third or modern era of liver surgery began with the lessons of

9

World War II, a better understanding of the vascular anatomy of the liver, and with successful reports of major hepatic lobectomy by Lortat-Jacob, Pack, and others. Although 30 years have gone by since the war we are still at the beginning of this modern era. This monograph is written to summarize how far we have advanced in the first century of liver resection.

THE ANCIENT ERA

The ancient Babylonians, 2000 years before Christ, created accurate models of the surface anatomy of animal livers (Fig. 2–1) and apparently used the livers of sacrificed animals to foretell the future. Hippocrates understood the seriousness of a liver wound, and the thoughts of Galen and Celsus about the liver as a nutritional storehouse were not far from the truth as we know it today.[41, 55] Paulus Aeginata is said to have cauterized protruding portions of the human liver after eviscerating injuries in the seventh century A.D.[55] Francis Glisson in his *Anatomia*

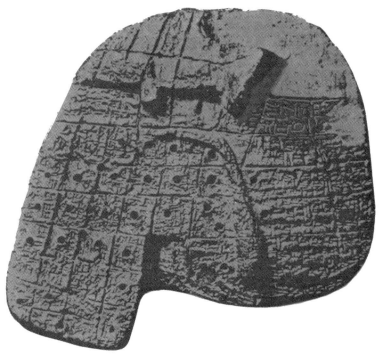

Figure 2–1.   Clay model of a sheep's liver, used in Babylonia about 2000 B. C. (British Museum).

Hepatis, published in London (1654), accurately portrayed the essential anatomy of the major vessels of the liver.[21]

The first documented case of removal of a portion of the human liver was recorded in 1716 by Berta, who treated a madman with a self-inflicted knife wound of the right hypochondrium through which part of the right lobe of the liver had prolapsed. On the day following injury Berta amputated the protruding portion, and the patient recovered.[11] John Thomson in his *Report after Waterloo* noted after one battle "twelve cases of wounds of the liver, in which considerable progress toward recovery had been made before our return from Belgium."[58] MacPherson (1846) reported a case of ligation and excision of a small portion of liver that was protruding from an abdominal spear wound in an aged Hindu, and cited a reference to another report of a soldier who had forceps removal of a small piece of his liver from a sword wound in 1688.[46] Samuel Cooper discussed liver wounds in his 1850 textbook of surgery and, although he noted that a serious wound of the liver was as bad as a heart wound, he also observed that bile leakage from liver wounds did not always have a fatal consequence.[41]

It is apparent that some of these early patients survived liver trauma, but it is not nearly so clear that the surgeons' effort contributed positively to the occasional happy outcome. The liver was too soft and too bloody an organ to deal with deliberately until better techniques had been worked out for the control of hemorrhage and peritoneal infection.

THE MIDDLE PERIOD

With the great advances pioneered by Morton in anesthesiology, by Pasteur in bacteriology, and by Lister in antisepsis came a reasonable chance for patient survival after elective opening of the abdominal cavity. The brilliant flowering of surgery in Germany and Austria under the leadership of Billroth, Bruns, von Mikulicz, and others that occurred in the decade beginning in 1880 saw a rapid advance in all types of abdominal operations. The first successful gastrectomy was done by Billroth in 1881, and the first cholecystectomy by Langenbuch in 1882. The liver, however, was so "friable, so full of gaping vessels, and so evidentally incapable of being sutured that it had always seemed impossible to successfully manage large wounds of its substance."[16] The tradition of animal experimentation soon became firmly established in the great European schools of Surgery, however, and the liver received considerable attention. Tillmans (1879),[80] Glück (1883),[22] Ponfick (1890),[63] and von Meister (1890)[56] developed the principles of liver resection in rabbits, cats and dogs and proved that transection of liver substance with survival was possible and that the liver had an amazing capacity to regenerate to replace resected volume.

In 1876, Kelsch and Kiener found only two cases of primary liver cancer,[35] but by 1901 Eggel of Munich was able to tabulate 160 cases of primary carcinoma from which he described microscopic features, types of metastasis, and the tendency of primary cancer to form tumor thrombi in large vessels.[15] The contributions of Hanot and Gilbert (1888) and Yamagawa (1911) were also important in establishing the pathologic basis of the modern classification of primary tumors (see Chapter 4).[26, 91]

Priority for the first elective formal liver resection is difficult to establish with certainty. The years 1886 to 1888 saw several papers published with descriptions of liver resection. Lius excised a solid tumor by ligating and cutting through a pedicled left lobe "adenoma" in November 1886. Attempts to suture the severed pedicle to the abdominal wall were unsuccessful, and the stump was returned to the abdomen. Death due to hemorrhage from the stump occurred six hours later.[40] Keen wondered whether the tumor removed by Lius was a constricted lobe rather than a true neoplasm.[32] It is perhaps just as likely that Lius' tumor was a malignant tumor, since the word "adenoma" had a very different usage in that era and often represented a localized malignant lesion by current criteria. The tumor was yellow-white, lobulated, and showed numerous septa from a fibrous capsule. The rest of the liver was described as normal.[40]

In 1888 Carl Von Langenbuch reported that he had successfully resected a pedicled tumor of the left lobe.[39] His patient was a 30-year-old woman who was hospitalized with diffuse erysipelas and who had suffered abdominal pain for eight years since her first pregnancy, at which time she discarded her tightly-laced corset and never used it again. At operation Langenbuch found that the epigastric mass that had been palpable preoperatively was a deformed left lobe with a constriction in the area of previous corset-pressure. Because he knew of a successful treatment of a right-sided deformed lobe by von Hacker of Vienna the previous year, Langenbuch went ahead and ligated the constricted area with several sutures, removed a 370 gm tumor, and returned the stump to the abdomen. (In 1886 von Hacker had indeed reported a case of constricted lobe of the liver, but apparently this tumor was fixed to the abdominal wall and not removed by Billroth.)[25] During the evening following operation, Langenbuch's patient fainted and had signs of internal bleeding that required reoperation for control of hemorrhage. She had a long and difficult postoperative course with development of ascites, but eventually recovered and was discharged. Langenbuch felt that the tumor was secondary to the tight constriction of the corset and to the release of this constriction during the eight years prior to operation. A subsequent editorial in the Lancet took note of the significance of what was thought to be the first successful planned liver resection, but also used the opportunity to decry the use of constrictive corsets.[66] Langenbuch's patient had indeed worn a tightly-laced corset, but she had discarded it eight years before the operation. This circumstance led the Lancet editorialist to the theory that it was the omission of tight lacing after a period of constriction that resulted in tumor formation, and led him also to the melancholy conclusion that, once the evil habit of corset-wearing was adopted, it had to be kept up if serious consequences were to be avoided. In the light of what we know today, one wonders whether this "corset-tumor" was really a liver cell adenoma (see Chapter 6).

Carl Garrè, reporting his own case of successful removal of an Echinococcus cyst in 1888, also cited three patients previously cared for by his chief, Prof. Victor von Bruns of Breslau.[20] The first case was that of a soldier who was wounded in the last days of the Franco-Prussian War of 1870–71. Bruns removed a small piece of liver that had prolapsed through an exit wound, and the patient was able to rejoin his regiment within two months. The second case was that of a 50-year-old man who had excision and cauterization of a small nodule of metastatic cancer from the edge of the right lobe. The patient survived the operation but the ultimate outcome was uncertain. Bruns' third patient was a lady with an Echinococcus cyst.

Many had aspirated echinococcal cysts in the 1870s, but it was Lawson Tait in 1880 who first made a formal entry into a cyst, drained its contents, and then sutured the cyst wound to the abdominal wall.[72] One year later he reported his sixth such operation,[73] and J. Knowsley Thorton and several others had reported various techniques of direct attack on echinococcal cysts of the liver in the 1880s, well before Garrè's report.[77]

L. McLane Tiffany of Baltimore gave the first American report of removal of a liver "tumor," but his description was very brief. His patient was a 25-year-old farmer with a history of four years of abdominal pain and chills, and the tumor was made up of biliary calculi and debris, suggesting residuals of stone disease rather than neoplasia. Tiffany excised this walnut-sized mass from the convex surface of the left lobe with curved scissors, and cauterized the wound.[78] He apparently was well prepared for this procedure (perhaps through studying the lessons of the European masters) because earlier in 1890 he had concluded in a paper on "Surgery of the Liver" that:

1. The surgery of the liver is to be considered as is the surgery of the rest of the body, not as surgery apart from everything else.
2. The liver may be cut, portions of it excised, tumors removed, bleeding arrested, and probably the flow of bile stopped, by means at present in the hands of the surgeon.

3. Inasmuch as the liver is an abdominal organ, rigid cleanliness must be observed lest peritoneal inflammation follow.

4. The portion of the liver subjected to operation should be shut off as soon as possible by suture or other methods from the general peritoneal cavity and healing induced by appropriate treatment.[79]

To W. W. Keen goes credit for the first report of the removal of a true neoplasm in the U.S. In the fall of 1892 he resected a 3½-inch cystic tumor from the edge of the right lobe of a 31-year-old white female. His description of the operation reflects an early appreciation of the usefulness of blunt technique. When the cautery led him into the wrong dissection plane he used his thumbnail to complete the dissection and resection of this tumor, which William H. Welch and Ewing both confirmed as a cystadenoma of biliary epithelium.[31] In addition to the cystadenoma, Dr. Keen resected an angioma in 1897 and a large primary carcinoma of the left lobe in 1899.

William Williams Keen was born in Philadelphia in 1837, graduated from Brown University and Jefferson Medical College, and served as a military physician in the Civil War with S. Weir Mitchell and George R. Morehouse. He continued his education in Europe, observing Langenbeck in Berlin and other surgical greats including Velpeau, Nelaton, Billroth, and the pathologist, Cohnheim. He returned to Philadelphia, where he served as Professor of Anatomy at the Pennsylvania College of Fine Arts (1876 to 1890) and Professor of Surgery at Women's Medical College (1884–1889). He edited Gray's Anatomy (1887) and did original work on the brain and other new areas of surgery. In 1889 he assumed the chairmanship of the Jefferson Medical College Department of Surgery and served with great distinction in that position until his retirement in 1907, when he was cited by his pupil DaCosta as the first man in American surgery.[10]

A man of boundless energy, Keen was respected by all who knew him as a superb craftsman, an innovator, a prolific writer and worker, and a medical statesman. He was president of the American Surgical Association, the American Medical Association, and several other medical organizations, and was presented with an honorary degree at the first Congress of the American College of Surgeons which was held in 1913.[51] He died in 1932 at the age of 95 years, revered as the Dean of American medicine.

Keen's first patient in 1891 was a 31-year-old mother-of-six with a right abdominal mass known to have been enlarging for two years. Preoperative evaluation led to a diagnosis of floating kidney for the fist-sized movable mass. Assisted by Dr. William J. Taylor and J. Chalmers DaCosta, Keen discovered a 3½-inch tumor hanging off the edge of the right lobe on a broad pedicle. Using the Paquelin cautery, individual ties for large veins, and his thumbnail, he quickly removed the tumor with the loss of only six to eight ounces of blood. Glass tube drainage was discontinued after 48 hours, and the patient's recovery was complicated only by a recurrence of malaria. She was kept in bed three weeks and discharged well 42 days after the operation.[31] When last reported, seven years later, she was still free of symptoms or other evidence of recurrent disease.[33]

Keen's second patient was a 53-year-old woman who had increasing symptoms associated with an epigastric mass known to be present for at least three years. At operation in 1897, a 7.5 cm angiomatous tumor with large feeding vessels was found on the lower edge of the left lateral segment of the liver. Fearing hemorrhage from attempts to excise the tumor, Keen cut through normal liver substance on either side of the tumor to develop a pedicle. He then placed a rubber tube around the base of the pedicle and drew it up as tightly as possible. The tumor was exteriorized and the wound closed around the pedicle. Six days later the tube was removed and the pedicle transected "without the loss of a drop of blood."[32] The patient had an uneventful course and was well more than two years later.[33]

Keen's third patient was a 50-year-old Englishman who had suffered several months of abdominal pain, anorexia, and weight loss when he was admitted to Jefferson Medical College Hospital in 1899. A large primary carcinoma involving most of the left lobe was found at operation, but there was no evidence of any disease in the right lobe or in the rest of the abdomen. Assisted again by Dr. DaCosta, Keen used the cautery and five catgut ligatures to transect the left lobe with the loss of only 8 to 10 ounces of blood. The patient did well after operation except for vomiting, which was unresponsive to ice, champagne, cocaine, and carbolic acid therapy.[33] Unfortunately the tumor recurred and death followed operation by five months.[3]

Keen admitted that during the third operation: "at no time was I anxious as to any particular hemorrhage, though I confess I was in constant dread lest alarming and possibly uncontrollable hemorrhage might occur; and I was conscious of a sigh of relief when the last portion of tissue had been cut through and the tumor lay free in my grasp without any notable loss of blood."[33] Three weeks later when he reported this case to the Pennsylvania State Medical Society at Johnstown, his confidence had increased, and he was ready to say: "in fact, after my experience with these three cases, I should hardly hesitate to attack almost any hepatic tumor without regard to its size."[33]

After each of these three resections, Keen published a separate paper developing his thoughts about liver resection. A unique feature of these three papers was the appended list (developed by successive assistants) which tabulated all the experience reported throughout the world. By 1899 this list had grown to 76 cases. Careful retrospective analysis of these case reports 77 years later still leaves uncertainty about the exact nature of many of the resected lesions. Most were benign, chiefly syphilitic gummata and echinococcal cysts, but as many as 30 may have been solid neoplasms. Some of the solid tumors were metastatic to the liver, but most were probably primary, and undoubtedly several were malignant by present criteria. Of the patients with solid tumors in Keen's collection only one had prolonged survival, and the nature of that tumor was uncertain.

Priorities for first operations performed for different diseases are difficult to establish with certainty in spite of a careful literature search. Probably Lücke (1891) resected the first cancer.[45] Although Kehr doubted the malignancy of this lesion and thought it may have been a gumma,[34] the patient died eight years after wedge resection of a fist-sized tumor, presumably from recurrence.[92] Yeomans tabulated all known patients operated upon for primary liver cancer in 1909, and completed this list in 1915 with a second article.[92, 93] Sir Berkeley Moynihan, in his 1914 *Abdominal Operations*, stated that he knew of no instance of successful extirpation of a primary cancer of the liver.[59]

The first metastatic carcinoma was probably resected by Bruns (see above),[19] and Grey Turner resected a metastatic tumor in 1894.[84] Many early partial liver resections for gallbladder carcinoma were done prior to 1900. Sheinfeld in a collected review (1947) cited 18 cases treated during the 19th century,[70] including early reports of Watson and Mayo Robson. Paschal reported drainage of a liver abscess in 1879,[55] and there were many other reports of trocar or open drainage within the next five years. Cysts of the liver were drained by Gloz (1864) and North (1882), and resected by Cousins (1874) and Kaltenbach (1885).[30] Konig (1889) treated an 11-year-old girl with a huge multiloculated cystic tumor that was lined with columnar epithelium. The patient was alive and well one year after removal of the cyst. Although the young age of this patient is quite atypical (see Chapter 7), this may be the first reported case of surgical management of a cystadenoma. Keen (1892) and Muller (1891) also successfully resected cystadenomas, and their patients were alive without signs of recurrence six and eight years after operation respectively.[30]

Although primary carcinoma was recognized in infants and children in the 19th century, and was fairly well defined pathologically by Yamagiwa and others as early as 1911, resection of a child's liver for cancer was rarely done. Griffith (1918) collected 57 cases of primary liver cancer in children, but only one resection had been attempted.[24] This was done by Castle in 1914 who operated upon a 10½-month-old male with a tumor that had been known to be present for five months. He resected a 651 gm pedicled malignant tumor by wedge excision, but unfortunately the patient died 16 days later with acute gastroenteritis.[6]

The first liver resections had been done for trauma, and the traumatized liver continued to demand more of the surgeon's attention than did the tumorous liver at the end of the 19th century, as it still does today. Edler reported a series of patients with liver trauma in 1887 who had an over-all mortality rate of 66 per cent.[13] Terrier and Auvray collected 45 trauma cases, all submitted to operation, with a mortality rate of 31 per cent (1896).[74] Benjamin Tilton collected ten years' experience with liver trauma in New York City hospitals (1895–1905) and found 25 cases. His over-all mortality was 44 per cent, a figure not much reduced by early laparotomy.[81] In each of these series of trauma cases, the mortality rate was higher after blunt trauma than it was after gunshot wounds or stab wounds—a situation that persists today.

Sporadic case reports of liver resection for various reasons continued into the first decade of the 20th century. Elliott, Thompson, and Freeman collected and nicely summarized much of this early experience,[16, 18, 76] and Terrier and Auvray (1898), Anschutz (1903), and Thöle (1912) published exhaustive monographs on the subject of liver tumors, injuries, and resection.[1, 74, 75]

The technical aspects of liver resection were largely worked out in the animal laboratory. The contributions of Kousnetzoff and Pensky[38] and of Auvray[2] clearly established the value of blunt technique in the passage of large ligatures which were placed as through-and-through mattress sutures. Cautery was often used, but most surgeons found that the hot knife was suitable only for smaller vessels. A number of ingenious methods for liver resection were used by these pioneer surgeons. Tumors on a stalk were brought out of the belly and held out with hat pins, knitting needles, and other convenient devices. Bulky removable ligatures and packs were used extensively to allow delayed slough and peritoneal exclusion of the tumor and its stalk. Occasionally clamps were left in the wound and removed days later when thrombosis was secure. Because any type of ligature tended to pull through soft liver tissue, Beck advocated securing the sutures with plates of decalcified bone or abdominal fascia.[3] Stamm used cartilage from the scapula of a calf (1905), Ceccherelli and Bianchi used whalebone (1894), and Payr and Martina used plates of magnesium to hold the liver sutures (1905).[59] Various types of intricate interlocking mattress sutures placed with blunt needles were advocated, and by 1900 most liver wounds were returned to the abdomen before closure of the abdominal wall.

In the U.S., early liver resections for tumors were done by John Wheelock Elliott at the Massachusetts General Hospital (1896),[16] Carl Beck in Chicago (1902),[3] Leonard Freeman in Denver Colorado (1903),[18] and Frank Yeomans in New York City (1906).[92]

In a Festschrift to Nicholas Senn in 1907, Carl Garrè of Breslau summarized the lessons that he had learned from two decades' experience with liver resection in man (six cases) with a confidence only exceeded by his good judgment.[20] Some comments from that article bear repeating. "If large hepatic vessels bleed, I consider it wrong to use the thermocautery. The operator unnecessarily loses time, the patient blood". . . . . "As soon as the operation has advanced from the edge to the central portions of the liver, it is hardly possible to apply clamps which compress the bulky liver sufficiently to secure a bloodless operation". . . . "The blood pressure in the vessels of the liver is low, therefore hemostasis easy. A frequent mistake is made by pulling too hard on ligature or suture in the liver." "The majority of operators prefer catgut as ligature material and incline to require it most of all in liver surgery. This is an error. I believe, on the contrary, that fine silk threads are of much greater service. However, for the deep sutures which go through the whole thickness of the liver, I prefer thick catgut because I consider thick firm sutures more correct and because I have a general dislike of burying thick silk threads". . . . . "As the records of my cases prove I have succeeded in all cases with these simple methods of isolated silk ligature of the large vessels and interrupted through sutures of the parenchyma with catgut. All of my resections of the liver have recovered." "While so far these simple means have been satisfactory in my practice, it does not follow that all of the other methods are useless. . . but I do not doubt that the simple and easily improvised methods will prove victorious."[20] Garrè's wisdom has stood the test of time, and his principles deserve more attention today (see Chapter 11).

J. Hogarth Pringle of Glasgow recommended digital compression of the hilar vessels to control bleeding from liver wounds in 1908,[64] and this maneuver has assisted many a biliary or hepatic surgeon out of a difficult situation in the ensuing 68 years.

The first four decades of liver surgery saw consolidation of knowledge and experience, but no striking new advances. Yeomans, in two papers, was able to tabulate 16 cases of liver resection for primary cancer with four operative deaths.[92, 93] Six of the 12 operative survivors died with disease from two months to eight years after resection, and six were alive at three to seven years. In the 1920s Frank Mann and others at the Mayo Clinic conducted a series of experiments that defined the physiology of liver and the possibilities of experimental resection.[49]

In 1923, at a single meeting of the Section of Surgery of the Royal Society of Medicine of Great Britain, a remarkable series of cases of liver resection were reported. Grey Turner began by detailing his resection in 1921 of a large "adenoma" from a 13-year-old boy who was alive and free of disease one year and eight months later.[84] This tumor, which was almost certainly a carcinoma by present criteria, was also reported by Shaw.[69] Garnett Wright then told how he had shelled out a multinodular primary cancer from a 16-year-old male who was well 2½ years later.[90] Philip Turner followed with what is probably the first report of spontaneous hemorrhage from a benign adenoma. His patient was a married 29-year-old woman with the sudden onset of severe abdominal pain. Although menses had been normal, the preoperative diagnosis was ruptured ectopic pregnancy. Massive hemoperitoneum was found. Although the source of the hemorrhage was a soft tumor that was resected from the edge of the right lobe of the liver, the patient died from hemorrhage about one hour after completion of the operation.[85] Frank Kidd then reported another "adenoma" found in a 57-year-old female who presented with symptoms of an appendiceal abscess, but who was found instead to have a cricket ball-sized tumor of the right lobe of the liver. Resection was accomplished successfully on July 5th, 1911, but the patient died "from heat stroke on July 10th of 1911 in company with many other victims of the heat lying in the wards of the hospital."[36] Subsequently Mr. A. J. Walton told of three liver resections for carcinoma of the gallbladder but doubted the wisdom of these procedures, saying that all the patients had recurrence of carcinoma within six months. Finally, Mr. Cyril Nitch presented his case of a resected "adrenal rest tumor" of the liver that had been resected from a 54-year-old female in 1910.[36] Death with recurrent disease occurred one year and eight months later. Almost certainly this tumor was what is described in Chapter Four as a clear cell variant of hepatocellular carcinoma. This meeting brought together all that was known about liver resection for tumor, and yet it illustrated clearly how little progress had been made in technique and in pathologic classification since the giant steps taken in the 1880s and 1890s.

Christopherson and Collier in 1953 reported a case contributed by Dr. Irvin Abell, Jr., of Louisville of a 1926 resection of an "adenoma" from a 13-month-old girl. The patient died 25 years later with multiple polyposis of the colon and two separate primary mucinous adenocarcinomas that were metastatic to the liver, but there was no evidence of primary liver neoplasia.[8] This may have been the first successful resection of a primary cancer in a child under two years of age.

Tull was one of the first to recognize the high incidence of primary liver cancer in Asians.[83] He studied 134 cases of primary liver carcinoma from Singapore in 1932, and made some important observations. However, none of his patients had undergone resection. Schrager's report of 1937 on "Surgical aspects of adenoma of the liver" was a gallant attempt to summarize what was known about the different types of solid liver tumors, but, in the light of present pathology classifications, his report can stand as an outstanding example of the confusion of terms and diseases that made a clear understanding of therapy and prognosis so difficult.[68] Tinker and Tinker summarized surgical experience in 1938,[82] and the general reviews of Charache (1939)[7] and Wallace (1941)[86] were useful in defining the nature of primary carcinoma of the liver and the role of the surgeon in its treatment. The monumental reviews of Warvi (1944 and 1945) about the clinical and pathologic aspects of liver tumors marked the end of the middle era of surgical therapy of liver tumors.[87, 88] It was impossible for me to tell from these reports exactly what had happened to many of the patients and what was the true nature of their diseases, but one can only admire the scholarship and industry of Warvi as he attempted to draw together the whole world's experience up to World War II.

THE MODERN ERA

The modern or "anatomic" era of liver resection for tumors began after World War II and was based on great improvements made in patient support, anesthesia, blood transfusion, and metabolic problems, as well as on a more widespread appreciation of the surgical anatomy of the liver. However, we must not give too much credit to the modern surgeon-anatomists, since much of their "new" information was available many decades earlier. Their contribution to our knowledge, although done with original techniques such as corrosion casts, simply reintroduced what had been demonstrated before but not widely accepted.

Glissons' drawings of 1654 show clearly the vascular divisions of the liver.[21] Rex (1888)[67] and Cantlie (1897)[4] reported on the "new" arrangements of the right and left lobes of the liver and nicely described the lobar anatomy as we know it today, and Martens (1920)[50] and McIndoe and Counseller (1927)[54] confirmed what was rediscovered in the 1940s and early 1950s as the "modern" surgical anatomy.

Madding and Kennedy, in a report of 3154 abdominal and thoracoabdominal war wounds of World War II[47] and in an excellent recent monograph on liver trauma,[48] emphasized several important points that have had a major influence on the development of safe liver surgery. They noted that hemorrhage would cease spontaneously from most liver lacerations and that suturing often aggravated, rather than alleviated, bleeding. They decried packing and pointed out the importance of adequate drainage—not for late hemorrhage, which was very rare, but for allowing egress of bile and devitalized tissue.

Perhaps the hallmark of the modern era was the shift away from resection without reference to vascular anatomy toward lobar resection through anatomic planes. Garrè stated in 1907 that "Langenbuch's proposal to produce preventive hemostasis by contemporary ligation of the portal vein cannot be accepted without grave objection."[20] Nonetheless, two years later Hans Von Haberer ligated the hepatic artery and removed the whole left lobe (probably the left lateral segment) of the liver to remove a cystic tumor with bile duct epithelium from a 34-year-old female who did very well thereafter.[30]

In 1910 Professor Walther Wendell resected a double-fist-sized liver cell "adenoma" from a 44-year-old woman after deliberately tying the right branch of the hepatic artery and the right hepatic duct at the liver hilum. He did not attempt ligation of the right portal vein because he worried about thrombosis of the vein extending into the remaining left branch. The patient did well, and was alive and free of apparent disease eight months later.[89]

In the modern era, credit for the first anatomic lobectomy based on vascular anatomy with preliminary hilar ligation is usually given to Lortat-Jacob and Robert (1952),[44] but McBride[52] credits Caprio (1931) with the first anatomic lobectomy.[5] Unfortunately, Caprio's paper was not available for confirmation, and the condition for which his operation was done is not known. Pettinari is said to have done an anatomic lobectomy in 1940,[62] perhaps for hypertrophic tuberculosis (see Dagradi and Brearley, case 5).[11] Donovan and Santulli in 1944 removed the lateral segment of the left lobe of a 6-year-old boy for a mesenchymoma after tying the branches of the left hepatic duct, portal vein, and left hepatic artery in the interlobar fissure.[12] Hershey performed a similar operation in Wheeling, West Virginia in 1945.[94] Fineburg et al. (1956) tabulated all the reported cases of right hepatic lobectomy, and it would appear that that of Lortat-Jacob and Robert may have been the fifth done with primary hilar ligation, rather than the first.[17] Fineburg credits Honjo and Araki with the resection of a right lobe for metastatic colon carcinoma in 1949, but when these Japanese authors reported their case in 1955 they claimed no priority over Lortat-Jacob, whom they cite.[29] However, the Japanese report was submitted for publication in 1953 and contained more than a year's follow-up information on their patient, so their operation may well have preceded that of the French.

Questions of priority aside, several major hepatic lobectomies for solid tumor were done in the first half of the 1950s, and the reports thereof stimulated a widespread acceptance of the procedures. Lortat-Jacob and Robert operated on a 42-year-old woman with multiple metastatic lesions involving her right lobe and the medial segment of the left lobe of the liver. Through a combined thoracoabdominal incision, a "controlled" hepatectomy was done after primary hilar ligation. The postoperative course was reasonably benign, but there was no late follow-up on this patient.[44] Pack and Baker reported total right hepatic lobectomy with primary hilar ligation for a female patient with cancer of the gallbladder in 1953. Unfortunately, the patient died with diffuse metastases in March 1954.[61] In Augusta, Georgia, Julian Quattlebaum resected a primary hepatoma from a 65-year-old woman in 1952 by right lobectomy after primary hilar ligation. The patient died 19 months later with recurrent disease. Quattlebaum had performed two other right lobectomies for angiomas in the 13 months prior to the hepatoma case, but these were done by guillotine transection.[65]

Quattlebaum in Georgia and Pack, Brunschwig, and Bowden of Memorial Hospital in New York performed most of the major hepatic lobectomies done in the U.S. that were reported from 1951 to 1954. Their work in the operating room and their writing and presentation did much to spread the knowledge of the possibility of safe liver resection. The anatomic studies of Healey, et al. and Goldsmith and Woodburne formed a sound basis for subsequent progress.[23, 27, 28] Longmire, McDermott, Mersheimer, Clatworthy, and their associates investigated and reported early successful liver resections, and their contributions to the subject continue to the present day.[9, 42, 43, 53, 57] The largest experience with primary liver cancer and its resection in the last two decades has been in Asia, and Lin, Ong, Tung, Honjo, and Balasegaram have added much of importance to our knowledge of liver tumors (see Chapters 1 and 4).

The first resection to alleviate symptoms of the malignant carcinoid syndrome was done in 1954.[37] Liver transplantation for primary carcinoma was first attempted in 1963 by Thomas Starzl of Denver. His patient was a 48-year-old male with cirrhosis and hepatoma who underwent orthotopic homotransplantation in 1963 and died 22 days later with pulmonary emboli and sepsis. Three other total hepatectomies with transplantation for primary carcinoma were done by the Starzl group in 1963, but all the patients succumbed postoperatively.[71] Moore and Birch also transplanted a liver for metastatic colon carcinoma in 1963, but postoperative survival was short.[71]

Armed with better techniques and with a better understanding of the physiology of the liver and its regeneration, the surgeon required only one more essential piece of basic information to define his role in the therapy of patients with solid tumors — an adequate pathologic classification. Although many contributed toward that classification, including Ewing, Willis, Steiner, Christopherson, and others, the monumental contribution was made by Hugh Edmondson in 1958 with the publication by the Armed Forces' Institute of Pathology of its Fascicle Number 25: *Tumors of the Liver and Intrahepatic Bile Ducts*.[14] Edmondson, by careful study of the liver tumors from his own institution and by collecting cases and reports from around the country, assembled enough material to organize a comprehensive picture of the problem. His classification, only slightly modified, is widely accepted today and forms the basis for this monograph.

Although not the most scientific, the most delightful article yet written about liver resection was published in the British Medical Journal in 1953. Sir Heneage Ogilvie reported the story of a young man with a rectal carcinoid tumor and a biopsy-proved 8-cm liver metastasis who had been given up as a hopeless case by another surgeon in 1949.[60] Ogilvie resected this liver metastasis in August 1951, well before the reports of Lortat-Jacob, Pack, and Quattlebaum. His prose merits direct quotation.

The accepted indications for partial hepatectomy are not many. . . Partial hepatectomy for malignant disease can very rarely be justified. . . . In the case here reported, the patient, a very fit young man of thirty who was about to be married, had a single large metastasis occupying the dome of his liver and bulging up the diaphragm a short distance in front of the opening for the inferior vena cava. The primary tumour in the rectum had been removed. The secondary deposit in the liver had been known to be there for about two years and had not increased greatly in size. Removal of this tumour with an adequate margin of surrounding liver tissue would in all probability remove the only malignant cells remaining in his body. The chance of turning the signals from red to green at the age of thirty seemed worth a considerable risk.

At the first operation in May 1951, when a transverse colostomy was done, "a round lump the size of a billiard ball" could be felt projecting upward from the dome of the right lobe of the liver, but could not be brought into view. At a second operation one month later, a low anterior resection of the distal colon and proximal rectum was done with removal of several enlarged lymph glands.

At a third operation in August 1951:

The metastasis in the liver was removed by the transthoracic transdiaphragmatic approach. . . A wedge removal of normal liver tissue varies from messy to alarming. . . The question was — how much blood?. . . The first incision into liver outside the edge of the swelling produced an alarming gush of blood, which was soon seen to be coming from a divided vessel. In securing this vessel it was clear that the haemostat cut through liver tissue like butter, but met with a resistance that could be appreciated when it reached the firmer tissue of Glisson's capsule in which the bleeding vessel lay. Thereupon the knife was laid aside. A fine-pointed haemostat was used, closed, for cutting the liver substance by very slow and gentle strokes. . . The instrument cut through liver parenchyma almost bloodlessly.

The patient did well postoperatively. . . He is now back at his work as a fruit farmer, playing games and feeling well. He has gained thirty pounds in weight. He has lost his fiancée who was more upset by the series of operations than he was, and threw him over. Perhaps he has gained more by his ordeal than he realises.

Having provided us with good technical advice and a bit of perspective, Ogilvie goes on to justify his report with a comment or two about medical reporting:

At a recent Colchester meeting we were discussing the surgery of the liver, and I learned for the first time that the method that proved so useful to me in this case was not known to the majority. For that reason, because the information may prove useful to others faced with a similar predicament, I venture to put out this unscientific communication. . . . I cannot claim to be familiar with the literature of partial hepatectomy, nor have I consulted more than the standard textbooks of operative surgery. I would, in any case, be out of place to burden a clinical report of a single case with references to the experience of others. The surgeon today is confronted with the almost impossible task of keeping in touch with a literature that increases in volume every year. He can read most of that which concerns the small branch in which he is particularly interested. For the rest he must be content to let others do the hard work at the coal face, and get the knowledge from them, picked, assorted, graded and delivered in clean sacks. The knowledge thus acquired gains in perspective from being unclogged by excessive detail, and it is laid down in the association centres of a mind clarified by idleness.[60]

What follows in this monograph is certain to clog the minds of many with excessive detail, but it is our hope that the minds of at least a few readers will be idle enough to allow entry of a new association or two.

REFERENCES

1. Anschutz, W.: Ueber die Resektion der Leber. Samml. Klin.-Vortr. Chir. *99*:451, 1903.
2. Auvray, M.: Étude expérimentale sur la resection du foie chez l'homme et chez les animaux. Rev. Chir. *17*:318, 1897.
3. Beck, C.: Surgery of the liver. J.A.M.A. *38*:1063, 1902.
4. Cantlie, J.: On new arrangement of right and left lobes of liver. *In* proceedings of the Anatomical Society of Great Britain and Ireland, June 1897. J. Anat. Physiol. *32*:i–xxiv, 1897–1898, iv–ix.
5. Caprio, G.: Un casa de extirpación de lóbulo izquierdo del higado. Bol. Soc. Cirurg. *2*:159, 1931.
6. Castle, O. L.: Primary carcinoma of the liver in childhood. Surg. Gynecol. Obstet. *18*:477, 1914.
7. Charache, H.: Primary carcinoma of the liver. Am. J. Surg. *43*:96, 1939.
8. Christopherson, W. M., and Collier, H. S.: Primary benign liver-cell tumors in infancy and childhood. Cancer *6*:853, 1953.
9. Clatworthy, H. W., Jr., Boles, E. T., Jr., and Newton, W. A.: Primary tumors of the liver in infants and children. Arch. Dis. Child. *35*:22, 1960.
10. DaCosta, J. C.: Papers and Speeches of John Chalmers DaCosta. Philadelphia, W. B. Saunders Co., 1931.
11. Dagradi, A., and Brearley, R.: The surgery of hepatic tumours. Postgrad. Med. J. *38*:670, 1962.
12. Donovan, E. J., and Santulli, T. V.: Resection of the left lobe of the liver for mesenchymoma. Ann. Surg. *124*:90, 1946.
13. Edler, L.: Die traumatischen Verletzungen der parenchymatösen Unterleibsorgane (Leber, Milz, Pankreas, Nieren). Archiv. Klin. Chir. *34*:343, 373, 738, 1886–1887.
14. Edmondson, H. A.: Tumors of the liver and intrahepatic bile ducts. Section VII-Fascicle 25 Atlas of Tumor Pathology, AFIP, 1958.
15. Eggel, H.: Primary carcinoma of the liver. Beitr. Pathol. *30*:506, 1901.
16. Elliot, J. W.: Surgical treatment of tumor of the liver with the report of a case. Ann. Surg. *26*:83, 1897.
17. Fineberg, C., Goldburgh, W. P., and Templeton, J. Y.: Right hepatic lobectomy for primary carcinoma of the liver. Ann. Surg. *144*:881, 1956.
18. Freeman, L.: Operations for primary carcinoma of the liver. Am. J. Med. Sci. *128*:611, 1904.
19. Garrè, C.: On resection of the liver. Surg. Gynecol. Obstet. *5*:331, 1907.
20. Garrè, C.: Contribution to surgery of the liver. Bruns Beitr. Klin. Chir. *4*:181, 1888.
21. Glisson, F.: Anatomia Hepatis. London, 1654.

22. Glück, T.: Ueber die Bedeutung physiologisch-chirurgischer Experimente an der Leber. Arch. Klin. Chir. (Berlin) 29:139, 1883.
23. Goldsmith, N. A., and Woodburne, R. T.: The surgical anatomy pertaining to liver resection. Surg. Gynecol. Obstet. 105:310, 1957.
24. Griffith, J. P. C.: Primary carcinoma of the liver in infancy and childhood. Am. J. Med. Sci. 155:79, 1918.
25. von Hacker, V., cited in Langenbuch, C.: Ein Fall von Resection eines linksseitigen Schnurlappens der Leber. Heilung. Klin. Wochenschr. 25:37, 1888.
26. Hanot, V., and Gilbert, A.: Études sur les Maladies du Foie. Paris, Asselin & Houseau, 1888, p. 334.
27. Healey, J. E., Jr., and Schroy, P. C.: Anatomy of biliary ducts within human liver, analysis of prevailing patterns of branching and major variations of biliary ducts. Arch. Surg. 66:599, 1953.
28. Healey, J. E., Jr., Schroy, P. C., and Sorenson, R. J.: The intrahepatic distribution of the hepatic artery in man. J. Int. Coll. Surg. 20:133, 1953.
29. Honjo, I., and Araki, C.: Total resection of the right lobe of the liver. J. Int. Coll. Surg. 23:23, 1955.
30. Jones, J. F. X.: Removal of a retention cyst from the liver. Ann. Surg. 77:68, 1923.
31. Keen, W. W.: On resection of the liver, especially for hepatic tumors. Boston Med. Surg. J. 126:405, 1892.
32. Keen, W. W.: Removal of an angioma of the liver by elastic constriction external to the abdominal cavity, with a table of 59 cases of operations for hepatic tumors. Pa. Med. J. 1:193, 1897.
33. Keen, W. W.: Report of a case of resection of the liver for the removal of a neoplasm with a table of seventy-six cases of resection of the liver for hepatic tumors. Ann. Surg. 30:267, 1899.
34. Kehr, V. H.: Cited in Freeman, L.: Primary carcinoma of the liver. Am. J. Med. Sci. 128:611, 1904.
35. Kelsh, and Kiener. Contribution à l'étude de l'adénome du foie. Arch. Physiol. 2–3, 622, 1876.
36. Kidd, F.: Case of primary tumor of the liver removed by operation. Proc. R. Soc. Med. 16:61, 1923.
37. Kincaid-Smith, P., and Brossy, J.: A case of bronchial adenoma with liver metastasis. Thorax 11:36, 1956.
38. Kousnetzoff, M., and Pensky, J.: Études cliniques et expérimentales sur la chirurgie du foie sur la résection partielle du foie. Rev. Chir. 16:954, 1896.
39. Langenbuch, C.: Ein Fall von Resection eines linksseitigen Schnurlappens der Leber. Heilung. Klin. Wochenschr. 25:37, 1888.
40. Lius, A.: Di un adenoma del fegato. Centralblatt fur chir 5:99, 1887. Abst. from Ganzy, delle cliniche, 1886, Vol. XXIII, No. 15.
41. Longmire, W. P.: Hepatic surgery: trauma, tumors and cysts. Ann. Surg. 161:1, 1965.
42. Longmire, W. P., Jr., and Marable, S. A.: Clinical experiences with major hepatic resections. Ann. Surg. 154:460, 1961.
43. Longmire, W. P., Jr., and Scott, H. W., Jr.: Benign adenoma of the liver. Surgery 24:983, 1948.
44. Lortat-Jacob, J. L., and Robert, H. G.: Hepatectomie droite régleé. Presse Med. 60:549, 1952.
45. Lücke, T.: Entfernung des linken Krebsiten Leber Lappens. Centralbl. Chir. 6:115, 1891.
46. Macpherson, J.: Cited in Mikeskey, W. E., et al. Int. Abstr. Surg. 103:323, 1956.
47. Madding, G. F., Lawrence, K. B., and Kennedy, P. A.: War wounds of the liver. Tex. State J. Med. 42:267, 1946.
48. Madding, G. F., and Kennedy, P. A.: Trauma to the Liver. 2nd ed. Philadelphia, W. B. Saunders Co., 1971.
49. Mann, F. C., and Graham, A. S.: Surgery of the liver with special reference to its removal. Int. Abstr. Surg. 47:176, 1928.
50. Martens, F.: Röntgenologische Studien zur arterieelen Gefässversorgung in der Leber. Arch. Klin. Chir. 114:1001, 1920.

51. Martin, F. H.: Fifty Years of Medicine and Surgery. Chicago, Surgical Publishing Co., 1934.

52. McBride, C. M., and Wallace, S.: Cancer of the right lobe of the liver. Arch. Surg. *105*:289, 1972.

53. McDermott, W. V., et al.: Major hepatic resection: diagnostic techniques and metabolic problems. Surgery *54*:56, 1963.

54. McIndoe, A. H., and Counseller, V. S.: Bilaterality of liver. Arch. Surg. *15*:589, 1927.

55. Meade, R. H.: Surgery of the Liver. *In* An Introduction to the History of General Surgery. Philadelphia, W. B. Saunders Co., 1968.

56. vonMeister, E.: Recreation des Lebergewebes nach Abtragung ganzer Leberlappen. Beitr. Pathol. Anat. *15*:1, 1894.

57. Mersheimer, W. L.: Successful right hepatolobectomy for primary neoplasm—preliminary observations. Bulletin, N.Y. Med. Coll., Flower & Fifth Ave. Hospitals *16*:121, 1953.

58. Mikesky, W. E., Howard, J. M., and DeBakey, M. E.: Injuries of the liver in three hundred consecutive patients. Int. Abstr. Surg. *103*:323, 1956.

59. Moynihan, B.: Abdominal Operations. 3rd ed. London, W. B. Saunders Co., 1914.

60. Ogilvie, H.: Partial hepatectomy. Br. Med. J. *2*:1136, 1953.

61. Pack, G. T., and Baker, H. W.: Total right hepatic lobectomy. Report of a case. Ann. Surg. *138*:253, 1953.

62. Pettinari, V.: La resezione epatica secondo la mia esperienza. Seizième Congrès Soc. Int. Chir. *1169*, 1955.

63. Ponfick, E.: Ueber Leber Resektion und Leber Recreation. Verh. Dtsch. Ges. Chir. *19*:28, 1890 (Congress).

64. Pringle, J. H.: Notes on the arrest of hepatic hemorrhage due to trauma. Ann. Surg. *48*:541, 1908.

65. Quattlebaum, J. K.: Massive resection of the liver. Ann. Surg. *137*:787, 1952.

66. Resection Editorial: Resection of left lobe of liver. Lancet *1*:237, 1888.

67. Rex (1888) cited in Hobsley, M.: The anatomical basis of partial hepatectomy. Proc. R. Soc. Med. Engl. *57*:550, 1964.

68. Schrager, V. L.: Surgical aspects of adenoma of the liver. Ann. Surg. *105*:33, 1937.

69. Shaw, A. F. B.: Primary liver-cell adenoma (hepatoma). J. Pathol. Bacteriol. *26*:475, 1923.

70. Sheinfeld, W.: Cholecystectomy and partial hepatectomy for carcinoma of the gallbladder with local liver extension. Surgery *22*:48, 1947.

71. Starzl, T. E.: Experience in Hepatic Transplantation. Philadelphia, W. B. Saunders Co., 1969.

72. Tait, L.: Case of hydatids of the liver, treated by abdominal section and drainage. Br. Med. J. Vol. 2:975, 1880.

73. Tait, L.: A case of hepatotomy for hydatids. Br. Med. J. Vol. 2:81, 1881.

74. Terrier, F., and Auvray, M.: Les traumatismes du foies et des voies biliaries. Rev. Chir. (Paris) *16*:717, 1896.

75. Thöle, F.: Die Verletzungen der Leber und der Gallenwege. (Neue Deutsch. Chir., IV) Stuttgart, Enke, 1912, p. 101.

76. Thompson, J. E.: The surgical treatment of neoplasm of the liver. Ann. Surg. *30*:284, 1899.

77. Thornton, J. K.: The surgical treatment of diseases of the liver. Br. Med. J. Vol. 2:901, 1886.

78. Tiffany, L. M.: Removal of solid tumor from the liver by laparotomy. Md. Med. J. *23*:531, 1890.

79. Tiffany, L. M.: Surgery of the liver. Bost. Med. Surg. J. CXXII *23*:557, 1890.

80. Tillmans, H.: Experimentelle und anatomische Untersuchugen über Wunden der Leber und Niere. Virchows Arch. *78*:437, 1879.

81. Tilton, B. T.: Some considerations regarding wounds of the liver. Ann. Surg. *41*:20, 1905.

82. Tinker, M. B., and Tinker, M. B., Jr.: Resection of the liver. J.A.M.A. *112*:2006, 1939.

83. Tull, J. G.: Primary carcinoma of the liver. J. Pathol. Bacteriol. *35*:557, 1932.

84. Turner, G. G.: A case in which an adenoma weighing 2lb, 3 oz was successfully removed from the liver; with remarks on the subject of partial hepatectomy. Proc. R. Soc. Med. *16*:43, 1923.
85. Turner, P.: Case of excision of an adenoma of the liver, which had ruptured spontaneously causing internal hemorrhage. Proc. R. Soc. Med. *16*:60, 1923.
86. Wallace, R. H.: Resection of the liver for hepatoma. Arch. Surg. *43*:14, 1941.
87. Warvi, W. N.: Primary neoplasms of the liver. Arch. Pathol. *37*:367, 1944.
88. Warvi, W. N.: Primary tumors of the liver. Surg. Gynecol. Obstet. *80*:643, 1945.
89. Wendell, W.: Beitrage zur Chirugie der Leber. Arch. Klin. Chir. *95*:887, 1911.
90. Wright, G.: Primary carcinoma of the liver excised by operation. Proc. R. Soc. Med. *16*:56, 1923.
91. Yamagiwa, K.: Zur Kenntniss des primaren parenchymatosen Leberkarcinoms. Virchows Arch. [Patholo. Anat.] *206*:439, 1911.
92. Yeomans, F. C.: Primary carcinoma of the liver. J.A.M.A. *52*:1741, 1909.
93. Yeomans, F. C.: Primary carcinoma of the liver. J.A.M.A. *64*:1301, 1915.
94. Hershey, C. D.: Partial hepatectomy in certain primary tumors of the liver. South. Surg. *12*:245, 1946.

Chapter Three

LABORATORY, RADIOGRAPHIC, RADIONUCLIDE, AND OTHER AIDS IN THE DIAGNOSIS OF SOLID LIVER TUMORS

INTRODUCTION

Fifteen years ago, an accurate diagnosis of primary liver cancer in most cases was not made until after the death of the patient. With the use of modern techniques, it is now possible to make an antemortem diagnosis in more than 85 per cent of such cases.[1, 59] Biopsy and histologic definition of tumor type will be necessary before any definite decision can be made about the therapy and prognosis of a patient found to have a solid liver tumor. However, when the possibility of a liver tumor has been raised by clinical evidence or by an unexpected result of a laboratory test, several other steps can be taken prior to biopsy to establish the nature and the extent of liver involvement.

The symptoms and signs of the different types of primary and secondary tumors will be discussed in the ensuing chapters devoted to specific lesions, but we have chosen to bring together in this introductory

Table 3–1. Abnormal Tests—1974 Liver Tumor Survey Patients

Test	Primary Epithelial Carcinoma — Adults Hepato-cellular 109	Cholangio. Ca. 18	Children 72	Benign Tumors Adenoma 37	FNH 63	Cystad. and cyst AdenoCa 8	Vascul. Tumors 6	Mesench. Hamartoma 5	Embryonal Sarcoma 12	Metastatic Tumors From colon and Rectum 126	Other Primary Source 50	Total Percentage Abnormal
Alkaline phosphatase	48/91*	11/15	15/43	5/26	5/40	4/7	2/5	1/4	3/7	38/82	16/28	43
SGOT	33/74	3/13	23/38	7/22	7/35	0/5	0/4	2/3	1/5	17/61	12/27	37
BSP	19/35	1/3	2/5	7/8	4/6	3/5	—	0/1	2/3	12/20	6/10	58
Bilirubin (2 mg)	4/83	1/10	10/45	1/24	0/36	1/7	0/5	0/4	0/8	0/64	0/22	6
CEA	0/1	—	—	—	—	—	—	—	—	1/1	—	
Alpha-fetoprotein	4/14	0/1	6/8	0/6	0/3	—	1/1	—	—	—	—	33
Radionuclide scan	51/56	9/10	28/30	14/16	12/16	2/2	3/3	2/2	6/6	26/34	19/20	88
Arteriogram	51/51	10/11	19/20	17/19	10/11	1/2	3/3	0	5/5	19/21	7/7	95

*Fractions are made as follows:
NUMERATOR—number of times test significantly abnormal *preoperatively*.
DENOMINATOR—number of times accurate *preoperative* information was available.

chapter some general information about the use of laboratory tests, of old and new techniques in radiology, of radionuclides, and of invasive techniques short of laparotomy in the discovery and differential diagnosis of liver tumors. A general summary from the viewpoint of a surgeon will be attempted, but the reader is encouraged to review the referenced sources for more complete information. Table 3–1 outlines the incidence of abnormal tests in the patients studied in the 1974 Liver Tumor Survey. Many, if not most, of these tumors were resected at a time before the measurement of alpha-fetoprotein and the use of some of the newer radionuclides became widespread. It also must be remembered that the patients included in the Survey represent a highly selected group of patients with resectable tumors.

LABORATORY AIDS TO DIAGNOSIS

The hemogram of most patients with resectable liver tumors is within the range of normal. Exelby, et al. reported abnormal red blood cell assays (usually anemia), in more than one-half of the children with primary epithelial cancers collected in a national survey, but many of these children had advanced disease.[25] Erythrocytosis is seen with primary liver cancer and may be more common with this disease than with primary renal cell cancer.[11, 42] Chan reported that 47 per cent of a group of Asian patients with primary liver cancer had thrombocyte counts below 150,000, and 32 per cent of the same group of patients had prolonged prothrombin times at the time their diagnosis was first made.[16] These abnormalities of coagulation may be more closely related to an associated cirrhosis than to the liver cancer, and they should alert the clinician to the probability of an unresectable situation.

Hypoglycemia[31] and hypercalcemia[59] are seen infrequently with primary liver tumors and may be related to abnormal hormone production by the neoplastic cells[42] (for further details about paraneoplastic syndromes, see Chapter 4).

LIVER FUNCTION TESTS

The serum alkaline phosphatase (AP), glutamic oxaloacetic transaminase (SGOT), and the glutamic pyruvic transaminase (SGPT), together with the Bromsulphalein retention (BSP) are among the commonly performed liver function tests that are most likely to alert the clinician to the possibility of liver tumor.

The serum alkaline phosphatase was elevated in 58 per cent of patients with liver metastases from primary sites outside of the liver in one series,[13] and in 49 per cent of 110 patients with resectable liver metastases in the 1974 LTS. However, elevation also may be seen in cancer patients without liver metastases,[13] so that this test cannot be used as absolute evidence of liver involvement.[5] Adult patients with primary carcinoma of the liver had elevations of alkaline phosphatase in 13 to 94 per cent of cases,[5, 24, 34, 41] and children showed elevations in 36 per cent of hepatoblastoma cases and 45 per cent of hepatocellular carcinomas.[25] The abnormally elevated isoenzymes produced by a primary liver cancer may be different from the usual isoenzymes of hepatic origin seen in other types of liver disease.[32] Adult patients with cholangiocarcinoma and with cystadenomas and cystadenocarcinomas (both lesions of bile duct origin) were more likely to have increased alkaline phosphatase than were patients with hepatocellular carcinomas in the 1974 LTS. Alkaline phosphatase was elevated in only 15 per cent of adult patients in the 1974 LTS with benign liver tumors, however large (see Table 3-1).

Although the SGPT is thought to be more liver-specific than the SGOT, the OT proved more often abnormal in patients with primary and secondary liver tumors. Castagna, et al. found elevation of SGOT in 29 of 48 patients with liver metastases from other primary sources, but they also found SGOT elevations in 10 of 48 patients with carcinoma not involving the liver.[13] Primary liver cancers were associated with increases in SGOT in 17 to 87 per cent of adult patients,[5, 8, 24, 34, 41] and in 42 per cent of children.[25] The children with hepatocellular carcinoma were more likely to have an elevation than the younger children with hepatoblastomas.

SGPT did not help to differentiate between patients with extrahepatic primary cancers who had liver metastases and those who did not,[13] and was not elevated as often as the SGOT in adults or in pediatric patients with primary cancer.[5, 8, 25] SGOT was elevated in 33 per cent of the 1974 LTS patients with resectable metastases, and in 38 per cent of the patients with resectable primary tumors. Of the 22 patients with resected hepatocellular adenomas who had preoperative evaluation of SGOT, only seven had elevations, and all of these presented with either intraperitoneal hemorrhage or severe pain—both undoubtedly associated with tumor necrosis. BSP was the standard test least often done but most often elevated in the resected 1974 LTS patients, and the percentage of abnormal values was higher with the benign lesions of adults than with the malignant. In the noncirrhotic patient, this test can be quite helpful in establishing the suspicion of primary or secondary involvement of the liver by tumor.

Ihde, et al. found an elevation of the serum bilirubin in 29 of 67 adult patients with hepatocellular carcinoma at the time of their presentation for therapy.[34] However, the serum bilirubin was elevated in only 6 per cent of patients with resectable tumors in the 1974 LTS, and most of these elevations occurred in pediatric patients. Exelby, et al. found an increase in serum bilirubin in 15 per cent of children with hepatoblastoma, and 25 per cent of those with hepatocellular carcinoma.[25] Ong believed that clinical jaundice is a contraindication to resection.[50] The five adult patients in the 1974 LTS who had preoperative elevation of bilirubin above 2 mg per cent all died after operation. However, seven of ten children with preoperative bilirubins above 2 mg per cent survived operation, and at least three went on to long-term survival. The only child with a preoperative bilirubin above 10 mg per cent did die, but of bleeding complications shortly after operation and not of liver failure.

The serum albumin concentration is often low in patients with primary liver cancer or with metastatic liver involvement. This test is of no help in differential diagnosis, however, and low values probably more truly reflect the wasting of advanced neoplastic disease or an associated cirrhosis. Lin reports that serum globulin levels and cholesterol esters were abnormal twice as often as were the SGOT and AP in noncirrhotic patients with liver cancer.[38] Neither of these tests was analyzed during the 1974 Liver Tumor Survey.

Various other enzyme tests have been recommended as more specific than the common ones discussed above. Lactic acid dehydrogenase was elevated in 13 of 19 patients with primary liver cancer and in five of six patients with metastatic disease in their liver.[8] Serum proline hydroxylase was elevated in approximately 70 per cent of Ugandan patients with hepatocellular carcinoma,[71] and serum isocitric dehydrogenase and serum leucine aminopeptidase levels usually were higher in patients with liver tumors than in those with other liver diseases.[38]

5′ nucleotidase was elevated in 45 of 51 adult patients with primary hepatocellular carcinoma who were tested in New York City,[34] and Smith, et al. found this enzyme to be considerably more sensitive and more specific than alkaline phosphatase.[63] Tsou, et al. found a unique fast-moving isoenzyme band of 5′ nucleotide phosphodiesterase after electrophoresis of the sera of six patients with histologically proved primary liver cancer. All six of these patients had negative alpha-fetoprotein by double immunodiffusion test.[70] This band was not seen in the serum of a patient with benign liver adenoma or in neonatal sera.

A suggestion that the Jirgl flocculation test might help to discover malignant transformation in the cirrhotic livers of Rhodesian patients was not borne out by the review of Gane.[27]

Although these sophisticated enzyme analyses may play an important role in our future understanding of liver cancer, they do not as yet add much to our ability to diagnose the type and extent of liver tumors.

ALPHA-FETOPROTEIN AND HEPATITIS-ASSOCIATED ANTIGEN

Two relatively recent developments have considerably enlarged our understanding of primary carcinoma of the liver. The identification of alpha-fetoprotein (AFP) as a specific biochemical marker that appears in the sera of many patients with hepatocellular carcinoma provides us with an exciting tool with which to study the disease. The additional observation that the Australia or hepatitis-associated antigen (HAA) could be found in the sera of many African patients with liver cancer has stimulated renewed interest in the role that viral infection may play in carcinogenesis. Because much of the information pertinent to the understanding of the usefulness of either or both tests is based on data that correlate the two, they will be discussed together in this section.

AFP

Pedersen first recognized AFP as a specific alpha-1-globulin that occurred in fetal calf serum in 1944. He called it "fetuin,"[52] but it was not until 1963 that Abelev confirmed that a tumor-specific antigen recovered from mouse hepatoma cells was identical to the fetal-specific serum protein of normal mice.[7] This finding was quickly confirmed in man and other animals, and the phenomenon was recognized as an example of "retroversion" or "derepression" of malignant cells toward an embryonal condition.

AFP is the major fetal globulin during early gestation, but its levels fall later in pregnancy and disappear during the first few weeks of newborn life. In several respects AFP does not act like other tumor-specific antigens. No autologous human antibody to AFP has yet been identified, no AFP-specific antibody has yet been recognized in patients with hepatocellular carcinoma, and, although AFP can be found in maternal sera near term, no maternal anti-AFP antibody has been found.[2]

AFP reappears in the sera of some patients with carcinoma arising from the hepatocyte (but not bile duct cells), and this is more apt to occur in areas where the instance of primary liver cancer is high. It has also been found in a few patients with embryonal cancers or teratomas of the gonads. As our ability to detect smaller amounts of this protein has increased with more sensitive tests, the number of diseases that have been associated with AFP has increased.

The quantitative aspects of the assay used are important. The standard immunodiffusion test by double diffusion in agar (DDA) detects amounts of AFP in excess of 1000 ng/ml.[7] Countercurrent immunoelectrophoresis (CCE) can detect levels as low as 200 to 250 ng/ml,[2] and radioimmunoassay techniques (RIA) can detect concentrations as low as

5 ng/ml.[10] A complement fixation technique that is said to be easier than RIA, and more sensitive than DDA or CCE, may share with the other quantitatively sensitive techniques a lack of specificity for tumor diagnosis.[22]

The absolute levels of AFP in patients with hepatocellular carcinoma has no apparent correlation with the histologic pattern of the tumor[17] or with cirrhosis, with symptoms, with liver function tests, or with the presence of antibodies to HAA.[72] In Ugandan patients with hepatocellular carcinoma, however, AFP was detected more often in patients who were young, male, and with HAA demonstrable in their sera.[71, 72] Changes in the level of AFP on serial examination may reflect response to therapy or progression of disease in an individual patient.[51]

The half-life of AFP is three to three and one-half days,[2, 55] so that changes should occur rapidly if therapy is effective. AFP levels fell in five Japanese patients after tumor resection and rose again in two with recurrent disease.[68] Matsumoto found good correlation of AFP levels with clinical response of a patient with hepatocellular carcinoma to chemotherapy,[44] but Ugandan patients with detectable levels of AFP showed little change after chemotherapy[45] (which, of course, may reflect ineffective therapy rather than failure of the test).

Most other reported surveys of patients with liver cancer have used the less sensitive and easier DDA method. By this technique, AFP has not been recognized in the sera of patients or of animals during periods of active liver regeneration after hepatectomy,[2] or in the sera of rats with liver cancers induced by aflatoxin. It may be that the more sensitive assays will pick up small amounts of AFP in most of these situations.[10] Miller, et al. found an AFP level above 500 ng/ml in a single patient among 90 with alcoholic hepatitis, and this level fell rapidly with clinical improvement.[47] Bloomer, using the very sensitive RIA technique, found detectable levels of AFP in 38 per cent of patients with active hepatitis—most commonly in those with bridging necrosis on liver biopsy.[10]

A mass screening trial in China tested the sera of 343,999 persons using DDA and CCE. Seventy-six per cent of 139 patients with proved hepatocellular carcinoma were "positive." Six of 52 patients with metastatic cancer of the liver, two of 2342 patients with noncancerous liver disease, and none of 791 control patients had detectable levels of AFP. Twelve of 14 patients in this series who had histologic proof of carcinoma, with no detectable AFP in their sera by DDA and CCE, were found to have significant levels of AFP when retested by the more sensitive RIA technique. Seven patients who were eventually shown to have hepatocellular carcinoma had positive AFP tests before any clinical symptoms were apparent.[19]

Although most authors have stated that Western patients with hepatocellular carcinoma are less likely to have detectable AFP in their

Table 3–2. Detection of Alpha-Fetoprotein
in Reported Series

		PATIENTS				
REFERENCE	CITY/COUNTRY	Heptao-cellular Carcinoma	Cholangio Carcinoma	Metastatic Carcinoma	Other Liver Disease	Controls
69	Japan	17/27	0/5	0/39		
4	Uganda	20/40		0/8	2/118	0/75
19	China	106/139		6/52	2/2342	0/791
36	South Africa	58/72				
38	Hong Kong	60/84	0/10	0/119	2/521	0/3682
72	Uganda	121/184				
15	Thailand	26/57				
5	Detroit	14/19	0/2			
41	Boston	5/10				
40	New York	5/19				
47	Miami	8/11		1/13		
51	Baltimore	16/25		0/25	0/7	
59	London	6/22	0/2			

sera,[2, 28] the data are not entirely consistent. Table 3–2 lists some of the reported incidences of detectable AFP measured by a number of different methods of varying sensitivity. Exelby, et al. found AFP present in the sera of 22 of 32 children with hepatoblastomas, and 11 out of 26 children with hepatocellular carcinomas.[25]

Clearly this test is extremely useful in diagnosis, *if* it is positive. Perhaps its most important role will be in the use of serial determinations of quantitative levels to follow the course of patients with liver cancer and certain gonadal tumors.[53]

There is no evidence yet available to suggest that patients with hepatocellular carcinoma unassociated with alpha-fetoprotein have a clinical course that is different from that of patients whose tumors produce AFP. However, specific antibody to AFP has been produced in the laboratory that will precipitate in hepatocellular carcinomatous tissue.[17] Parks, et al. suggest that a highly specific anti-AFP might function as a carrier of tumoricidal agents and/or that passive humoral immunotherapy of liver cancer may be possible in the future.[51]

AFP was present in only 11 of 33 patients tested in the 1974 LTS. One 3-day-old child (Case 1 – Table 7–3) with an infantile hemangioendothelioma was positive, but whether this was due to his age or his tumor cannot be determined. Six children 2 years of age or younger, all with hepatoblastoma, had AFP measured, and five showed evidence of the protein in their sera by DDA. AFP was found in the serum of the only pediatric patient with hepatocellular carcinoma who was tested (a 2½-year-old girl).

All of the four adult patients who were AFP-positive had hepatocellular carcinoma. Two had cirrhosis and two did not, but otherwise their clinical presentation and postoperative course had nothing to set them apart from other patients who were AFP-negative or who were not tested.

HEPATITIS-ASSOCIATED ANTIGEN (AUSTRALIA ANTIGEN)

The discovery that many African patients with liver cancer had hepatitis-associated antigen (HAA) in their sera has renewed interest in a possible relationship between infection with hepatitis B virus and carcinogenesis. Purified HAA seems to contain RNA-dependent DNA polymerase, an enzyme that is a common constituent of experimental oncogenic viruses.[14]

Anthony has tabulated recent reports of the frequency of HAA in patients with cirrhosis and hepatocellular carcinoma.[7] HAA was found in 3 per cent of control patients and in 40 per cent of patients with hepatocellular carcinoma in Uganda. However, there was no difference between the frequency of a positive serologic test for antibody to HAA in control patients or in patients with carcinoma or cirrhosis, suggesting a high rate of exposure to HAA in Uganda.[71] Forty per cent of Bantu patients had HAA in their sera compared to a 7 per cent incidence in 18,377 controls, but there was no correlation of AFP positivity to HAA positivity in this Bantu population.[36]

The weight of evidence from other areas suggests little or no correlation between the incidence of hepatocellular carcinoma and the presence of HAA in the serum. Smith collected data from Hong Kong, East Africa, and the U. S.,[62] and more recent studies from Detroit,[5] Boston,[3] Singapore,[60] London,[59] Great Britain,[57] Thailand,[15] and New York[40] suggest that either there is no correlation or that the correlation may be closer with cirrhosis than with liver cancer.

The reports of certain kindreds or clusters of patients with cirrhosis and liver cancer who have had persistent levels of HAA suggest a genetic factor that may relate to susceptibility to both persistent antigenemia and carcinogenesis.[14] In Thailand HAA seems to correlate with liver carcinoma in cirrhotic patients, but not in noncirrhotic patients.[15]

Thus, the question whether the hepatitis B virus is related to liver cancer entirely through its ability to produce chronic liver injury leading to cirrhosis, or whether the virus can cause cancer in an undamaged liver, remains to be answered. HAA was tested in very few of the patients collected in the 1974 LTS, and there are no lessons to be learned from that brief experience.

Carcinoembryonic Antigen (CEA)

First described by Gold and Freedman in 1965, carcinoembryonic antigen (CEA) has been the subject of innumerable investigations in the last decade.[29] The recent report of Martin, et al. brings together most of what is known about this protein–polysaccharide complex.[43] The initial hope that CEA would prove to be a specific indicator for the presence of colorectal carcinoma has not been realized. CEA levels may be elevated in patients with extracolonic gastrointestinal cancer, with many nondigestive cancers, and with a host of benign conditions including colon polyps, inflammatory bowel disease, cirrhosis, and even pancreatitis and chronic lung disease. About 20 per cent of the patients who do have colorectal carcinoma will not show elevation in CEA levels. The quantitative aspects of CEA determination may eventually prove more important than the qualitative.

Patients with benign and malignant conditions of the liver may show elevated levels of CEA. Martin, et al. found elevations of CEA in two of five patients with primary liver carcinoma.[43] The only patient with a hepatocellular carcinoma who was tested in the 1974 LTS had normal levels of CEA. One patient with a colonic carcinoma who underwent synchronous resection of a solitary liver metastasis had preoperative elevations of CEA, but postoperative levels of CEA were not available.

CEA has little, if any, role to play in the differential diagnosis of liver tumors. Serial CEA measurements may be of great prognostic value. A drop of CEA to zero level after tumor resection should reassure the surgeon, whereas persistent levels of CEA or a change from normal to increased levels, even in asymptomatic patients, almost always is associated with recurrent or persistent carcinoma.

RADIOLOGIC AIDS TO DIAGNOSIS

Although angiography is the mainstay of the radiologist's ability to help the clinician in diagnosis and planning therapy for patients with solid liver tumors, there is much to be learned from noninvasive techniques.

The chest x-ray of patients with bulky lesions in the right lobe of the liver may show an elevated right hemidiaphragm, with or without basal atelectasis of the right lung (Fig. 3–1). Pulmonary nodules were evident at the time of first diagnosis in 10 per cent of children with primary epithelial tumors in one series,[25] and in 21 per cent of adults

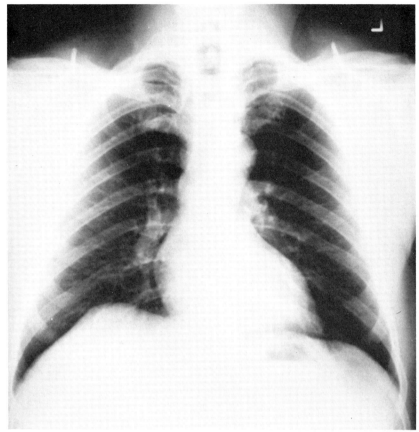

Figure 3-1. Chest film. Posteroanterior chest radiograph of a 53-year-old male with a huge cholangiocarcinoma of the right lobe which has tented up the right diaphragm. At laparotomy no extracapsular tumor involvement of the diaphragm was found.

with hepatocellular carcinoma in another series.[40] Tomography of the chest is perhaps the most important examination to perform to rule out metastatic disease in a patient who is being considered for liver resection for metastatic carcinoma, and who is clinically free of disease otherwise. Tomographic evidence of pulmonary disease not evident on regular chest films has stayed our hand in several instances. Cardiomegaly is seen occasionally in association with vascular tumors of children.[21]

A regular flat film of the abdomen will show abnormalities in 85 per cent of children with liver tumors.[25] This usually is an enlargement of the liver and/or spleen, but calcification may be seen in the tumor or there may be displacement of other organs. Liver tumors classically push the colon down and to the left, whereas renal tumors push it forward. The second portion of the duodenum remains in its normal position with both of these lesions.[23, 65] The stomach may be displaced to the left and the right kidney may be pushed down (Fig. 3–4, A).[65, 74] Cephalad displacement of the right kidney by a low-lying tumor of the right lobe of the liver is rare, but does occur.[74] Tumor calcification is unusual but may be seen in neoplasms of vascular origin,[21] in pediatric epithelial tumors,[18, 23, 26, 49, 65] and in cysts.[23, 65] Sorsdahl and Gay have distinguished patterns of calcium deposition peculiar to each of these lesions.[65]

Generalized osteoporosis may be seen with liver tumors in children or with other types of liver disease.[65] In adult patients with liver tumors, enlargement of the spleen was seen in 17 patients with primary liver tumors and in 18 with metastatic liver disease, so that this finding is not particularly helpful in differential diagnosis.[74]

Total body opacification with urographic contrast material, when combined with tomography, may opacify the liver and reveal areas of avascular tumor or necrosis in children.[30, 65]

Angiography

Although splenoportography and inferior venacavography occasionally may add useful information, selective arteriography is clearly the most useful test in supplying information to the physician caring for a patient with a liver tumor. In addition to providing evidence about the type, size, and number of lesions, arteriography can confirm clinical impressions about portal vein involvement, and it will give a "road map" of the arterial supply to tumors of the liver—a supply where anomalies are very common and important to a surgeon contemplating liver resection or arterial ligation for tumor control. Water-soluble contrast material usually is used, but Lipiodol injected through the superior mesenteric artery may produce an hepatogram that persists for up to four hours and which may reveal lesions as small as 1 cm in diameter. The diagnostic accuracy of the Lipiodol technique is reported as 95 per cent, but arteriovenous fistulas contraindicate its use, and most primary liver tumors demonstrate such fistulas.[12] Lipiodol may prove to be most helpful in detecting metastatic tumors that are avascular.

Arteriographic changes of the left lobe of the liver may be more difficult to see than those of the right, because the lobe is thinner, it overlies the spine, and details may be obscured by superimposition of vessels to the stomach, pancreas, and spleen.[74]

Among those arteriographic changes that give information about a tumor are:

(1) Dilatation of the hepatic artery (present in 100 per cent of 50 adult patients with primary carcinoma of the liver).[76]

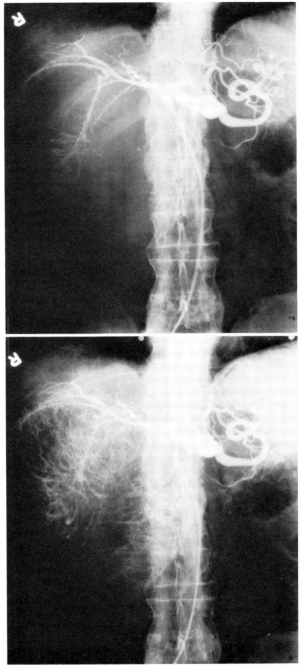

Figure 3–2. Hepatocellular carcinoma. A huge but resectable primary hepatocellular carcinoma of the right lobe is seen by celiac arteriography. Distortion of surrounding vessels, a central feeding artery and radiating tumor vessels are seen on serial views of this 57-year-old male patient.

(2) Distortion and displacement of vessels (which can result from any mass lesion).

(3) Hypervascularity (more common with primary tumors than with secondaries and more common with lesions of hepatocellular origin than those of bile duct origin).

(4) Tumor blush—an increased capillary blush in the area of the tumor which is seen in the late phases after injection.

(5) Tumor vessels—bizarre forms characteristic of neovascularity in malignant lesions.

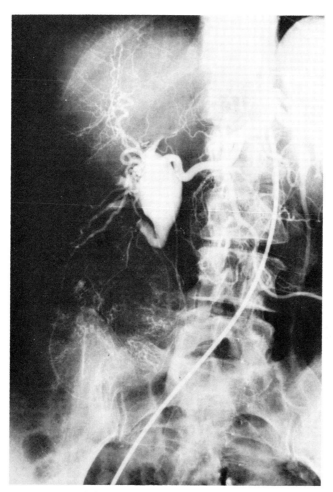

Figure 3–3. Hepatocellular carcinoma. A large hepatocellular carcinoma of the lower edge of the right lobe which had descended into the lower abdomen is demonstrated by selective arteriography. Note that the arterial neovascular supply comes from peripheral elongated vessels. Resection was easily accomplished through a thinned-out pedicle (see Figure 4–1). The tumor had apparently partly blocked the right ureter, although it had not broken out beyond the liver capsule.

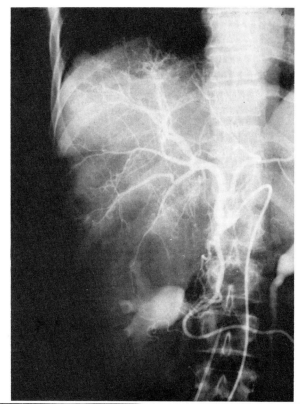

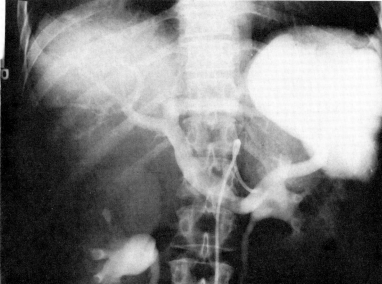

Figure 3-4. Hepatocellular carcinoma. A selective arteriogram shows elongated and distorted arteries in the area of a large tumor of the lower half of the right lobe. Note the absence of portal blood supply to the same area on the splenoportogram. The right kidney has been displaced downward by the liver mass.

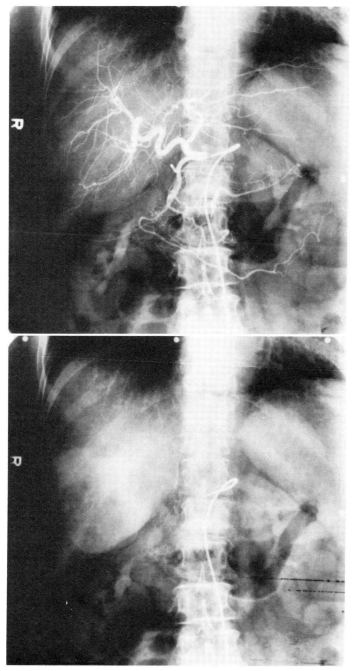

Figure 3–5. Cholangiocarcinoma. There appears to be reduced arterial supply to a large cholangiocarcinoma of the lower edge of the right lobe. In a later film the edge of the tumor nearest normal liver shows a pronounced tumor "blush" (Case 123, Appendix IV).

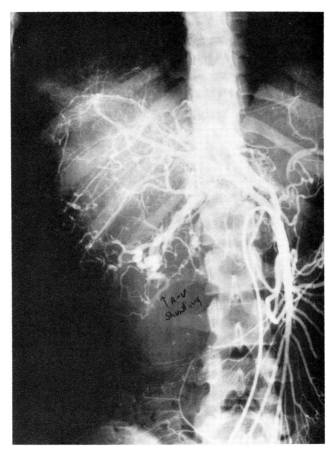

Figure 3–6. Hepatocellular carcinoma. Abnormal vessels and arteriovenous shunting are seen in a large hypovascular tumor of the lower right lobe.

(6) Arteriovenous shunting—usually thought to signify malignant change, but often seen with focal nodular hyperplasia (see Chapter 6).

(7) Vessel encasement—more characteristic of neoplasm than inflammation, but may be seen with both.

(8) Pooling—where contrast material remains in abnormal vascular spaces after the rest of the liver is cleared.

(9) Marginal changes at the border of the lesion which, when sharp, suggest benign tumor and which, when poorly defined, suggest malignancy.[49, 76]

Figures 3–2 through 3–8 illustrate typical changes demonstrated by arteriography.[49, 76]

Increased vascularity is probably the most important sign in the differential diagnosis of mass lesions of the liver, and is characteristic of most hepatocellular carcinomas and hepatoblastomas.[59, 74] With metastatic lesions, increased vascularity is most apt to be seen with the carcinoid and islet cell tumors, with leiomyosarcomas, and with lesions of

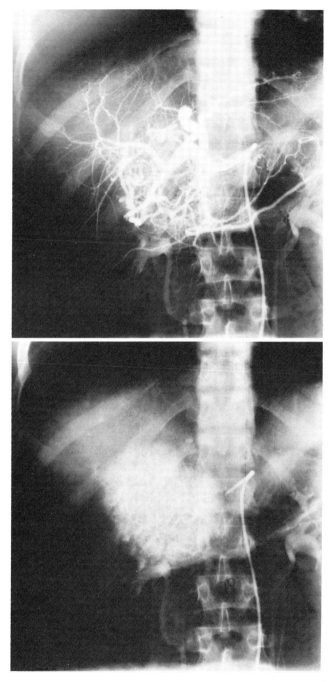

Figure 3-7. Focal nodular hyperplasia. Arteriography demonstrates striking arterial enlargement, distortion, and arteriovenous fistulization in a tumor of the quadrate lobe in a 16-year-old girl (Case 10, Appendix VI-A). A later film reveals a pronounced "blush" in this benign tumor which was difficult to see on a 99^m Tc liver scan (see Figure 3-16).

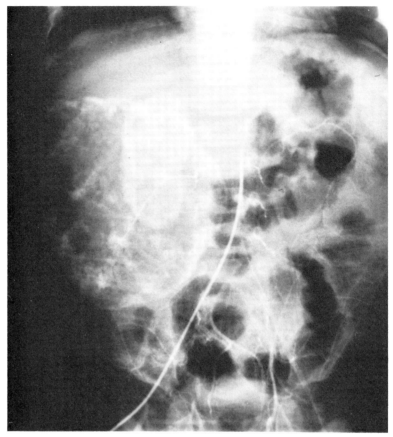

Figure 3–8. Hemangioendothelioma. Vascular puddling is seen in a solitary tumor of a four-month-old male. The lesion was resected by right lobectomy.

renal origin.[64, 74] Focal nodular hyperplasia often shows very prominent vascular changes, and these may relate to its etiology (see Fig. 3–7 and Chapter 6). Enlargement of major vessels is seen with avascular, poorly vascularized, and hypervascular lesions, and is found associated with metastatic as well as primary disease.[74]

In spite of its limitations in differential diagnosis, selective arteriography is very helpful in establishing the presence and size of liver tumors and is moderately helpful in defining whether the lesions are solitary or multiple. When angiogram, scan, and laparotomy were done for 118 patients with a mixed group of liver lesions, the angiograms demonstrated the disease in 93 per cent of the patients and were accurate about the specific location and number of lesions in 69 per cent.[37] The usefulness of arteriography is increased by combining its findings with those derived from radionuclide scanning. Few lesions of significant size should escape detection by both techniques.

Venography

Splenoportography has been supported by Balasegaram and Ong[8, 50] as a useful way of demonstrating primary and secondary liver tumors and of confirming intrahepatic spread of tumor. The technique also allows measurement of portal vein pressure, and this may indirectly provide evidence of unresectability due to tumor involvement of the portal vein in a noncirrhotic patient. However, my own experience and the reports of others suggest that evidence provided by portal vein filling and flow on splenoportography, and/or by late-phase portal venous filling after selective arteriography, is not very reliable.[1, 74] The common simultaneous occurrence of hepatocellular carcinoma and cirrhosis compounds this difficulty of accurate delineation of intrahepatic portal vein changes. Intraoperative palpation probably is more accurate than intraoperative portal venography in detecting small tumor nodules, but the venogram may be more reliable than the surgeon's fingers in finding soft tumor thrombus in the portal vein (Fig. 3–9).

An inferior venacavogram will often be abnormal in patients with primary liver carcinoma. Exelby, et al. found changes in 22 of 27 children with hepatoblastomas, and in 14 of 22 children with hepatocellular carcinomas.[25] Balasegaram noted changes in the inferior vena cava of 15 of 22 adult patients, which helped him to rule out their need for laparotomy.[8] Total occlusion of the intrahepatic cava or demonstration of tumor at the hepatic vein-inferior vena cava junction probably should rule out the possibility of resection but compression or partial occlusion of the inferior vena cava is often seen with resectable tumors and should not preclude exploration. (Fig. 3–10).

Total hepatic parenchymal visualization by injection of the hepatic veins via a transjugular route has been advocated by Skalkeas, et al. based on animal work,[61] but it is difficult to see how this would add much to the information derived from selective arteriography. However, selective hepatic venography often provides very important information about the resectability of bulky liver tumors,[75] and should be attempted whenever inferior venacavography is done. In the author's experience, the demonstration of intraluminal tumor or extraluminal compression at the hepatic vein-inferior vena cava junction has avoided operation in two patients whose arteriograms still left open the question of resection.

Various types of angiograms were completed in at least 153 patients in the 1974 LTS (see Table 3–3). Ninety-five per cent of the arteriograms showed at least one lesion. Fourteen out of 16 pediatric epithelial malignancies showed increased vascularity, as did 38 of 44 primary hepatocellular carcinomas in adults. Three of five adult patients with cholangiocarcinoma, and both patients with mixed hepatocellular and cholangiocarcinoma in adults who had arteriography,

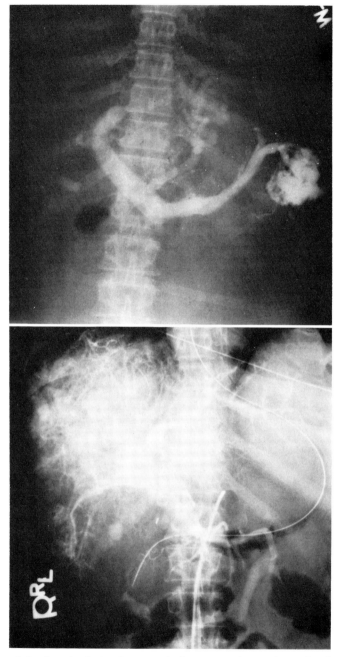

Figure 3–9. Portal vein involvement. Ascites recurred several months after side-to-side portacaval shunt operation in a 50-year-old man with cirrhosis and bleeding esophageal varices. On a pre-shunt splenoportogram the portal vein was seen to be patent, but on a repeat venogram done through the patent shunt several months later, the portal vein is seen to be full of tumor, which has grown retrograde down the portal vein.

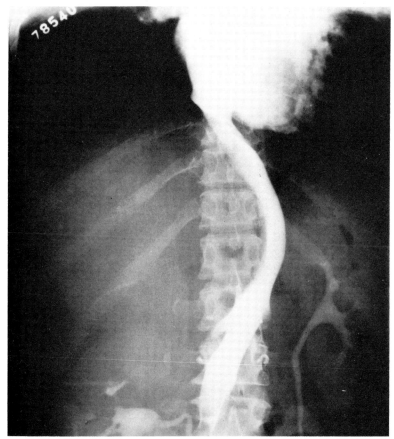

Figure 3-10. Inferior vena cavography. Marked distortion with partial occlusion of the intrahepatic vena cava is demonstrated by vena caval injection of contrast agent in a patient with metastatic carcinoma of the colon.

showed an increased, rather than a decreased, vascularity. All of the focal nodular hyperplasia tumors and most of the hepatocellular adenomas showed increased vascularity, but only three of 22 metastatic liver lesions showed an increased blood supply. Two of the three metastatic lesions with increased vascularity were primary in the colon.

Three patients with primary tumors of vascular origin who had arteriography all showed increased vascularity, whereas patients with benign myxoma, mesenchymal hamartoma, and cystadenocarcinoma all showed decreased vascularity by arteriography. Two of four patients with embryonal sarcomas showed increased vascularity, and the other two had decreased vascularity.

An inferior venacavogram showed obstruction of the inferior vena cava in at least four patients in the 1974 LTS, when resection sub-

Table 3–3. Results of Angiography–1974 Liver Tumor Survey

	PRIMARY EPITHILIAL CANCER		BENIGN TUMORS		METASTATIC TUMORS	MISCELLANEOUS TUMORS	TOTAL
	Adults	Children	Adenoma	FNH			
Arteriography: Patients	62	20	19	11	28	10	150
Lesion Visualized	61	19	17	10	26	9	142(95%)
*Increased Vascularity	43	14	10	10	3	5	84
Decreased Vascularity	8	2	6	0	19	4	40
Lesion Not Visualized	1	1	2	1	2	1	8(5%)
Inferior Vena Cavogram: Patients	2	2	0	2	0	2	8
Lesion Visualized	1	1		0	0	2	4
Lesion Not Visualized	1	1		2	0	0	4
Splenoportography	0	1**	0	0	0	0	1

*Discrepancy between total of increased and decreased vascularity and number of lesions visualized is because vascularity was not reported in some records.

**Did not visualize lesion.

sequently was proved possible because of noninvolvement of the inferior vena cava by direct invasion of tumor.

CHOLANGIOGRAPHY

Cholangiography, done preoperatively by a percutaneous transhepatic route or by endoscopic retrograde cannulation of the bile duct, can be most helpful in demonstrating lesions of the distal right and left hepatic ducts or their confluence. Cholangiography also will demonstrate the rare papillomas of the bile ducts that may be seen in association with cystadenomas or cystadenocarcinomas (see Chapter 7). It has been recommended as being helpful in the diagnosis of liver tumors,[56] but other techniques are more useful in demonstrating the size and number of most hepatic tumors, and cholangiography probably has a small role to play for most patients with solid liver tumors.

RADIOISOTOPE SCANNING AS AN AID TO DIAGNOSIS

In 1954 Stirret, et al. reported that space-occupying lesions of the liver could be demonstrated by scintillation scanning after radioisotope injection,[67] and remarkable advances in scanning technology have been made since that time. Scanning is probably more effective than any laboratory test in picking up primary and secondary liver tumors, and it is easier to do and more comfortable for the patient than invasive techniques. It is said that lesions as small as 1 to 2 cm in diameter can be picked up by modern equipment. The comprehensive review of Spencer summarizes current knowledge, and Figures 3–11 to 3–17 illustrate typical patterns.[66]

Radionuclides are picked up by the Kupffer cells of the reticuloendothelial system (gold-198-colloid, technetium-99M-sulfur colloid), by the hepatocyte (I-131-Rose Bengal), by amino acid transporting sites (selenium-75-methionine), or by neoplastic or inflammatory cells (gallium-67-citrate). Abnormal vascular pooling may be defined with I-131-human serum albumin (IHSA), with technetium-99m-albumin, or with 113m In-transferrin. Dynamic tracer study can add to information derived from static scans.[66]

Liver scans usually are positive with primary liver tumors. Table 3–1 demonstrates that 93 per cent of primary malignant tumors and 82 per cent of primary benign tumors of the liver collected in the 1974 LTS were shown by liver scan, and most other reports confirm this accuracy.[9, 25, 59, 69] However, information about whether scans can pick up multiple nodules of primary malignant disease, or can demonstrate

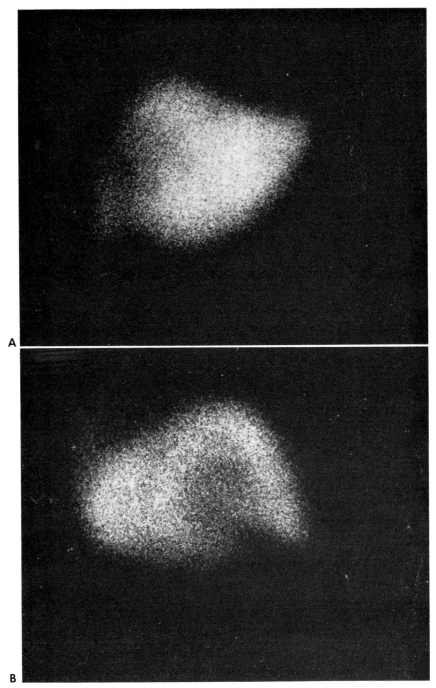

Figure 3–11.

See legend on opposite page.

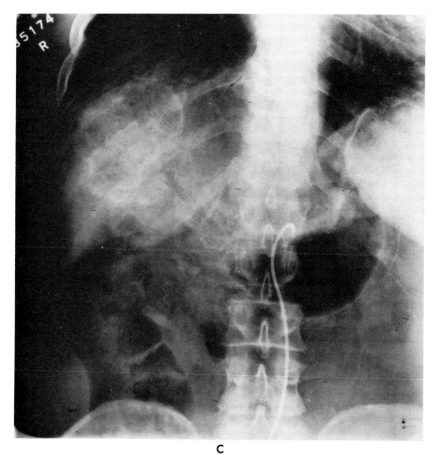

C

Figure 3–11. Large cholangiocarcinoma in a 53-year-old man. The right lobe appears almost completely replaced on the anterior Technetium 99^m sulfurcolloid (99^m Tc) scan *(A)*. A large defect is seen in the right lateral scan projection and in the late phases of a selective arteriogram *(B)*. The angiographic appearance is shown in *(C)*. Laparotomy revealed extension of this solitary tumor to involve the umbilical fissure, precluding resection.

the smaller metastatic lesion, is not so comforting. Although Watson and Torrance believe that scans are of much greater value than liver function tests and even exploratory laparotomy in picking up liver metastases from primary gastrointestinal cancer,[73] others provide evidence that false-positive and false-negative scan reports are common with metastatic tumors.[13, 54, 58] Most would probably agree that if there is no clinical or laboratory evidence of chronic benign liver disease, and if the metastatic deposit is at least 2.5 cm in diameter, the liver scan will pick it up.

Use of more than a single radionuclide may be helpful.[6, 48, 66] For reasons that remain unclear, gallium uptake was greater in one report

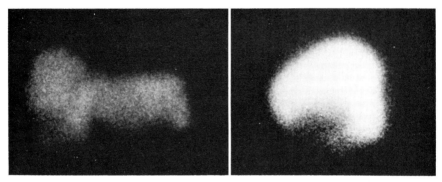

Figure 3–12. Technetium scan of primary liver cancer. A 68-year-old female with a solitary cholangiocarcinoma of the lateral inferior aspect of the right lobe (Case 123, Appendix IV). Tumor resected by right lobectomy. Anterior view, *A;* right lateral view, *B.*

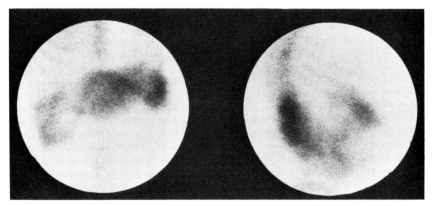

Figure 3–13. Primary hepatocellular carcinoma. Anterior and right lateral views of a 99^m Tc liver scan of a 47-year-old patient with cirrhosis and a large multifocal hepatocellular carcinoma.

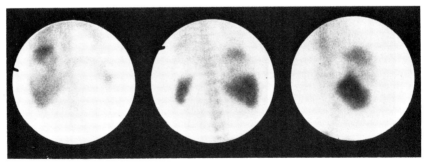

Figure 3–14. Metastatic breast cancer. Composite photo of anterior, posterior, and right lateral 99^m Tc liver scan of a 54-year-old woman.

Extensive involvement of both lobes of the liver with metastatic breast carcinoma is seen, and there is obvious activity in the skeletal system.

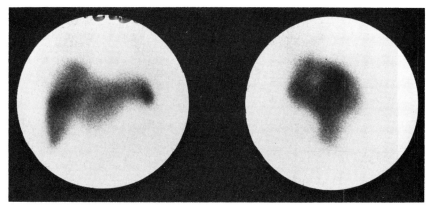

Figure 3–15. Metastatic colon cancer. Anterior and right lateral views of a 99ᵐ Tc scan of a solitary 3-cm. nodule of metastatic colon carcinoma occurring in a 64-year-old woman.

for 10 patients with liver cancer who had no serum AFP than it was in 17 patients with demonstrable AFP.[69] The differential diagnosis between cyst and liver tumor may be aided by the fact that neoplastic liver cells may take up selenium and/or gallium. Differentiation between benign and malignant solid tumors of the hepatocyte may be more difficult with present-day techniques.[20]

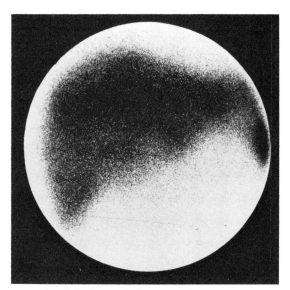

Figure 3–16. Focal nodular hyperplasia. 99ᵐ Tc liver scan of a 16-year-old girl with a 7-cm. nodule of focal nodular hyperplasia in her quadrate lobe (Case 10, Appendix VI-A). The nodule is considerably more difficult to appreciate on the scan than on an angiogram (see Figure 3–7).

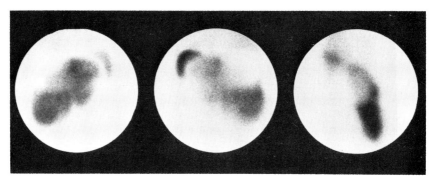

Figure 3–17. Liver cyst. Anterior, posterior, and right lateral views of 99ᵐ Tc liver scan of a 66-year-old woman with a huge simple cyst in the superior-posterior segment of her right lobe. The cyst was unroofed and its cavity filled with omentum.

Recent personal experience, and the fact that four of 16 focal nodular hyperplasia tumors collected in the 1974 LTS were not revealed by technetium scan, suggest that a negative scan should not rule out this lesion, even though it is large. Failure to visualize by scanning could be explained if the reticuloendothelial system and hepatocytes of focal nodular hyperplasia tumors function near the level of normal liver tissue. Whether the spontaneous "disappearance" of focal nodular hyperplasia tumor on serial scans represented a true fading away of a tumor, or simply the maturation of its functional capabilities, must remain an unanswered question (see Chapter 6, case 11, Appendix VI-A).

ULTRASOUND AND COMPUTERIZED TOMOGRAPHY

Ultrasound has been used recently to differentiate liver tumors,[30] and is particularly helpful in diagnosing cystic lesions.[30, 46, 77] Computerized tomography undoubtedly will play a very important role in the future diagnosis of solid and cystic liver tumors. These techniques were employed infrequently before 1974, and little information about their effectiveness is available from the 1974 LTS.

INVASIVE TECHNIQUES

Needle Biopsy

Needle biopsy is an effective method of establishing a histologic diagnosis of the nature of the liver tumor in many patients. It is contraindicated in patients suspected of having Echinococcus cyst, hemangiomas, or bleeding tendencies. With a cooperative patient and normal levels of circulating hemostatic factors, aspiration biopsy with a

Menghini needle usually can be done safely and will establish the diagnosis in 40 to 82 per cent of cases.[56] Biopsy with a thin-walled 18 to 22 gauge fine needle has been advocated recently for palpable nodules,[33] and peritoneoscopy and/or preliminary liver scanning will help to guide the needle into a tumor in patients without palpable disease.[16, 59]

There are limitations to needle biopsy, however. Many liver tumors are very vascular. Linder, et al. report three deaths due to intra-abdominal hemorrhage following needle biopsy in 27 patients.[39] Needle biopsy may or may not reveal the presence of an associated cirrhosis if a biopsy has been taken from an obvious tumor nodule. Finally, a needle biopsy taken from liver cell adenomas or focal nodular hyperplasia may be interpreted as normal liver. Because of these difficulties with interpretation of limited histologic material, because most liver tumors in young women are vascular and occur in noncirrhotic livers, and because resectability can be determined in most such patients only at laparotomy, it is recommended that needle biopsy of demonstrated masses not be done for most female patients in the menstruating age-group. Open biopsy at laparotomy, together with careful gross evaluation of the tumor, is a more effective and safer way to establish the diagnosis in this group.

Peritoneoscopy

Chan[16] and Balasegaram[8] are strong advocates of peritoneoscopy to help in establishing a diagnosis and in evaluating operability in patients with primary liver cancer. The left lobe of the liver and part of the anterior surface of the right lobe can be visualized through a peritoneoscope in most patients who have not had previous upper abdominal surgery. The presence of cirrhosis can be determined and the biopsying needle can be guided to a focus of obvious tumor under peritoneoscopic control.[35] Peritoneoscopy was rarely done in patients collected in the 1974 LTS, but this probably reflects the highly selected sample of resectable patients. Many patients who were determined to be unresectable may have been spared laparotomy by this technique, and this group would not have been collected in the Survey.

Perhaps the greatest value of peritoneoscopy lies in its ability to determine resectability. It will make laparotomy unnecessary in many patients for whom clinical and laboratory evidence suggest diffuse disease or associated cirrhosis.

Thoracic Duct Cannulation

Raffucci, et al. recommend cannulation of the thoracic duct in combination with cervical lymph node biopsy for patients suspected of having primary liver carcinoma.[56] Malignant cells may be found in the lymph, but their presence has not been yet shown to rule against the advisability of liver resection. The discovery of an unsuspected microscopic focus of metastatic carcinoma in the cervical lymph nodes would certainly contraindicate laparotomy and liver resection, but cervical node metastasis is rare with liver cancer. It is an interesting idea, but I know of no reports of the clinical effectiveness of this approach.

SUMMARY AND RECOMMENDATIONS

When a child or an adult patient presents with an upper abdominal mass, the initial evaluation probably should include liver function tests, a technetium liver scan, chest x-ray, coagulation studies, and an assay for alpha-fetoprotein.

Liver function tests will often be within the range of normal for patients with tumors that are still resectable. AP, SGOT, and BSP most often are abnormal with primary and secondary liver cancer, and a low serum albumin should raise the question of an associated cirrhosis. None of the standard liver function tests, however, will define the nature and extent of liver involvement by tumor. Coagulation studies that do not quickly revert to normal should represent an absolute contraindication to elective resection for liver tumor, since the surgeon's ability to resect safely depends to an enormous extent on the patient's own ability to control hemorrhage from minor vessels. Serum alpha-fetoprotein determination will help to confirm a diagnosis of primary carcinoma of hepatocellular origin, but will not assist in determining the extent of the disease or prognosis unless done serially. Both CEA and AFP determinations probably will have their greatest value in following the course of a patient during and after therapy.

When a clinician wishes to investigate the possibility of occult metastases in the liver of a patient without liver enlargement or palpable mass, the standard liver function tests (including BSP) and a liver scan should be done. If both are within normal limits, further studies usually will not be rewarding. If metastases are found for which resection is contemplated, tomography of the chest and bone scan should be done to rule out hidden disease.

REFERENCES

    1. Albacete, R. A., Matthews, M. J., and Saini, N.: Portal vein thromboses in malignant hepatoma. Ann. Intern. Med. 67:337, 1967.

2. Alpert, E.: Alpha-1-fetoprotein: serologic marker of human hepatoma and embryonal carcinoma. Natl. Cancer Inst. Monogr. *35*:415, 1972.
3. Alpert, E., and Isselbacher, K. J.: Hepatitis-associated antigen and hepatoma in the U. S. Lancet *2*:1087, 1971.
4. Alpert, M. E., Uriel, J., and de Nechaud, B.: Alpha-fetoglobulin in the diagnosis of human hepatoma. N. Engl. J. Med. *278*:984, 1968.
5. Al-Sarraf, M., Kithier, K., and Vaitkevicius, V. K.: Primary liver cancer. Cancer *33(2)*:574, 1974.
6. Anderson, J. E., and Perlmutter, G. S.: Diagnosis of hepatoma using a multiple radionuclide approach. Radiology *102*:387, 1972.
7. Anthony, P. P.: Carcinoma of the liver in man. Bull. Int. Pathol. *29*:44, 1974.
8. Balasegaram, M.: Hepatic surgery: present and future. Ann. R. Coll. Surg. Engl. *47*:139, 1970.
9. Baum, S., Silver, L., and Vouchides, D.: The recognition of hepatic metastases through radioisotope color scanning. J.A.M.A. *197*:83, 1966.
10. Bloomer, J. R., et al.: Relationship of serum α-fetoprotein to the severity and duration of illness in patients with viral hepatitis. Gastroenterology *68*:342, 1975.
11. Brownstein, M. H., and Ballard, H. S.: Hepatoma associated with erthrocytosis. Am. J. Med. *40*:204, 1966.
12. Caron, J., et al.: Arteriographic exploration of secondary cancers of the liver; interest of Lipiodol by arterial injection. Sem. Hop. Paris *49*:3367, 1973.
13. Castagna, J., et al.: The reliability of liver scans and function tests in detecting metastases. Surg. Gynecol. Obstet. *134*:463, 1972.
14. Castleman, B., Scully, R. E., and McNeely, B. U.: Case records of the Mass. General Hospital, case 23 – 1973. N. Engl. J. Med. *288(23)*:1230, 1973.
15. Chainuvati, T., Viranvatti, V., and Pongpipat, D.: Relationship of hepatitis B antigen in cirrhosis and hepatoma in Thailand. Gastroenterology *68*:1261, 1975.
16. Chan, K. T.: The management of primary liver carcinoma. Ann. R. Coll. Surg. *41*:253, 1967.
17. Chu, M. L., et al.: Demonstration of alpha-fetoglobulin in hepatoma tissue by fluorescent antibody technique. Cancer *34*:268, 1974.
18. Clatworthy, H. W., Schiller, M., and Grosfeld, J. L.: Primary liver tumors in infancy and childhood. Arch. Surg. *109*:143, 1974.
19. The Coordinating Group for the Research of Liver Cancer. People's Rep. of China. Application of serum alpha-feto-protein assay in mass survey of primary carcinoma of liver. Am. J. Chin. Med. *2(3)*:241, 1974.
20. Danais, S., et al.: Radiopertechnetate flow study and liver scan in a case of benign hepatoma (liver cell adenoma). Am. J. Roentgenol. Radium Ther. Nucl. Med. *118(4)*:836, 1973.
21. Dehner, L. P., and Ishak, K. G.: Vascular tumors of the liver in infants and children. Arch. Pathol. *92*:101, 1971.
22. Division of Cancer Research, National Vaccine and Serum Institute, Peking. Complement fixation test for detection of alpha-fetoprotein in the diagnosis of primary liver cancer. Chin. Med. J. *8*:100, 1973.
23. Edmondson, H. A.: Progress in pediatrics: differential diagnosis of tumors and tumor-like lesions of liver in infancy and childhood. A.M.A. J. Dis. Child. *91*:168, 1956.
24. Ervasti, J.: Primary carcinoma of the liver. Acta Chir. Scand. (Suppl.) 334, 1964.
25. Exelby, P. R., Filler, R. M., and Grosfeld, J. L.: Liver tumors in children in the particular reference to hepatoblastoma and hepatocellular carcinoma. American Academy of Pediatrics Surgical Section Survey – 1974. J. Pediatr. Surg. *10*:329, 1975.
26. Gandhi, R. K., Deshmukh, S. S., and Bhalerao, R. A.: Hepatoblastoma in children. Indian Pediatr. *10*:259, 1973.
27. Gane, N. F. C.: Malignant hepatoma. J. Clin. Pathol. *26*:384, 1973.
28. Geography of primary liver cancer. Br. Med. J. *6*:381, 1970.
29. Gold, P., and Freedman, S. O.: Specific carcinoembryonic antigens of the human digestive system. J. Exp. Med. *122*:467, 1965.
30. Grossman, H.: The evaluation of abdominal masses in children with emphasis on noninvasive methods. A roentgenographic approach. Cancer *35*:884, 1975.

31. Handa, S. P.: Hypoglycemia in primary carcinoma of the liver. Am. J. Dig. Dis. *11*:898, 1966.
32. Hersh, T., et al.: Hepatocellular carcinoma. Am. J. Gastroenterol. *58*:162, 1972.
33. Hurwitz, A. L., Gueller, R., and Pugay, P.: Fine-needle aspiration of malignant hepatic nodules for cytodiagnosis. J.A.M.A. *229*:814, 1974.
34. Ihde, D. C., et al.: Clinical manifestations of hepatoma; a review of six years' experience at a cancer hospital. Am. J. Med. *56*:83, 1974.
35. Jori, G. P., and Peschle, C.: Combined peritoneoscopy and liver biopsy in the diagnosis of hepatic neoplasm. Gastroenterology *63*:1016, 1972.
36. Kew, M. C., et al.: Hepatitis -B antigen and cirrhosis in Bantu patients with primary liver cancer. Cancer *34*:539, 1974.
37. Kim, D. K., et al.: Tumors of the liver as demonstrated by angiography, scan and laparotomy. Surg. Gynecol. Obstet. *141*:409, 1975.
38. Lin, T. Y.: Primary cancer of the liver; quadrennial review. Scand. J. Gastroenterol. (Suppl.) *6*:223, 1970.
39. Linder, G. T., Crook, J. N., and Cohn, I., Jr.: Primary liver carcinoma. Cancer *33*:1624, 1974.
40. Mabogunje, O., Rosen, P. P., and Fortner, J. G.: Liver cell carcinoma during the prime of life. Surg. Gynecol. Obstet. *140*:75, 1975.
41. Malt, R. A., Van Vroonhoven, T. J., and Kakumoto, Y.: Manifestations and prognosis of carcinoma of the liver. Surg. Gynecol. Obstet. *135*:361, 1972.
42. Margolis, S., and Homcy, C.: Systemic manifestations of hepatoma. Medicine *51*:381, 1972.
43. Martin, E. W., et al.: Carcinoembryonic antigen, clinical and historical aspects. Cancer *37*:62, 1976.
44. Matsumoto, Y., et al.: Response of alpha-fetoprotein to chemotherapy in patients with hepatoma. Cancer *34*:1602, 1974.
45. McIntire, K. R., et al.: Effect of surgical and chemotherapeutic treatment on alpha-fetoprotein levels in patients with hepatocellular carcinoma. Cancer *37*:677, 1976.
46. Melki, G.: Ultrasonic patterns of tumors of the liver. J. Clin. Ultrasound *1*:306, 1973.
47. Miller, A. I., Moral, M. D., and Schiff, E. R.: Presence of serum α-1-fetoprotein in alcoholic hepatitis. Gastroenterology *68*:381, 1975.
48. Muroff, L. R., and Johnson, P. M.: The use of multiple radionuclide imaging to differentiate the focal intrahepatic lesion. Am. J. Roentgenol. Radium Ther. Nucl. Med. *121(4)*:723, 1974.
49. Novy, S., et al.: Angiographic evaluation of primary malignant hepatocellular tumors in children. Am. J. Roentgenol. Radium Ther. Nucl. Med. *120(2)*:353, 1974.
50. Ong, G. B., and Leong, C. H.: Surgical treatment of primary liver cancer. J. R. Coll. Surg. *14*:42, 1969.
51. Parks, L. C., et al.: Alpha-fetoprotein: an index of progression or regression of hepatoma and a target for immunotherapy. Ann. Surg. *180*:599, 1974.
52. Pedersen, K. O.: Fetuin, new globulin isolated from serum. Nature (Lond.) *154*:575, 1944.
53. Perlin, E., et al.: The value of serial measurement of both human chorionic gonadotropin and alpha-fetoprotein for monitoring germinal cell tumors. Cancer *37*:215, 1976.
54. Poulose, K. P., and Reba, R. C.: Liver scanning in hepatic metastases. Lancet *1*:517, 1974.
55. Purtilo, D. T., et al.: Alpha-fetoprotein: diagnostic and prognostic use in patients with hepatomas. Am. J. Clin. Pathol. *59*:295, 1973.
56. Raffucci, F. L., and Ramirez-Schon, G.: Management of tumors of the liver. Surg. Gynecol. Obstet. *130*:371, 1970.
57. Reed, W. D., et al.: Detection of hepatitis B antigen by radioimmunoassay in chronic liver disease and hepatocellular carcinoma in Great Britain. Lancet *2*:690, 1973.
58. Rosenthal, S., and Kaufman, S.: The liver scan in metastatic disease. Arch. Surg. *106*:656, 1973.
59. Sharpstone, P., et al.: The diagnosis of primary malignant tumors of the liver. Findings in 48 consecutive patients. Q. J. Med. New Series *41(161)*:99, 1972.
60. Simons, M. J., et al.: Australia antigen in Singapore. Chinese patients with hepatocellular carcinoma. Lancet *1*:1149, 1971.

61. Skalkeas, G., et al.: Hepatography. Am. J. Surg. *131*:235, 1976.
62. Smith, J. B., and Blumberg, B. S.: Viral hepatitis, postnecrotic cirrhosis, and hepatocellular carcinoma. Lancet *2*:953, 1969.
63. Smith, K., et al.: Serum 5' nucleotidase in patients with tumor in the liver. Cancer *19*:1281, 1966.
64. Smrcka, J., et al.: Arteriographic demonstration and successful removal of metastatic islet cell tumors in liver. Diabetes *16*:598, 1967.
65. Sorsdahl, O. A., and Gay, B. B., Jr.: Roentgenologic features of a primary carcinoma of the liver in infants and children. Am. J. Roentgenol. Radium Ther. Nucl. Med. *100*:117, 1967.
66. Spencer, R. P.: Radionuclide liver scans in tumor detection. Cancer *37*:475, 1976.
67. Stirret, L. A., Yohl, E. T., and Cassen, B.: Clinical application of hepatic radioactivity surveys. Am. J. Gastroenterol. *21*:310, 1954.
68. Sugahara, K., et al.: Serum alpha-fetoprotein and resection of primary hepatic cancer. Arch. Surg. *106*:63, 1973.
69. Suzuki, T., et al.: Serum alpha-fetoprotein and Ga citrate uptake in hepatoma. Am. J. Roentgenol. Radium Ther. Nucl. Med. *120(3)*:627, 1974.
70. Tsou, C., Ledis, S., and McCoy, M. G.: 5' nucleotide phosphodiesterase isoenzyme pattern in the serum of human hepatoma. Cancer Res. *33*:2215, 1973.
71. Vogel, C. L., and Linsell, C. A.: Highlights: international symposium on hepatocellular carcinoma, Kampala, Uganda. J. Natl. Cancer Inst. *48*:567, 1972.
72. Vogel, C. L., et al.: Serum alpha-fetoprotein in 184 Ugandan patients with hepatocellular carcinoma. Cancer *33*:959, 1974.
73. Watson, A., and Torrance, B.: Liver scanning and hepatic metastases (letter to editor). Lancet *1*:1352, 1974.
74. Watson, R. C., and Baltaxe, H. A.: The angiographic appearance of primary and secondary tumors of the liver. Diagnost. Radiol. *101*:539, 1971.
75. Williams, R. D., and Peterson, C., Jr.: Selective hepatic venography in primary liver cell carcinoma. Am. J. Surg. *131*:350, 1976.
76. Yu, Chun: Primary carcinoma of the liver (hepatoma), its diagnosis by selective celiac arterography. Am. J. Roentgenol. Radium Ther. Nucl. Med. *99*:142, 1967.
77. Goldberg, B. B., et al.: Diagnostic Uses of Ultrasound. New York, Grune & Stratton, 1975.

Chapter Four

PRIMARY EPITHELIAL
CANCER IN ADULTS

Primary carcinoma of the liver is a disease with a character all its own. The striking differences in its incidence around the world, its relationship to several etiologic agents, and its ability to produce a unique serum protein marker make it most unusual.

Perhaps this should not be surprising, since this large organ manages the most complex of metabolic functions within the simplest of histologic frameworks. The liver's unique ability to regenerate and its role as a detoxifier may combine to render it more susceptible to neoplastic change when exposed to any number of injury-producing substances. Yet, at least in the Western world, primary carcinoma of the liver is a rare disease, so rare that few surgeons have had enough experience with it to provide a basis for recommending therapy.

This chapter will consider those primary solid epithelial cancers of the liver that arise in adults from the hepatocyte or from the intrahepatic bile ducts. Tumors arising from mesenchymal elements, cystadenomas, and cystadenocarcinomas will be considered in Chapter Seven.

The separation of childhood cancers is arbitrary and perhaps not justified, since much evidence suggests that at least the hepatocellular carcinomas of childhood behave much like the adult disease. However, there are important differences, and our choice is to consider all primary cancers in children less than 16 years of age in Chapters Five and Seven.

Table 4-1. Primary Epithelial Cancer of Liver in Adults: Incidence, Sex, Age, and Cirrhosis

REF.	YEAR	CITY OR COUNTRY	DURATION OF STUDY	CASES	MEAN AGE	MALE / FEMALE	HEPATOCELLULAR / CHOLANGIOCELLULAR	PERCENTAGE INCIDENCE AT POST MORTEM	PERCENTAGE ALL CANCER	PERCENTAGE CIRRHOSIS
98	1932	Singapore	–	134	43 yrs	133/1	99/35	0.76	–	73
87	1948	New Orleans	16 yrs	55	–	41/14	29/13	0.31	–	71
23	1961	Liverpool	21 yrs	109	–	82/27	80/21	0.145	–	60
101	1963	China	20 yrs	336	41 yrs	273/63	296/27	–	–	98
33	1964	Finland	10 yrs	100	65 yrs	56/37	45/29	0.6	2.9	48
72	1965	Glasgow	15 yrs	49	–	43/6	45/2	–	–	86
66	1966	Los Angeles	11 yrs	144*	–	–	121/10	0.12	–	53
21	1967	Singapore	4 yrs	108	–	84/24	98/10	–	–	59
64	1970	Taiwan	16 yrs	271	–	68**/14	262/8	–	3.2	31
59	1971	Japan	42 yrs	89	57 yrs	78/11	57/7	2.28	19.5 (males)	61
14	1971	Sweden	11 yrs	92	–	60%/40%	50%/33%	–	–	48
24	1971	Richmond	18 yrs	65	53 yrs	2.3:1	49/4	0.23	–	47–60
71	1972	Boston	25 yrs	51	–	4:1	44/6	–	–	60
10	1973	Uganda	–	282	40 yrs	227/55	263/19	–	–	84
84	1973	Boston	13 yrs	98	64 yrs	80/18	71/12	0.7	–	81
76	1973	India	10 yrs	59*	–	49/10	50/2	1.29	14.6	78
8	1974	Detroit	11 yrs	64	–	43/21	53/9	–	–	67***
26	1974	England	7 yrs	85	56 yrs	64/21	only hepatocell. Ca.	–	–	58
65	1974	New Orleans	22 yrs	164	–	5:1	98/19	–	–	56
83	1974	Thailand	10 yrs	511	–	–	–	2.43	–	17[64]
79	1975	Hong Kong	11 yrs	406	–	5:1	81/15	–	–	84

*Includes some children.
**Resected cases only.
***20/30 patients with hepatocellular Ca.

ETIOLOGY AND EPIDEMIOLOGY

Table 4-1 details the incidence of primary liver cancer in various parts of the world, and correlates incidence with various clinical factors.

Many factors have been implicated in liver carcinogenesis, and the reader is referred to the excellent recent reviews of Anthony,[9] Higginson and Svoboda,[51] and Lin[64] for more complete information than is outlined briefly below.

Malnutrition has been implicated because the areas of higher incidence of liver cancer are those of extreme poverty and protein deprivation. However, no specific deficiency has been clearly related to malignant change and, if there is a relationship, it may be that the liver injury of malnutrition may render the hepatocyte more susceptible to the influence of a specific carcinogen.

Cycasin has been shown to be carcinogenic in animals but the incidence of liver cancer in Guam, where this substance is consumed as a starch substitute, is low.[51] Various Senecio alkaloids ingested as "bush tea" in the Caribbean area are definitely related to hepatic veno-occlusive disease, but probably are not associated with an increased risk of malignancy.[9] The mycotoxins, particularly those produced by the fungus Aspergillus flavus, have come under great suspicion in recent years, but a clear demonstration of their relation to liver cancer in man has yet to be made. Aflatoxins will produce hepatocellular carcinoma in rats and other animals, but monkeys and apes are particularly resistant to malignant change when fed moldy foodstuffs containing aflatoxins. Interestingly, when tumors do occur, they do not produce alpha-fetoprotein. Epidemiologic studies in Africa and Taiwan have shown a close correlation between areas with heavy contamination of foodstuffs with aflatoxins and the incidence of liver cancer.[9, 64]

However, blacks living in America and Caucasians living in South Africa have an incidence and presentation of liver carcinoma that do not differ from those of other patients in the Western world. In general, the age at which Africans and Asians develop liver carcinoma is a decade or two younger than patients reported from the Western world.[7]

Clonorchis sinensis infestation has been associated with liver carcinoma in China and the Far East,[42, 55] but Tull found Clonorchis in only two of 134 cases of liver carcinoma from Singapore,[98] and Lin reported no parasites in 271 cases of liver cancer from Taiwan.[64] Stitnimankarn reported liver cancers in 42 patients with Opisthorchis viverrini infestation, 83 per cent of which were cholangiocarcinomas or mixed tumors.[64] Clonorchis sinensis was found in the bile duct of a single patient in the 1974 Liver Tumor Survey, but he was a Chinese man with a trabecular hepatocellular carcinoma (Case 7, Appendix IV).

In Western countries liver cirrhosis is the most commonly associated disease. Tables 4-1 and 4-2 document this impressive association, and

Table 4–2. Primary Epithelial Carcinoma in Adults
Cirrhosis Versus Histologic Pattern

REFERENCE (YEAR)	HEPATO-CELLULAR CARCINOMA		CHOLANGIO-CELLULAR CARCINOMA		MIXED CARCINOMA	
	Cases	Cirrhosis (%)	Cases	Cirrhosis	Cases	Cirrhosis (%)
10 Uganda (1973)	138	84.7	19	1 patient biliary cirrhosis	—	—
26 England (1974)	85	58	—	—	—	—
33 Finland (1964)	45	60	29	38%	7	29
87 New Orleans (1948)	29	86	13	38%	5	60
98 Singapore (1932)	99	75	35	66%	—	—
21 Singapore (1967)	98	64	10	0	—	—
8 Detroit (1974)	30	67	—	—	—	—
59 Japan (1971)	82	63	7	29%	0	0
1974 LTS	109	21	13	1 patient Thorotrast	5	40

cancer is as likely to occur in the patient with nutritional or posthepatic cirrhosis as in the patient with alcoholic cirrhosis. Fisher, et al. make the point that the use of ethyl alcohol may correlate more closely with liver carcinoma than with the presence of cirrhosis,[36] but most others believe that the liver destruction and subsequent push toward regeneration in chronic diffuse liver injury may escape from normal "control" and proceed to neoplasia. With cirrhosis, the ability to regenerate may be limited by scar tissue, and the as yet poorly understood drive toward regeneration may continue unabated—a circumstance not found after post-resection regeneration of the normal liver. Mori attempts to differentiate between the type of cirrhosis and the coincidence of cancer,[75] and Anthony and Higginson and Svoboda both noted that cancer is more commonly associated with livers with fine fibrosis and large macronodules than with livers with small nodules and coarse fibrosis.[9, 51]

The interval between the diagnosis of cirrhosis and the development of liver carcinoma in 17 patients averaged 47 months in one series, and one patient was known to have cirrhosis for at least 17 years.[94] Purtilo and Gottlieb reported an interval averaging eight years between a diagnosis of cirrhosis and the development of liver carcinoma.[84]

Whatever the theoretic considerations, the fact of limited regenerative ability and decreased hepatocellular reserve of the cirrhotic liver is of major practical importance in the ability of the physician and/or surgeon to effect the course of patients with liver cancer.

Most series have noted a preponderance of male patients, and the

Table 4–3. Primary Epithelial Cancer in Adults — 1974 LTS:
Age, Sex, and Cirrhosis

	MALE	FEMALE
AGE		
16–29 years	5	13
30–39 years	3	7
40–49 years	10	8
50–59 years	16	10
60–69 years	25	14
70 and older	12	4
Total	71	56
CIRRHOSIS	23	3
With Thorotrast Fibrosis	1	2
With Hemochromatosis	2	0

disease most commonly occurs late in life. However, in the 1974 LTS, 70 per cent of resectable primary liver cancers in adults under 40 years of age occurred in females, whereas two-thirds of patients over 50 years of age were male (see Table 4–3). Table 4–9 documents that, among Caucasian Americans, the number of resections done was about equally divided between males and females, and in noncirrhotic patients the females actually outnumbered the males. There must be an as yet unappreciated significance in the fact that both benign and malignant solid liver tumors occur more frequently in Caucasian females during their child-bearing years.

Is there a familial incidence of liver carcinoma? Lin reports two siblings with primary cancer,[64] Kaplan and Cole found hepatocellular cancer in three adult male siblings,[57] and Fraumeni, et al. reported the first such relationship in children.[39] Hepatoblastoma occurred in two infant sisters found during the 1974 LTS (Cases 34 and 35, Appendix V).

Although Al-Sarraf, et al. found an increased incidence of type B blood serotype in Negro patients with hepatocellular carcinoma,[8] no such relationship was found between ABO blood groupings and liver cancer in the larger series reported from China and Africa.[22, 89]

Thorotrast may produce chronic progressive liver injury over a period of years, as pointed out first by MacMahon, et al.[69] Rare cases continued to be reported of this association, occurring as long as 33 years after Thorotrast ingestion. Most of these Thorotrast-induced tumors are cholangiocarcinomas and angiosarcomas, although a few hepatocellular carcinomas also have been reported.[25, 93, 96, 99]

Two patients in the 1974 LTS developed primary liver cancer many years after irradiation of the liver for other diseases. One patient had 2550 Rads of irradiation for a hemangioma in 1947 and developed liver cancer in 1967 (Case 96, Appendix IV). The other patient had radiation therapy to a "fibrosarcoma" of the right lobe of her liver at age 12 in 1939. Thirty years later she had resection of a primary malignant tumor from the right lobe, and she was dead with disease 12 months later (Case 98, Appendix IV). Both patients had an anaplastic form of hepatocellular carcinoma. However, there was no apparent increase in the incidence of liver cancer in Nagasaki and Hiroshima 25 years after World War II.[92]

Galdabini discusses the relationship between chronic cholangitis and the development of carcinoma.[41] Cholangiocarcinoma developed after ten years of intermittent cholangitis in a single patient in the 1974 LTS.

Rawlings, et al. described the occurrence of hepatocellular carcinoma in two patients with alpha-1-antitrypsin deficiency and cirrhosis in 1974,[85] and Eriksson and Hagerstrand reported six liver cancers in nine patients with the homozygous (ZZ) deficiency and cirrhosis.[32] A mixed hepatocellular and cholangiocellular carcinoma has been reported recently as an incidental autospy finding in a patient without cirrhosis who had the homozygous alpha-1-antitrypsin deficiency.[90] Farber has summarized some of what is known about carcinogenesis in animal livers, and has related these findings to man.[35]

The perhaps confusing and varied array of relationships briefly summarized above may have some common factor that eventually will become known. For the present, however, one must conclude that neoplastic change of the liver cells in man is probably encouraged by a number of environmental, toxic, and genetic factors. The field remains a fascinating one for future study.

THE PATHOLOGY OF EPITHELIAL LIVER CANCER IN ADULTS

Historical Background

Primary liver cancer as a pathologic entity was first recognized in the early 19th century. Although earlier anatomists, including Morgagni, observed tumor masses within the liver, they did not distinguish their origin. Rokitansky noted the relative frequency of cancer involving the liver, but it was Virchow who finally established the liver as a primary site for the origin of cancer. Late in the 19th century, Hanot and Gilbert classified liver cancer according to its gross appearance. They identified three patterns which they called "massive," "nodular," and "diffuse." They also described a fourth variant termed "carcinomatous cirrhosis" (cancer avec cirrhose) which represented a combination of the nodular and diffusely infiltrative patterns.[45] Their gross classification has persisted to the present day.

In 1911, Goldzieher and von Bokay advanced the concept that liver carcinoma originated in the hepatocyte.[43] Herxheimer,[48] on finding tubular carcinoma with columnar epithelium, considered bile duct epithelium also to be a site of origin. Yamagiwa, in 1911, first clearly separated liver cancer into liver cell (hepatocellular) and intrahepatic bile duct (cholangiocellular) types,[106] and Ewing in 1919 recognized a "mixed" pattern with both liver cell and bile duct features as a rare but distinct category.[34]

GROSS PATHOLOGY

The gross appearance of primary hepatocellular carcinoma may have a massive, a nodular, or a diffuse configuration. The massive type consists of a single large predominant mass that may have associated satellite nodules; the nodular type consists of an aggregate of clusters of similarly sized nodules; and the diffuse type, which is very rare, is characterized by a widespread, finely nodular pattern that may involve the entire liver. The disease may have a multicentric origin, particularly in the cirrhotic, but in the normal liver it usually starts from a single focus and grows in a fashion similar to most cancers, forming nodules and satellites as it enlarges. The fact that it often is massive when recognized reflects the hidden position of the liver behind the rib margin, the enormous functional reserve of the liver, and the fact that liver cancer probably remains within the capsule of its mother organ longer than most other cancers before widespread metastasis occurs. Most reports indicate that all types of primary liver tumors occur more frequently in the right lobe, and this undoubtedly is correct if "right lobe" means that fraction of the liver to the right of the umbilical fissure. However, the distribution of tumors on either side of the central plane, as defined by the inflow vessels (see Chapter 11), may be more nearly equal. Hepatocellular carcinomas usually are soft, very vascular, and dull gray to tan-yellow in color. In a liver grossly distorted by cirrhosis, it may be difficult to differentiate malignant from regenerative nodules, but the cancer often is more vascular and softer than the adjacent surrounding nodules. Umbilication is rare. Necrosis of the tumor is common and, if associated with invasion of Glisson's capsule, may lead to intraperitoneal hemorrhage. Invasion of the portal and/or hepatic veins may be a prominent feature.[5] Involvement of the inferior vena cava is less common. Regional lymph node metastasis is uncommon, but does occur. The underlying liver frequently shows an associated cirrhosis that most often is macronodular (see Table 4–2). Pulmonary metastases due to venous involvement may be present upon initial presentation.

Cholangiocellular carcinomas also exhibit massive, nodular, and/or diffuse patterns of liver involvement; but they usually are gray-white, firm to hard, less vascular, and more nodular. Necrosis of the tumor mass is uncommon. Infiltration of Glisson's capsule by the tumor frequently results in an umbilicated external appearance. Venous invasion is rare. Cirrhosis is an uncommon occurrence, although diffuse portal fibrosis and bile duct proliferation associated with Thorotrast deposition is seen. Distant metastases at initial presentation are uncommon, but involvement of the regional portal, peripancreatic, and celiac lymph nodes is often present. Rarely, cholangiocellular carcinoma arising in the hilum of the liver may present with a wedge-shaped configuration.

Mixed hepatocellular and cholangiocellular carcinomas show no distinct gross pathologic features. Their appearance is variable, depending on the combination and proportion of cell types.[6]

Microscopic Pathology

Higginson and Steiner emphasized that the gross appearance and size of liver tumors may vary in different geographic regions.[50] However, the microscopic patterns of primary liver carcinoma have a similar appearance world-wide,[16] and, ultimately, classification is dependent on histologic appearance.

Primary liver carcinoma is characterized by two distinct cell types: (1) hepatocellular carcinoma, resembling liver cells and cords; and (2) cholangiocellular carcinoma, which resembles bile duct structures. Winternitz distinguished these categories by comparing cell type, structural patterns, and stromal reaction,[104] and these criteria generally have been utilized by successive authors.[9, 15, 28, 30, 50]

Hepatocellular carcinomas characteristically are composed of cells with abundant granular eosinophilic cytoplasm and nuclei with a prominent membrane and large eosinophilic nucleoli, but many variations occur. Edmondson and Steiner recognized two variants: a trabecular type with adult and an embryonal differentiation and a giant cell type.[30] Higginson and Steiner recognized a common trabecular pattern, and less common variant forms including adenoid, giant cell, anaplastic, and pseudoepitheliomatous patterns.[50] Anthony, reviewing the histopathology of liver carcinoma in Uganda, additionally identified a rare "clear cell" variety.[10] The reported increasing preponderance of hepatocellular carcinomas, compared to cholangiocellular carcinomas, may

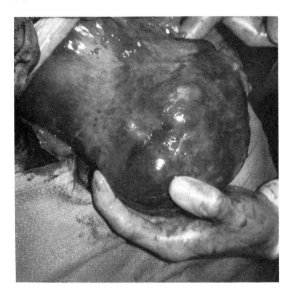

Figure 4–1. Large hepa-
tocellular carcinoma in a 62-
year-old female which had
dragged down and thinned
out the center of the right
lobe of the liver.

be due to the recognition and acceptance of a classification that implies
an hepatocellular origin for most of the variant patterns.

The cholangiocellular carcinomas commonly are composed of
tubules and ductular structures of well or moderately differentiated
cuboidal epithelium embedded in a dense, fibrous stroma. The abun-
dance of connective tissue usually associated with these ductular car-

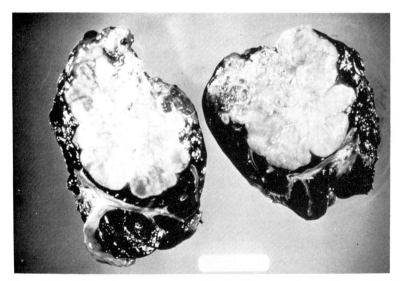

Figure 4–2. Cholangiocarcinoma resected by left lobectomy from a 52-year-old white
female. Tumor was hard, white, and nodular. (Photo provided courtesy of R. Freeark,
M.D., and E. Orfei, M.D., of Loyola University, Chicago.)

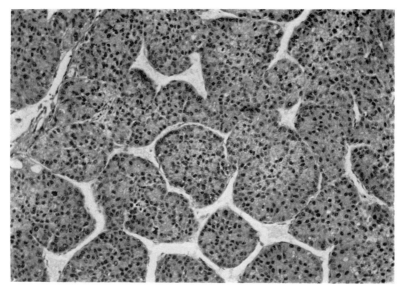

Figure 4–3. Hepatocellular carcinoma, trabecular type. The most common and characteristic pattern with broad trabecular cords of cells closely resembling normal hepatocytes.

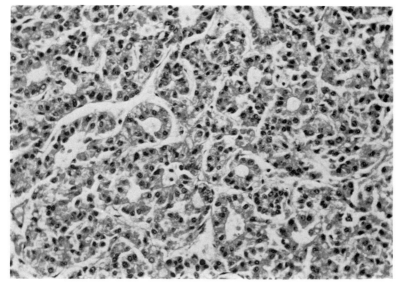

Figure 4–4. Hepatocellular carcinoma, adenoid type. A pseudoglandular pattern composed of multiple acinar-shaped structures. This type may be confused with cholangiocellular carcinoma.

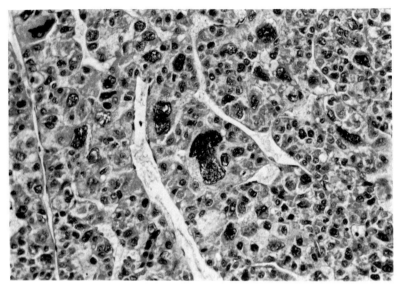

Figure 4–5. Hepatocellular carcinoma, syncytial type. Histologic pattern predominated by prominent large bizarre malignant hepatocytes.

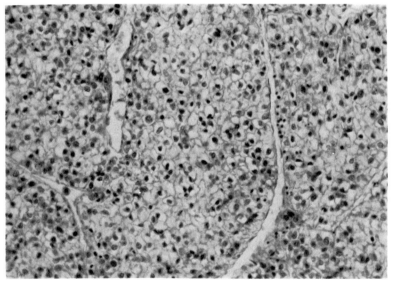

Figure 4–6. Hepatocellular carcinoma, clear cell type. Broad cords of carcinoma cells with clear cytoplasm, which resemble renal cell carcinoma.

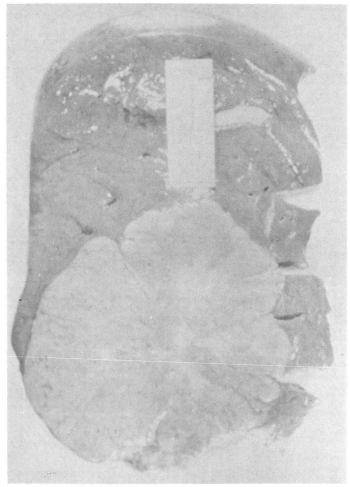

Figure 4-7. Large primary hepatocellular carcinoma resected from 15-year-old boy (polygonal cell with fibrous stroma variant). Alive, free of disease, ten years later.
Case 81 – Appendix IV).

cinomas explains their characteristic firm gross appearance (see Figs. 4-10, 4-11).

The mixed hepatocellular-cholangiocellular carcinomas show the distinct histologic features of both types, either in combination or separately. Many liver cell tumors exhibit more than one histologic pattern and more than one grade of malignancy.

A more detailed discussion of a unique histologic variant of primary hepatocellular carcinoma, polygonal cell with fibrous stroma (PCFS) is included in the discussion of the findings of the 1974 LTS (see pages 86-87 and Figs. 4-7 through 4-9).

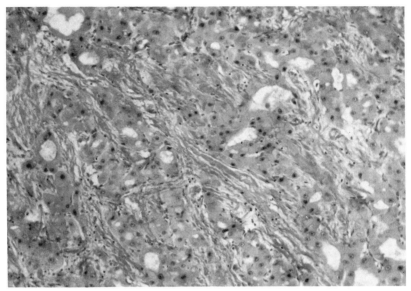

Figure 4-8. Hepatocellular carcinoma with solid and adenoid groups of polygonal type hepatic cells enmeshed in fibrillar bands of acellular fibrous stroma. (PCFS variant. See pages 86–87. Case 81 – Appendix IV.)

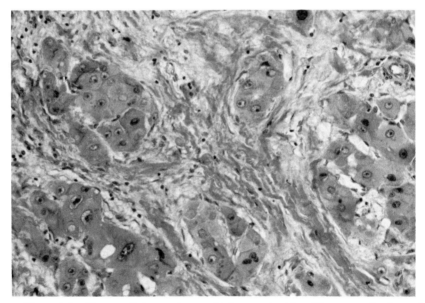

Figure 4-9. Hepatocellular carcinoma (high power) with solid groups of polygonal cells with associated fibrous stroma. Note the atypical large nuclei with prominent and irregular nucleolar structures. (PCFS variant. Case 81 – Appendix IV.)

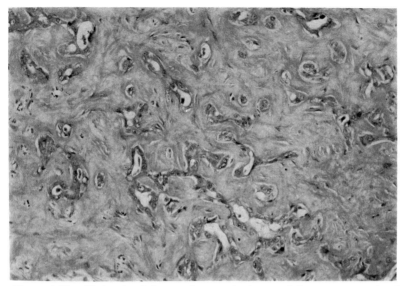

Figure 4-10. Cholangiocellular carcinoma. A characteristic appearance showing moderately well-differentiated acini embedded in a dense fibrous stroma.

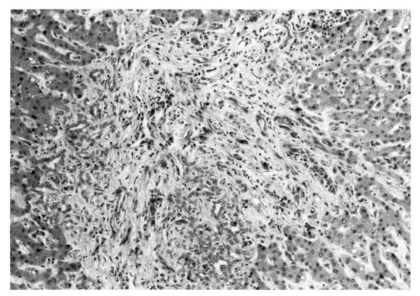

Figure 4-11. Intrahepatic Thorotrast. Note the atypical proliferation of bile ducts and the presence of granular Thorotrast material in a portal area adjacent to, but uninvolved by, cholangiocarcinoma.

THE NATURAL HISTORY OF LIVER CANCER

Most reports have painted a dismal picture for patients with histologically proved liver cancer. Table 4–4 outlines the details from several centers, and it is clear that many, if not most, patients die within a few months after liver cancer is diagnosed. However, the author's own experience, the findings of the 1974 LTS, and several other reports suggest that, with or without therapy, a few patients may live a long time with histologically proved liver carcinoma.[26]

Author's experience: Figure 4–1 depicts an enormous hepatocellular carcinoma resected for palliation in a 62-year-old female ten months after a histologic confirmation of the diagnosis has been made at laparotomy. Tumor was left behind in the retroperitoneum and at the dome of the right lobe of the liver after resection of the major tumor mass with the lower portion of the right lobe, yet this patient survived an additional 19 months, or a total of 32 months, since she first noted the mass. Another patient, a 19-year-old girl with upper abdominal pain and fullness for one and one-half years, was found to have a large hepatocellular carcinoma with lymph node metastasis that was not resected. The mass did not shrink with chemotherapy, but she lived an additional 29 months or approximately four years after the mass was first noted.

Table 4–4. Primary Epithelial Cancer in Adults:
Natural History – Survival After Diagnosis

REFERENCE	PATIENTS	SURVIVAL
98 Singapore	134	None lived more than 2 months after hospital admission
87 New Orleans	55	Onset symptom to death average 2.8 months (4 days–13 months)
33 Finland	100	Onset symptom to death average 5.6 months (longest 19 months)
82 Thailand	273	Onset symptom to death average 4.1 months
14 Sweden	92	1 month (0–12 months)
21 Singapore	108	Symptoms to death, 5.8 months; Diagnosis to death 3.6 months
71 Boston	51	38/51 dead in less than 3 months
101 China	394	Onset of symptoms to death, 4.3 months (average)
59 Japan	89	82% dead 6 months after first symptom

Perhaps the most remarkable example of the variable natural course of these tumors is provided by Case 65, Appendix IV. In September, 1968 this 67-year-old woman was found to have an unsuspected hepatocellular carcinoma in her left lateral segment, which was not resected because of histologically proved metastasis to an excised solitary celiac lymph node. Re-exploration was made eight months later because the patient was doing well, and revealed multiple tumor nodules in the left lobe. Again, resection was not done, and the patient went elsewhere and had a left lobectomy in June, 1969. She is presently alive and free of any evidence of disease 70 months later. Her tumor had an adenoid pattern with considerable fibrous stroma.

Fifty-four of the 100 adult patients with primary epithelial carcinoma in the 1974 LTS who survived operation are known to be dead with their disease. Figure 4–12 outlines the interval between resection and death in these patients, and it can be seen that many lived a long time after resection in spite of the fact that disease was advanced when first treated.

Heaton cites the case of a 40-year-old African female who had resection of a solitary pulmonary metastasis two years after liver resection for primary carcinoma. Four years later an ovarian metastasis was

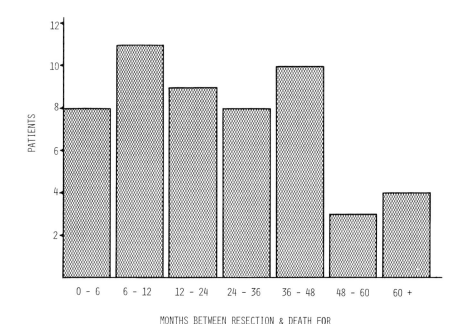

MONTHS BETWEEN RESECTION & DEATH FOR
53 PATIENTS WHO DIED WITH RECURRENT CANCER

Figure 4–12. Survival of adult patients in 1974 Liver Tumor Survey who eventually died with disease after liver resection.

Table 4–5. Primary Epithelial Cancer of Liver in Adults:
Incidence of Extrahepatic Metastases at Autopsy

REFERENCE	AUTOPSIED PATIENTS	PATIENTS WITH EXTRAHEPATIC METASTASIS	
76 India	32	21	65%
98 Singapore	134	31	23%
87 New Orleans	55	40	73%
10 Uganda	137	83	61%
33 Finland	93	58	62%
65 New Orleans	120	66	55%
59 Japan	89	53	60%
23 Liverpool	88	35	40%
	748	387	52%

resected during a gynecologic operation for benign disease. She eventually died of liver cancer seven years after her initial liver resection.[47]

Hoffman notes the death of a patient six to seven years after enucleation of a liver carcinoma.[52] Wilson reports the death of an Australian woman who finally succumbed 14 years and four months after resection of her primary liver cancer. In the interval she had undergone 13 operations for the removal of 71 intra-abdominal metastases![103] Davidson, et al. report that, of 85 patients with histologically proved hepatocellular carcinoma, 12 survived more than two years, only four of whom had resection.[26]

More cases could be cited, but the lesson is clear that not all liver cancers pursue a rapid course. How long does the disease remain within the capsule of the liver? Table 4–5 reports autopsy findings on patients with liver cancer, and, even in these most advanced cases, it is surprising and encouraging to find that in 48 per cent of patients no extrahepatic metastases were found at the time of death. Al-Sarraf, et al. document that from 30 to 70 per cent of patients with liver cancer have metastases at the time of diagnosis,[8] but it must follow that 70 to 30 per cent do not, a more favorable situation than with many other carcinomas, and a situation that should improve with a higher index of suspicion based on some optimism about effective therapy and the better diagnostic techniques available today. When the disease does spread, it usually goes to regional lymph nodes, lung, and bone. Direct invasion of diaphragm is common, but omental metastasis or diffuse peritoneal spread is quite rare. The propensity of hepatocellular carcinoma to grow down the portal vein, or up into the hepatic veins and inferior vena cava as fas as the right auricle, has already been mentioned. A single case has been reported of hepatocellular carcinoma developing in a retroperitoneal ectopic liver.[70]

DIAGNOSIS

Symptoms

The classic report of Rosenberg and Ochsner[87] and more recent reviews[7, 20, 21, 56, 65, 94] outline the symptoms and signs of patients with primary hepatocellular carcinoma. Table 4–6 outlines the symptoms in the more selected group of patients undergoing resection that was studied in the 1974 LTS. Pain is usually the primary symptom of patients with liver cancer, but in the resectable group the patient presented more often with an asymptomatic mass.

Fifteen of 127 patients in the 1974 LTS presented with signs and symptoms of intraperitoneal hemorrhage. Balasegaram reported such a presentation in ten cases (10.2 per cent) of hepatocarcinoma from

Table 4–6.   Primary Epithelial Cancer in Adults
1974 Liver Tumor Survey:
Symptoms and Signs on Hospital Admission

Mass	60
Pain	51
Weight loss	29
Epigastric Distress	16
Intraperitoneal hemorrhage	15
Hepatomegaly	14
Fever	9
Incidental at laparotomy for other disease	7
Diarrhea	6
Anorexia	6
Nausea and vomiting	6
Weakness, malaise	5
Misdiagnosis — cholecystitis	5
Endocrine symptoms	3
Pruritus	3
Jaundice	2
Calcification on x-ray	1
Needle biopsy for benign disease	1
Abnormal liver function tests	1
Abnormal scan	1

Malaysia,[13] and Ong found it in 61 of 460 patients from Hong Kong.[79, 81] Chan found intraperitoneal hemorrhage as the presenting symptom in eight of 108 patients with hepatocellular carcinoma, all of whom had cirrhosis.[21] Many others[20, 49, 76] have reported one or more such cases. When spontaneous intraperitoneal hemorrhage occurs from a cirrhotic liver, it should be considered as a sign of malignant change, since cirrhosis with portal hypertension rarely produces intraperitoneal hemorrhage, and metastatic tumors seldom rupture.

Several types of paraneoplastic syndromes have been reported in patients with primary liver carcinoma. Margolis and Homcy, in an excellent review article,[73] state that about 11 per cent of patients with hepatoma will have erythrocytosis, and they and others[18] believe that such a finding in a cirrhotic patient is a reliable indicator of neoplastic transformation. Increased serum calcium is another manifestation of abnormal hormone production by a liver tumor. Hypoglycemia, hyperlipidemia, and dysfibrogenemia also have been described,[44, 73] as well as porphyria cutanea tarda[94] and osteoporosis. Liver tumors also may produce virilizing and feminizing effects that disappear with appropriate resection.[61 73] Neuropathy in association with hepatocellular carcinoma has been reported by Walter, et al.[100] Paraneoplastic syndromes were noted in at least three patients in the 1974 LTS. Palliative resection was done to relieve hypoglycemic attacks in one patient (Case 15, Appendix IV), and another patient, a 20-year-old female, had amenorrhea, decrease in breast size, and hirsutism for one year prior to resection of a polygonal cell hepatocellular carcinoma (Case 85, Appendix IV). Symptoms due to hypercalcemia led to the diagnosis and resection of an adenoid hepatocellular carcinoma in a 67-year-old male (Case 62, Appendix IV).

PHYSICAL EXAMINATION

A palpable mass or liver enlargement is the only important physical sign to be found in adult patients without paraneoplastic syndromes who are still curable. When weight loss, wasting, ascites, jaundice, an enlarged spleen, or palpable lymphadenopathy are found, the disease is in a preterminal state. A bruit or venous "hum" over liver tumors is heard occasionally.

Tumors in the left lateral segment of the liver present as epigastric masses that descend with respiration and may be tender. Right-sided tumors may extend into the pelvis and still be resectable. Tumors of the medial segment of the left lobe usually present to the right of the midline and may be mistaken for an enlarged gallbladder. Cholangiocarcinoma may feel firmer than hepatocellular carcinoma on physical examination, and central umbilication suggests secondary rather than primary liver tumor.

DIAGNOSTIC TESTS

The various radiographic, laboratory, and isotopic techniques used to assist the clinician in the differential diagnosis of liver tumors are described in Chapter Three. Liver function tests are seldom markedly abnormal when malignant solid tumors are resectable for cure. Isotopic scanning, angiography, and ultrasonography should differentiate solid from cystic conditions. Cystic lesions such as pyogenic abscess, hydatid cyst, and amebic disease can be suspected on the basis of the well-known clinical signs and symptoms and standard laboratory tests.

Needle biopsy is to be discouraged with vascular tumors, and most primary liver tumors are vascular. Linder, et al. describe three fatal hemorrhages after 27 percutaneous needle biopsies of liver cancers.[65] If laparotomy is required to determine resectability, biopsy should be delayed. If cirrhosis is present or if the tumor clearly is not resectable, percutaneous needle biopsy or biopsy under peritoneoscopic control should be done, in spite of the risk, to spare the patient the discomforts of laparotomy. Perhaps the most important tests to be done prior to laparotomy are those that rule out involvement of the bone marrow, the lungs (tomography), and the inferior vena cava and portal vein (venography).

OPERATION

The details of preoperative preparation, choice of incision, and operative evaluation for resection are considered in Chapter Eleven. Operative biopsy should be done early. When hepatocellular or cholangiocarcinoma are proved in a patient with adequate hepatocellular reserve, and when the surgeon has satisfied himself that the disease has not spread beyond the capsule of the liver, the tumor should be excised. Enough evidence has accumulated to indicate clearly that resection is the only method leading to cure, and may well be the most effective means to provide palliation for patients with primary carcinoma of the liver.

How often is liver cancer resectable? The 1974 LTS cannot provide an answer to this critical question because it considered only those patients with resected tumors. Table 4–7 attempts to catalog the experience of others to answer this question. Important to this issue are the

Table 4–7.   Primary Epithelial Cancer of Liver in Adults:
Resectability

REFERENCE	PATIENTS WITH LIVER CANCER	LAPAROTOMIES	RESECTIONS
64 Taiwan	271	197	82
46 Uganda	120	36	10
83 Thailand	511	138	23
21 Singapore	108	27	7
14 Sweden	92	50	5
66 Los Angeles	144	33	9
80 Hong Kong	180	110	30
53 Japan	76	71	21
65 New Orleans	164	49	6
11 Malaysia	232	–	16
68 New York City	43	17	10
101 China	261	261	55

surgeon's individual criteria for resectability, which must vary widely. "Palliative resection" is a term used by Honjo, et al.,[53] but it is the surgeon-author's opinion that this is rarely indicated except to control intraperitoneal hemorrhage.

The risk of operation varies enormously in collected reports. Fac-

Table 4–8.   Primary Epithelial Cancer in Adults:
Reported Operative Mortality – Series Only

REFERENCE	PATIENTS	OPERATIVE DEATHS
38	296	70
31	18	5
74	2	0
102	4	0
78	7	0
24	6	0
37	7	1
66	4	1
14	5	1
53	10	2
65	6	3
46	10	3
3, 11, 12, 64, 67, 79*	128	18
	503	104 (21%)

*Experience of Adson, Balasegaram, Lin, Longmire, and Ong included in Ref. 38 updated with new reports.

tors of operative technique are certainly the most important determinant of immediate morbidity, and are discussed more fully in Chapter Eleven. Associated conditions such as cirrhosis play an important role, as does the extent and technique of resection. Table 4–8 outlines mortality rates following resection of primary adult cancer from reported series. Individual case reports are not included. It is remarkable that the reported operative mortality rate from many centers is exactly the same as that experienced in the 1974 LTS (21 per cent).

The questions of how much liver to resect, and whether resection alters the natural history of the disease, must be answered by looking at long-term survival. The 1974 LTS data will be presented first, followed by a summary of the reports of others.

1974 LIVER TUMOR SURVEY

THE PATIENT SAMPLE

The records of 127 patients 16 years of age and older who had undergone liver resection for primary solid epithelial cancers were reviewed from 49 hospitals or medical centers. The mean age of the patients was 53 years. The noncirrhotic patients averaged 51 years of age, and the cirrhotic patients 60 years of age. 16 patients were more than 70 years of age when they underwent liver resection. Tables 4–3, 4–9, 4–10, and 4–11 document age, sex, race, and pathology correlations. The preponderance of females in the younger age-groups is remarkable. Appendix IV documents this experience and notes the 18 cases previously reported that are included in the 1974 LTS.

The histologic sections were reviewed by both authors for 119 patients, and a histopathologic classification given. An additional eight patients with no available tissue sections were classified on the basis of an adequate pathology report in which a primary hepatocellular or cholangiocellular carcinoma could be clearly identified. Cases with insufficient written or histopathologic material were excluded. Nine cases originally submitted as hepatocellular carcinoma were reclassified as hepatocellular adenoma, and four cases of hepatocellular adenoma were reclassified as carcinoma. Cases in which the histology strongly suggested metastatic carcinoma or metastatic carcinoid or islet cell carcinoma were also excluded.

Primary liver carcinoma was classified as hepatocellular, cholangiocellular, or mixed hepato-cholangiocellular. Hepatocellular carcinoma was further subdivided by its architectural pattern into trabecular, adenoid, syncytial, clear cell, and polygonal cell type with fibrous stroma. These were also evaluated by histologic grading from I to IV according to the method of Broder.[17]

Table 4–9. Primary Epithelial Cancer in Adults: 1974 Liver Tumor Survey

	CAUCASIAN		BLACK		CHINESE	OTHER	TOTAL	
	54	53	9	3	6	2	71	56
	Males	*Females*	*Males*	*Females*	*Males*	*Males*	*Males*	*Females*
Cirrhosis	12	3		8	2	1	26	
Mean age (years)	58	47		51	49	54	53	
Operative mortality	26%	13%		42%	17%	0	21%	
2-Year survival*	22/36 61%	25/35 71%		4/7	4/4	1/2	56/84 – 67%	
5-Year survival*	9/32 28%	9/30 30%		0/6	2/3	0/1	20/72 – 28%	

*Excludes operative deaths.

Table 4–10. Primary Epithelial Cancer in Adults — 1974 LTS: Age and Sex

| | UNDER 50 YEARS OF AGE | | 50 YEARS AND OLDER | |
	Male	*Female*	*Male*	*Female*
Patients	18	28	53	28
Cirrhosis	3	1	20	2
Operative deaths	1	2	19	5
2-Year survival*	7/14	14/20	23/32	12/18
	50%	70%	72%	67%
5-Year survival*	3/11	4/16	8/31	5/14
	27%	25%	26%	36%

*Excludes operative deaths.

Table 4–11. Primary Epithelial Cancer in Adults—
1974 Liver Tumor Survey:
Survival after Resection for Cure*

	91 NONCIRRHOTIC PATIENTS	10 CIRRHOTIC PATIENTS	TOTAL
1 Year	64/77 – 83%	6/10 – 60%	70/87 – 80%
2 Year	52/72 – 72%	2/8 – 25%	54/80 – 68%
3 Year	39/65 – 60%	0/8 – 0	39/73 – 53%
4 Year	26/62 – 42%	0/8 – 0	26/70 – 37%
5 Year	20/59 – 34%	0/8 – 0	20/67 – 30%

*Excludes operative deaths and palliative resections.

Sections of liver parenchyma adjacent to the carcinoma were evaluated for the presence or absence of cirrhosis, which was classified as macronodular or micronodular type.

Of the 127 cases of histologically classified primary liver carcinoma in adults, 109 were hepatocellular, 13 were cholangiocellular, and five were mixed hepatocholangiocellular. Primary hepatocellular carcinoma was further classified by the predominating pattern as trabecular (49 cases), adenoid (19), clear cell (7), syncytial (4), and polygonal cell with fibrous stroma (7 adult cases). Of two miscellaneous cases, one showed a peritheliomatous pattern and the other a totally undifferentiated appearance. Histologic grading of hepatocellular carcinomas showed the vast majority to be either Grade II or III. Grade IV was noted only once in the trabecular group and not at all in the other types. Grade I differentiation was relatively uncommon, being found in six instances of trabecular carcinoma and one instance of adenoid carcinoma. The extremely well differentiated Grade I trabecular carcinoma proved difficult to distinguish from the hepatocellular adenoma, especially in the presence of foci of liver cell dysplasia. A single case of Grade I trabecular carcinoma showed a focus of vascular invasion as the sole determinant for classification as carcinoma.

Figures 4–3 through 4–11 illustrate some of these histologic patterns, and their legends describe characteristic features. Abundant fibrous stroma is an uncommon feature of most hepatocellular carcinomas. However, during an initial histopathologic survey of all primary liver cancers in the 1974 LTS, a type of hepatocellular neoplasm not previously encountered was noted both in the adult and pediatric age groups, that was characterized by a prominent fibrous stroma. The ten patients (seven adults, three children) with this unique histologic pattern formed a group with distinct clinical differences in presentation and prognosis. For that reason we have utilized a new term "polygonal cell with fibrous stroma" (PCFS) to describe the features of

87

this variant of hepatocellular carcinoma, which is characterized by an epithelial component comprised of clusters of liver cells, liver cords, or acinus formation, and a prominent but variable fibrous stroma. The epithelial cells were large and of polygonal shape; the cytoplasm was strikingly eosinophilic, occasionally containing coarse fatty vacuoles and bile pigment. Nuclei were large with prominent nucleoli. Atypical variations in nuclear chromatin and the nuclear membrane were noted, but mitoses were not a significant feature. The stromal component consisted of broad hypocellular fascicles of mature collagen interdigitating with the hepatocellular component to form a separate pattern (see Figs. 4–8, 4–9). This pattern was very different from the other varieties of hepatocellular carcinoma in adults and children, and resembles a case illustrated by Edmondson (AFIP Fascicle 25, Fig. 87).[29] His case was that of a 14-year-old female who was alive and well five years after resection—a clinical history paralleling that of our own cases (see below).

The 13 cases of cholangiocellular carcinoma showed a relatively uniform pattern with similar moderate cellular differentiation. Of the five cases of mixed hepatocellular-cholangiocellular carcinoma, only one showed separate and discrete nodules, one of which was hepatocellular carcinoma and the other cholangiocellular carcinoma. The remaining cases showed a merging of the patterns with trabecular differentiation of the hepatocellular component.

An underlying cirrhosis that was macronodular in most instances was identified in 26 cases. Two cirrhotic patients had hemochromatosis, one associated with a trabecular hepatocellular carcinoma and the other with a mixed hepato-cholangiocellular tumor. Three patients had histologic evidence of previous Thorotrast administration—two with cholangiocellular carcinoma and one with an anaplastic trabecular variant of hepatocellular carcinoma. Only two of the three Thorotrast patients had a grossly evident fibrotic process in the liver. The third patient, therefore, has been included with the noncirrhotics in the tabulations that follow. Twenty-three of the 26 cirrhotic patients had hepatocellular carcinomas with no predominance of any particular histologic variant.

Of the 26 cirrhotic patients, eight were black, one was from the Philippine Islands, and the rest were Caucasian. Their average age was 60 years, and only three were female. Seven patients had a definite history of excessive alcohol intake, and several others probably were heavy drinkers. One patient had been exposed to carbon tetrachloride many years before his hepatocellular carcinoma was resected. Six of the 26 cirrhotic patients presented with intraperitoneal bleeding, and only three of these six survived operation.

The tumor originated in the right lobe of the liver in 79 patients, in 14 of whom growth had extended to the left of the central plane, requiring resection of part of the left lobe to encompass all the disease.

40 tumors originated in the left lobe, 21 of which were confined to the left of the falciform ligament. Five tumors were "central," i.e., involving a significant part of both lobes near the gallbladder but sparing the lateral portion of both lobes, and one tumor originated in the caudate lobe. Finally, there were two patients in whom discrete tumor nodules were present in both lobes, and it was not possible to determine which was primary.

In 87 patients the tumor was solitary — defined as a single mass or a large nodule with or without a few very small satellite nodules within the immediate vicinity of the mother tumor. In 40 patients there were multiple nodules, often occurring close to the mother tumor, but in 18 instances involving both anatomic lobes of the liver.

RESULTS OF THERAPY

Operative mortality refers to death occurring during operation, or at any time thereafter during the same hospitalization. Two patients died of vascular disease less than five years after liver resection for primary cancer, and at postmortem examination were proved to have no residual cancer. However, they are included as deaths in the mortality figures that follow.

Chapter Eleven more carefully considers the causes of operative mortality, and the conclusion is unavoidable that operative technique and the presence of cirrhosis, rather than the extent of the disease, determined the operative mortality rate in these resected cases. Therefore, Tables 4–9 through 4–17 exclude operative deaths when reporting long-term survival. Mean and median figures for long-term survival were calculated using the actual postoperative survival at the time of last known follow-up, so that a patient dying with disease at ten months would have the same effect on median and mean figures as a patient alive and free of disease after ten months. Thus, with time and additional follow-up information, these survival figures can only improve. The yearly survival figures are calculated by counting only the patients at risk. For example, if there were 100 operative survivors and 16 were alive less than two years postoperatively, the two-year survival rate would be calculated by dividing the number of patients who survived more than two years by 84.

Tables 4–3, 4–9, 4–10, and 4–11 categorize the experience of the 1974 LTS. It is interesting to note that the resectable tumors in Caucasian patients were about equally divided between male and female. Thirty-four per cent of the noncirrhotic patients who survived operation lived five years or more, but no cirrhotic patient had survived as long as three years. The high incidence of operative mortality in

Table 4–12. Primary Epithelial Cancer in Adults—1974 Liver Tumor Survey: Operative Mortality

	NONCIRRHOTIC PATIENTS		CIRRHOTIC PATIENTS		ALL PATIENTS	
	Number	*Deaths*	*Number*	*Deaths*	*Number*	*Percentage Deaths*
Extended right lobectomy	10	1	3	2	13	23
Right lobectomy	39	10	10	8	49	37
Left lobectomy	20	0	5	2	25	8
Left lateral segmentectomy	11	0	2	1	13	8
Wedge	19	0	6	3	25	11
"Middle" lobectomy	1	0	0	—	1	—
Unspecified	1	0	0	—	1	—
Over-all:	101 – 12%		26 – 58%		127 – 21%	

Table 4–13. Primary Epithelial Cancer in Adults – 1974 Liver Tumor Survey: Survival versus Operation in Noncirrhotic Patients*

	PATIENTS SURVIVING RESECTION	SURVIVAL Mean (months)	Median (months)	5-Year
Extended right lobectomy	9	23	28	0/6
Right lobectomy	29	32	27	6/19
Left lobectomy	20	36	35	5/17
Left lateral segmentectomy	11	44	15	2/6
Wedge	19	59	55	7/11
Over-all:	88	38 months	34 months	20/59

*Excludes operative deaths.

blacks and in males over 50 years of age probably is directly related to the presence of cirrhosis in both groups (Tables 4–9 and 4–10). Otherwise, sex, race, and age seem to have no significant effect in either operative mortality or long-term survival. Five-year survival for patients under 50 years of age was 26 per cent (7/37) and for those over 50 was 29 per cent (13/45). This is not a significant difference, but it suggests that in the preponderantly younger female group the disease is at least as bad as in older males. That we found not a single case of recurrent or metastatic hepatocellular adenoma, a condition which almost exclusively affects younger females (see Chapter 6), suggests that carcinoma and adenoma are two separate and very different diseases, and are not simply "shades of gray" that blend gradually one into the other.

Tables 4–12 and 4–13 relate the extent of operation to immediate mortality and long-term survival. Operative mortality was prohibitive in the cirrhotic patients and low in noncirrhotic patients, except for those undergoing right lobectomy. The details will be discussed more fully in Chapter Eleven, but three of the ten patients dying after right lobectomy exsanguinated on the operating table, and four others died as a direct result of technical complications of the operation. Improvements in technique should lower mortality rates significantly when elective operation is done for liver tumor in noncirrhotic patients. Wedge resection refers to all sublobar resections, and includes at least six instances in which a large segment of the right lobe was taken. Some authors have used "segmentectomy" to define these large wedge resections, but we have reserved that term for anatomic segmental resections that are based on individual ligation of feeding and draining vessels at the liver hilum and diaphragm. There were no such resections in this series.

Table 4–14 relates maximum tumor diameter to immediate and late survival. The numbers are small in each group, but it is clear that size makes little difference when related to outcome. There were two opeative deaths in noncirrhotic patients with 4 cm tumors, both of whom underwent right lobectomy and both of whom died during the third postoperative week of liver failure and jaundice with bile fistula (Cases 119 and 27, Appendix IV).

Forty patients had multiple tumor nodules, and Table 4–15 compares their progress with that of 87 patients with solitary nodules. The differences are not as great as might be expected. Of the 40 patients with multiple tumor nodules, 18 had tumor in both anatomic lobes. The over-all five-year survival rate of patients with multiple nodules is the same as for patients with solitary nodules.

In 11 patients the tumor was fixed to the diaphragm, and in at least seven, a piece of diaphragm was excised together with the liver

Table 4–14. Primary Epithelial Cancer in Adults – 1974 Liver Tumor Survey: Tumor Size versus Survival

			MAXIMUM TUMOR SIZE		
	Less than 5 cm	5–9.9 cm	10–14.9 cm	15–19.9 cm	More than 20 cm
Patients	7	35	51	23	11
Operative deaths	2	7	12	3	3
Survival*					
Mean (months)	42	25	43	35	37
2-Year	3/3	13/24 – 54%	23/33 – 70%	11/16 – 69%	4/6
5-Year	1/3	2/18 – 11%	11/30 – 37%	4/13 – 31%	2/5

*Excludes operative deaths.

Table 4–15. Primary Epithelial Cancer in Adults—
1974 Liver Tumor Survey:
Solitary versus Multiple Nodules of Tumor

	SOLITARY	MULTIPLE Unilobar	Bilobar
Patients	87	22	18
Cirrhotics	14	4	8
Operative deaths	16	5	6
Survival*			
Mean (months)	36	40	26
2-Year	40/56 – 71%	8/17 – 47%	6/9 – 67%
5-Year	13/45 – 29%	5/16 – 31%	2/7 – 29%

*Excludes operative deaths.

tumor. Four died after operation, five were dead of disease within 16 months postoperatively, and two are alive 24 and 61 months after resection without evidence of disease.

Three patients were found to have tumor in the portal vein at the time of transection during lobectomy. They died with disease at 5, 8, and 11 months postoperatively. Hepatocellular carcinoma often is quite soft and difficult to palpate within the portal vein at operation. Preoperative or operative portal venography is more helpful and should be done, particularly in patients with portal hypertension. Two patients had tumor in the hepatic veins at the site of transection near the inferior vena cava, and both died in the immediate postoperative period.

HISTOLOGIC TYPE VERSUS CLINICAL COURSE

Although the numbers are small in some groups, an attempt was made to investigate the correlation between the histologic patterns of liver cancer and certain clinical factors. Table 4–16 outlines this data, and no obvious differences are noted with the exception of the cholangiocarcinomas, the mixed hepato-cholangiocellular tumors, and the small group of ten patients showing the PCFS pattern of liver cell cancer. Three children with this pattern are included in Appendix IV and with the experience in Table 4–16 but, even excluding the pediatric patients, the average age of the adult patients was only 22 years. Seven of nine patients with the PCFS pattern who survived operation are still alive from nine to 172 months after operation. Six of the seven adult patients with this histologic pattern were female, which brings to mind

Table 4–16. Primary Epithelial Cancer in Adults—1974 Liver Tumor Survey: Histologic Type versus Clinical Course

	Cases	Mean Age (Range)	% Female	% Cirrhosis	Operative Deaths	Mean Tumor Size	Survival (Months) Mean	Survival (Months) Median	AFD† at Report Time
Hepatocellular carcinoma									
Trabecular	49	56(21–82)	24.5	24.5	9	12 cm	40	31	14(6–144 months)
Adenoid	19	57(22–75)	37	19	5	11 cm	38	34	6(15–70 months)
Clear cell	7	48(16–67)	71	33	1	12 cm	30	33	2(33+36 months)
Syncytial	4	61(37–70)	50	25	1	11 cm	36	30	3(4–73 months)
PCFS*	10	19(5–28)	70	10	1	14 cm	52	34	7(9–172 months)
Unclassified	23	47(19–73)	48	16	5	13 cm	31	39	3(19–74 months)
Cholangiocellular carcinoma	13	57(37–70)	77	8	3	8 cm	16	12	5(4–23 months)
Mixed hepato-cholangiocellular carcinoma	5	55(35–71)	40	40	2	9 cm	19	11	1(11 months)

*PCFS = Polygonal cell with fibrous stroma.
†AFD = Alive, free of disease.

Table 4–17. Primary Epithelial Cancer in Adults—1974 LTS:
Survival versus Histologic Grade: Operative Survivors
with Hepatocellular Carcinoma

| | GRADE | | | |
	I	II	III	IV
Patients	6	29	26	3
Mean survival (months)	47	44	42	5
2-Year survival	5/5	19/27	19/24	0/3
	100%	70%	79%	
5-Year survival	1/4	9/22	7/20	0/3
	25%	41%	35%	

the high incidence of hepatocellular adenomas in young women. However, the histologic features of PCFS tumors are markedly different from those of hepatocellular adenomas. These are clearly two different lesions. Our findings concur with those of Buchanan and Huvos,[19] that patients with clear cell carcinomas fared as poorly as the over-all group. The 18 patients with cholangiocarcinoma or mixed liver cell and bile duct patterns were all over 35 years of age. These tumors were smaller than the hepatocellular tumors, and yet their median and mean survival figures were lower. The mixed tumors behaved like cholangiocarcinomas rather than hepatocellular carcinomas.

Pathologic grading was done for 83 patients with liver cell carcinoma. When more than one grade was seen in a single tumor, the higher grade was used for this tabulation. Sixty-five patients survived operation and had enough follow-up information to construct Table 4–17, which shows no significant correlation with long-term survival and Grades I, II, and III. There were too few Grade IV patients or anaplastic tumors to be of significance, but it is interesting to note that all three patients with grade IV tumors were dead within eight months of resection.

INTRAPERITONEAL HEMORRHAGE FROM LIVER CELL CANCER

Seventeen patients, all with hepatocellular carcinoma, had ruptured their tumors with intraperitoneal hemorrhage prior to resection. In four, rupture with shock occurred in the hospital during a period of diagnostic evaluation for abdominal pain. Fourteen patients underwent emergency laparotomy for diagnosis and to control hemorrhage. Eight resections were done immediately, and one patient had packing and required reoperation and resection one day later. Five patients had

Table 4-18. Primary Epithelial Cancer of Adults — 1974 LTS: Re-resection for Recurrent Cancer

	AGE/SEX	LOCATION OF RECURRENCE	INTERVAL BETWEEN FIRST AND SECOND OPERATION	OPERATION FOR RECURRENCE	OUTCOME (SURVIVAL AFTER FIRST LIVER RESECTION)
1.	55 M	Omentum	36 months	Omental excision	AFD 144 months
2.	57 M	Abdominal incision	28 months	Local excision	DWD 35 months
3.	68 M	Abdominal incision	5 months	Local excision	DWD 8 months
4.*	28 F	(1) Left lung	33 months	Left lower lobectomy	
		(2) Liver, right lung	34 months	Left liver lobectomy	AFD 172 months
		(3) Right lung	38 months	Right lower lung lobectomy / Right middle lobectomy (lung)	
5.	44 M	(1) Quadrate lobe liver	46 months	Wedge, quadrate lobe	DWD 63 months
		(2) Lung, left	47 months	Left upper lobectomy (lung)	DWD 59 months
		(3) Cerebellum	52 months	Removal cerebellar tumor	
6.	43 F	Subhepatic	46 months	Local excision	AWD 9 months
7.	47 M	Lesser sac and bile ducts	8 months	"Palliative" local excision	DWD 43 months
8.	25 M	Liver	10 months	Wedge excision	AFD 109 months
9.	63 F	Abdominal incision	6–7 years	Local excision	AFD 14 months
10.	57 M	Chest incision	10 months	Local excision	

*Lawrence, et al. J.A.M.A. *191*:139, 1965 (Case 89, Appendix IV).[62]

temporary control of hemorrhage followed by transfer to another center where resection was done 13 days to two months later. Three patients underwent a primary elective resection, 2, 10, and 30 days after an episode of acute pain with intraperitoneal hemorrhage which was treated with blood transfusion and other supportive therapy. Five of the 17 patients with intraperitoneal hemorrhage died after resection, including three of six cirrhotic patients. Three surviving patients were dead of disease within a year of resection, but the remaining nine patients have done surprisingly well. Three are dead with disease at 14, 46, and 54 months after resection; five are alive at 22, 28, 39, 55, and 55 months after resection; and the last patient died of a traumatic rupture of the spleen eight years after cautery wedge excision of a 4 cm adenoid, grade II ruptured hepatocellular carcinoma from the dome of the right lobe of the liver. At postmortem examination this patient's liver weighed 5700 gm and was filled with tumor, but there was no tumor outside the liver capsule. Thus, intraperitoneal hemorrhage is not a sign of incurability.

Packing may provide transient control of bleeding, but a subsequent attempt at definitive resection should be done when possible in the patient with a noncirrhotic liver. If transfer to another center for resection is contemplated, the surgeon obtaining temporary control on an emergency basis should assess resectability as completely as possible to aid subsequent planning for a second operation.

Re-Resection for Recurrent Disease

Ten patients with primary liver cancer in the 1974 LTS developed evidence of recurrent tumor and underwent another operation (or operations) for its removal. Table 4–18 outlines the details of these cases, and it is clear that an aggressive attack on localized recurrent disease is justified in certain cases.

LITERATURE SURVEY ON LONG-TERM RESULTS OF RESECTION FOR PRIMARY LIVER CANCER

It is often difficult to abstract from reports that discuss all aspects of hepatic cancer the specific details needed to develop accurate survival information. However, an attempt was made in 1970.[38] To that collected experience 28 new reports have been added, and the total experience is reported in Tables 4–19 and 4–20. Every attempt was made to exclude from these tabulations patients who are included in the 1974

Table 4–19. Primary Epithelial Cancer in Adults:
Survival After Operation: Literature Review*

Patients	<12	12–23	24–35	36–47	48–59	60+
			Months			
Alive	64	29	17	16	4	33
Dead	164	45	20	9	1	3
Totals	228	74	37	25	5	36

*References: 1, 14, 24, 27, 37, 38, 40, 46, 47, 53, 58, 60, 64–66, 77–79, 83, 86, 88, 91, 94, 95, 97, 102, 104, 105.

LTS. Operative mortality was calculated by considering only those reports in which the total experience of a surgeon or institution was included (39 series). Long-term survival figures include case reports as well as larger series. The experience of Ong,[79] Lin,[64] Balasegaram,[11] Longmire,[67] and Adson,[3] part of which was included in the 1970 collected review, has been updated by the inclusion of information from more recent reports.

There was reasonably accurate information on 405 patients who survived operation. Of 309 who were dead or were followed for at least two years, 102 (33 per cent) were living 24 months after resection. Thirty-six of 273 resected patients (13 per cent) who were followed until death or for at least 60 months were alive. At least three and probably more of these five-year survivors subsequently died of their disease.

These unhappy survival figures are considerably worse than the experience reported in the 1974 LTS. Separation of the Asian from the non-Asian patients (Table 4–20) helps to explain the difference. The

Table 4–20. Primary Epithelial Cancer in Adults:
Survival After Resection: Literature Review*

	Asian Patients	Non-Asian Patients
Operative mortality**	76/365 – 21%	28/149 – 19%
2-Year survival***	54/230 – 23%	48/79 – 61%
5-Year survival***	15/213 – 7%	21/60 – 35%

*References: 1, 2, 11, 14, 24, 27, 37, 38, 40, 46, 47, 53, 58, 60, 64, 65, 66, 77, 78, 83, 86, 88, 91, 94, 95, 97, 102, 103, 105.
**Series only.
***Excludes operative deaths.

Asian patient five-year survival of approximately one-third of the operative mortality rate is in sharp contrast with the survival rate of non-Asian patients, which is almost double the rate of operative deaths. Most Asian patients had cirrhosis of the liver, and perusal of Asian reports suggests that the disease was more often multinodular and widespread, although still contained within the capsule of the liver. The comparable operative mortality figures suggest that Asian surgeons were highly skilled in bringing cirrhotic patients through major operations. However, the rapid long-term decline in survival of Asian patients suggests that the disease acts differently from resectable "western" liver cancer, which occurs largely in noncirrhotic livers. The "western" cirrhotic patients in the 1974 LTS fared no better than their reported Asian counterparts.

At least 22 patients, five of whom are also in the 1974 LTS, are added to the previous collection of five-year survivors (see Table 4–21). An additional 15 patients from the 1974 LTS are listed in Appendix IV, bringing the total of collected five-year survivors to at least 56 patients. At least 11 of the 56 five-year survivors eventually died of recurrent disease.

SUMMARY AND RECOMMENDATIONS FOR THERAPY

Most reports of large experience with liver cancer have come from Africa and Asia, and only the Asian surgeons have resected enough tumors to provide useful survival information—and that information has been discouraging. This review has attempted to look at the disease as it occurs in Western patients and as it is treated by Western surgeons. The picture that emerges is considerably more encouraging.

The natural history of the disease in the noncirrhotic patient may be prolonged, with or without therapy. The male dominance in the Asian series is not repeated in Western noncirrhotic patients and, for patients under 50 years of age, resectable liver cancer is actually more common in females.

Most liver cancers remain confined within Glisson's capsule for a long period before metastasis and, unfortunately, before diagnosis. Newer diagnostic techniques and a higher index of suspicion should uncover many tumors while they are still within the bounds of cure.

Operative mortality remains too high, but this is attributable almost entirely to the technical failure to control hemorrhage at operation and to the selection of cirrhotic patients. Experience should correct both factors and result in an operative mortality rate well below 10 per cent.

Table 4–21.   Primary Epithelial Cancer in Adults: 5-Year Survivors[+]: Literature Review

	AUTHOR	AGE/SEX	TUMOR	RESECTION[**]	RESULTS
1.	Bengmark, et al.[14]	N.S.	Liver cancer	N.S.	AFD 126 months
2–3.	Honjo[53]	54M	HCCa	LLS	Dead 17 years, 5 months
3.	Lin[64]	62M	HCCa	XRL	AFD 88 months
4–8.		8 cases[*]	HCCa		3 AFD 8–10 years
					3 AFD more than 5 years
					2 dead more than 5 years
9.	Curutchet[24]	52F	HCCa	PRL	Dead at 64 months
10.	Warren and Hardy[102]	59M	HCCa	Wedge	Left lung lobectomy 7 years later for metastatic hepatoma. DWD 113 months (1974 LTS, Case 104, Appendix IV)
11.	Ochsner[78]	33M	HCCa	RL	DWD 62 months (Case 96, Appendix IV)
12–15.	Adson[3]	6 patients[**]	HCCa		6 lived 5 years, but only 4 still alive
		44M	HCCa	Wedge	DWD 64 months (Case 11, Appendix IV)
		63F	HCCa	PRL	AFD 128 (Case 29, Appendix IV)
		22M	HCCa	RL	AFD 60 (Case 3, Appendix IV)
16.	Heaton[47]	40F	HCCa	Lobectomy	Pulmonary metastasis resected 2 years, ovarian metastasis resected 6 years. DWD at 7 years
17.	Wilson, et al.[103]	37F	HCCa	Wedge	DWD 14 years and 4 months postop. after 13 other operations for 71 abdominal metastases.
18–19.	El-Domeiri, et al.[31]	4 patients[***]	HCCa	RL	"Survived more than 5 years"
20.	Ong[79]	2 patients[****]	HCCa		AFD 9 years. AFD 6 years
21–22.	Balasegaram[11]	2 patients	HCCa		"Lived 5 years after surgery"

[+]In addition to ref. 38.
[++]N.S. – not stated
LLS – left lateral segmentectomy
XRL – extended right lobectomy

[*]3 of 8 cases included in ref. 38.
[**]2 of 6 cases included in ref. 38.
[***]May include 2 cases from ref. 38.
[****]Probably includes 1 case from ref. 38.

When primary epithelial carcinoma is found in a noncirrhotic liver and when no evidence of spread beyond liver capsule is evident, it should be resected if tumor anatomy allows. Neither the size of the tumor, the presence of multiple nodules (if confined to one lobe), nor the histologic type or grade should influence the decision. Diaphragmatic invasion or peritoneal rupture does not exclude the possibility of cure, and patient age and sex have no correlation with immediate or prolonged survival. Resection should *not* be done for tumors occurring in cirrhotic livers unless it is necessary to control hemorrhage.

The amazing capacity of the liver to regenerate, the variable natural history of primary epithelial cancer of the noncirrhotic liver, and the knowledge that more than one-third of noncirrhotic patients will live more than five years after "curative" resection should allow us a cautious optimism when we encounter a patient with liver cancer.

REFERENCES

1. Adam, Y. G., Huvos, A. G., and Hajdu, S. I.: Malignant vascular tumors of liver. Ann. Surg. *175(3)*:375, 1972.
2. Adson, M. A., and Jones, R. R.: Hepatic lobectomy. Arch. Surg. *92*:631, 1966.
3. Adson, M. A., and Sheedy, P. F.: Resection of primary hepatic malignant lesions. Arch. Surg. *108*:599, 1974.
4. Adson, M. A.: Major hepatic resections: elective operations. Mayo Clin. Proc. *42*:791, 1967.
5. Albacete, R. A., Matthews, M. J., and Saini, N.: Portal vein thrombosis in malignant hepatoma. Ann. Intern. Med. *67*:337, 1967.
6. Allen, R. A., and Lisa, J. R.: Combined liver cell and bile duct carcinoma. Am. J. Pathol. *25*:647, 1948.
7. Alpert, M. E., Hutt, M. S. R., and Davidson, C. S.: Primary hepatoma in Uganda. Am. J. Med. *46*:794, 1969.
8. Al-Sarraf, M., Kithier, K., and Vaitkevicius, V. K.: Primary liver cancer. Cancer *33(2)*:574, 1974.
9. Anthony, P. P.: Carcinoma of the liver in man. Bull. Int. Pathol. *29*:44, 1974.
10. Anthony, P. P.: Primary carcinoma of the liver: a study of 282 cases in Ugandan Africans. J. Pathol. *110*:37, 1973.
11. Balasegaram, M.: Hepatic surgery: a review of a personal series of 95 major resections. Aust. N.Z.J. Surg. *42*:1, 1972.
12. Balasegaram, M.: Hepatic surgery: present and future. Ann. R. Coll. Surg. Engl. *47*:139, 1970.
13. Balasegaram, M.: Spontaneous intraperitoneal rupture of primary liver-cell carcinoma. Aust. N.Z.J. Surg. *37*:332, 1968.
14. Bengmark, S., Borjesson, B., and Hafstrom, L.: The natural history of primary carcinoma of the liver. Scand. J. Gastroenterol. *6*:351, 1971.
15. Berman, C.: Primary Carcinoma of the Liver. London, H. K. Lewis & Co., Ltd., 1951.
16. Bras, G.: Nutritional aspects of cirrhosis and carcinoma of the liver. Fed. Proc. *7*:353, 1961.
17. Broders, A. C.: Carcinoma grading and practical application. Arch. Pathol. *2*:376, 1926.
18. Brownstein, M. H., and Ballard, H. S.: Hepatoma associated with erythrocytosis. Am. J. Med. *40*:204, 1966.

19. Buchanan, T. F., and Huvos, A. G.: Clear-cell carcinoma of the liver. Am. J. Clin. Pathol., *61*:529, 1974.

20. Cartia, Q.: Emorragia massiva intra peritoneale da carcinoma primitive del fegato. Minerva Med. *64*:3667, 1973.

21. Chan, K. T.: The management of primary liver carcinoma. Ann. R. Coll. Surg. *41*:253, 1967.

22. Chew, B. K., et al.: ABO blood groups in primary carcinoma of the liver. Aust. N.Z.J. Med. *3*:129, 1973.

23. Cruickshank, A. H.: The pathology of 111 cases of primary hepatic malignancy collected in the Liverpool region. J. Clin. Pathol. *14*:120, 1961.

24. Curutchet, H. P., et al.: Primary liver cancer. Surgery *70*:467, 1971.

25. DaSilva Horta, J., et al.: Malignancy and other late effects following administration of thorotrast. Lancet *2*:201, 1965.

26. Davidson, A. R., et al.: The variable course of primary hepatocellular carcinoma. Br. J. Surg. *61*:349, 1974.

27. Duckett, J. W., and Montgomery, H. G.: Resection of primary liver tumors. Surgery *21*:455, 1947.

28. Edmondson, H. A.: Progress in pediatrics: differential diagnosis of tumors and tumor-like lesions of liver in infancy and childhood. A.M.A. J. Dis. Child. *91*:168, 1956.

29. Edmondson, H. A.: Tumors of the liver and intrahepatic bile ducts. Section VII, Fascicle 25, Atlas of Tumor Pathology, AFIP, 1958.

30. Edmondson, H. A., and Steiner, P. E.: Primary carcinoma of the liver; a study of 100 cases among 48,900 necropsies. Cancer *7*:463, 1954.

31. El-Domeiri, A. A., et al.: Primary malignant tumors of the liver. Cancer *27*:7, 1971.

32. Eriksson, S., and Hagerstrand, I.: Cirrhosis and malignant hepatoma in alpha-1 antitrypsin deficiency. Acata Med. Scand. *195*:451, 1974.

33. Ervasti, J.: Primary carcinoma of the liver. Acta Chir. Scand. (Suppl.) *334*:1–65, 1964.

34. Ewing, J.: Neoplastic diseases. 1st ed. Philadelphia, W. B. Saunders Co., 1919.

35. Farber, E.: Pathogenesis of liver cancer. Arch. Pathol. *98*:145, 1974.

36. Fisher, R. L., Schever, P. J., and Sherlock, S.: Primary liver cell carcinoma: alcohol and chronic liver disease. Br. Soc. Gastroenterol. *15*:343, 1974.

37. Fortner, J. G., et al.: Vascular problems in upper abdominal cancer surgery. Arch. Surg. *109*:148, 1974.

38. Foster, J. H.: Survival after liver resection for cancer. Cancer *26*:493, 1970.

39. Fraumeni, J. F., Jr., et al.: Hepatoblastoma in infant sisters. Cancer *24*:1086, 1969.

40. Freeman, B. S., and Moreland, R. B.: Primary carcinoma of the liver: report of a case treated by lobectomy. Ann. Surg. *127*:1240, 1948.

41. Galdabini, J. J.: Case records of the Massachusetts General Hospital. Case 27–1974. N. Engl. J. Med. *291*:88, 1974.

42. Geography of primary liver cancer. Br. Med. J. *6*:381, 1970.

43. Goldzieher, M., and von Bokay, Z.: Der primare Leberkrebs. Virchows Arch. [Pathol. Anat.] *203*:75, 1911.

44. Handa, S. P.: Hypoglycemia in primary carcinoma of the liver. Am. J. Dig. Dis. *11*:898, 1966.

45. Hanot, V., and Gilbert, A.: Etudes sur les Maladies du Foie. Paris, Asselin & Houseau, 1888, p. 334.

46. Harrison, N. W., et al.: The surgical management of primary hepatocellular carcinoma in Uganda. Br. J. Surg. *60(7)*:565, 1973.

47. Heaton, A.: Hepatocellular carcinoma: prolonged survival following resection. S. Afr. J. Surg. *12*:61, 1974.

48. Herxheimer (1902): Cited in Kaufman, E. Textbook of Pathological Anatomy. Philadelphia, Blakiston & Son & Co., 1929.

49. Heupel, H. W.: Liver metastases simulating acute surgical abdomen. Arch. Surg. *92*:273, 1966.

50. Higginson, J., and Steiner, P. E.: Definition and classification of malignant epithelial neoplasms of the liver. Acta Un. Int. Cancer *17*:593, 1961.

51. Higginson, J., and Svoboda, D. J.: Primary Carcinoma of the Liver as a Pathologist's Problem. Path. Annual 1970. New York, Appleton-Century-Crofts, 1970, pp. 65–90.

52. Hoffman, H. S.: Benign hepatoma; review of the literature and report of a case. Ann. Intern. Med. *17*:130, 1942.
53. Honjo, I., and Mizumoto, R.: Primary carcinoma of the liver. Am. J. Surg. *128*:31, 1974.
54. Horivchi, N., et al.: Hepatoma originated in the retroperitoneal space. Oncology *27*:235, 1973.
55. Hou, Pao-Chang: The relationship between primary carcinoma of the liver and infestation with Clonorchis sinensis. J. Pathol. Bacteriol. *72*:239, 1956.
56. Ihde, D. C., et al.: Clinical manifestations of hepatoma. A review of six years' experience at a cancer hospital. Am. J. Med. *56*:83, 1974.
57. Kaplan, L., and Cole, S. L.: Fraternal primary hepatocellular carcinoma in three male adult siblings. Am. J. Med. *39*:305, 1965.
58. Kappel, D. A., and Miller, D. R.: Primary hepatic carcinoma; a review of 37 patients. Am. J. Surg. *124*:798, 1972.
59. Kojiro, M.: Pathological studies on primary carcinoma of the liver. Kurume Med. J. *18*:205, 1971.
60. Lannon, J.: Seventeen cases of hepatectomy. S. Afr. J. Surg. *12*:227, 1974.
61. Lannon, J.: Endocrine liver tumors. S. Afr. J. Surg. *11*:39, 1973.
62. Lawrence, G. H., and Bashant, G. H.: Bilateral pulmonary resection for metastatic hepatoma. J.A.M.A. *191*:139, 1965.
63. Lawrence, G. H., et al.: Primary carcinoma of the liver. Am. J. Surg. *112*:200, 1966.
64. Lin, T. Y.: Primary cancer of the liver; quadrennial review. Scand. J. Gastroenterol. *6*:223, 1970.
65. Linder, G. T., Crook, J. N., and Cohn, I., Jr.: Primary liver carcinoma. Cancer *33*:1624, 1974.
66. Longmire, W. P., Passaro, E. P., and Joseph, W. L.: The surgical treatment of hepatic lesions. Br. J. Surg., *53*:852, 1966.
67. Longmire, W. P., et al.: Elective hepatic surgery. Ann. Surg. *179*:712, 1974.
68. Mabogunje, O., Rosen, P. P., and Fortner, J. G.: Liver cell carcinoma during the prime of life. Surg. Gynecol. Obstet. *140*:75, 1975.
69. MacMahon, H. E., Murphy, A. S., and Bates, M. I.: Sarcoma of the liver. Rev. Gastroenterol. *14*:155, 1947.
70. Makk, L., et al.: Clinical and morphologic features of hepatic angiosarcoma in vinyl chloride workers. Cancer *37*:149, 1976.
71. Malt, R. A., VanVroonhoven, T. J., and Kakumoto, Y.: Manifestations and prognosis of carcinoma of the liver. Surg. Gynecol. Obstet. *135*:361, 1972.
72. Manderson, W. G., Patrick, R. S., and Peters, E. E.: Primary carcinoma of liver. Scott. Med. J. *10*:60, 1965.
73. Margolis, S., and Homcy, C.: Systemic manifestations of hepatoma. Medicine *51*:381, 1972.
74. McDermott, W. V., and Ottinger, L. W.: Elective hepatic resection. Am. J. Surg. *112*:376, 1966.
75. Mori, W.: Cirrhosis and primary cancer of the liver. Cancer *20*:627, 1967.
76. Murthy, D. P., and Reddy, D. B.: Primary carcinoma of liver (a clinicopathological study of 59 cases both from autopsy and biopsy). Indian J. Cancer *10*:60, 1973.
77. Nystrom, T. G.: Liver resection in primary malignant hepatoma. Acta Chir. Scand. *103*:241, 1952.
78. Ochsner, J. L., Meyers, B. E., and Ochsner, A.: Hepatic lobectomy. Am. J. Surg. *121*:273, 1971.
79. Ong, G. B., and Chan, P. K. W.: Primary carcinoma of the liver. Surg. Gynecol. Obstet. *143*:31, 1976.
80. Ong, G. B., and Leong, C. H.: Surgical treatment of primary liver cancer. J. R. Coll. Surg. *14*:42, 1969.
81. Ong, G. B., and Taw, J. L.: Spontaneous rupture of hepatocellular carcinoma. Br. Med. J. *21*:146, 1972.
82. Plengvanit, V., et al.: Treatment of primary carcinoma of the liver by hepatic artery ligation. Tijdschr. Gastroenterol. *106*:491, 1967.
83. Plengvanit, V., Viranuvatti, V., and Chearanai, O.: Treatment of primary liver cancer. Med. Chir. Dig. *3*:301, 1974.
84. Purtilo, D. T., and Gottlieb, L. S.: Cirrhosis and hepatoma occurring at Boston City Hospital (1917–1968). Cancer *32(2)*:458, 1973.

85. Rawlings, W., Jr., et al.: Hepatocellular carcinoma and partial deficiency of alpha-1-antitrypsin (mz). Ann. Intern. Med. *81*:771, 1974.

86. Raynor, A. C., Fitts, C. T., and Hennigar, G. R.: Long-term survival after massive liver resection for hepatocellular carcinoma. South Med. J. *67*:977, 1974.

87. Rosenberg, D. M. L., and Ochsner, A.: Primary carcinoma of the liver. Surgery *24*:1036, 1948.

88. Sanguilly, J., and Calderin, V. O.: Partial resection of the liver for primary cholangiocarcinoma. Am. J. Surg. *128*:603, 1974.

89. Sankale, M., et al.: Distribution of blood groups in 120 African patients with primary cancer of the liver. Pathol. Biol. *16*:1071, 1968.

90. Schleissner, L. A., and Cohen, A. H.: Alpha-1-antitrypsin deficiency and hepatic carcinoma. Am. Rev. Resp. Dis. *111*:863, 1975.

91. Schottenfeld, L. E.: Surgery of the liver. Am. J. Dig. Dis. *22*:139, 1955.

92. Schreiber, W. M., Kato, H., and Robertson, J. D.: Primary carcinoma of the liver in Hiroshima and Nagasaki, Japan. Cancer *26*:69, 1970.

93. Selinger, M., and Koff, R. S.: Thorotrast and the liver: a reminder. Gastroenterology *68*:799, 1975.

94. Sharpstone, P., et al.: The diagnosis of primary malignant tumours of the liver. Findings in 48 consecutive patients. Q. J. Med. New Series *41(161)*:99, 1972.

95. Shaw, A. F. B.: Primary liver-cell adenoma (hepatoma). J. Pathol. Bacteriol. *26*:475, 1923.

96. Suckow, E. E., Henegar, G. C., and Baserga, R.: Tumors of the liver following administration of thorotrast. Am. J. Pathol. *38*:663, 1971.

97. Sugahara, K., et al.: Serum alpha-fetoprotein and resection of primary hepatic cancer. Arch. Surg. *106*:63, 1973.

98. Tull, J. G.: Primary carcinoma of the liver. J. Pathol. Bacteriol. *35*:557, 1932.

99. Visfeldt, J., and Poulsen, H.: On the histopathology of liver and liver tumours in thorium-dioxide patients. Acta Pathol. Microbiol. Scand. Sect. A. *80*:97, 1972.

100. Walter, E. P., Hanaver, F. A., and Kent, D. C.: Primary liver carcinoma in young men. Am. J. Med. Sci. *252*:675, 1966.

101. Wang, C., and Li, K.: Surgical treatment of primary carcinoma of liver. Chin. Med. J. *82*:65, 1973.

102. Warren, K. W., and Hardy, K. J.: A review of hepatic resection at the Lahey Clinic 1923–1967. Lahey Clin. Fed. Bull. *16*:241, 1967.

103. Wilson, E.: Malignant hepatoma: repeated resection of metastases with survival for 15 years. Med. J. Aust. *2*:889, 1966.

104. Winternitz, M. C.: Primary carcinoma of the liver. Johns Hopkins Hosp. Reps. *17*:148, 1916.

105. Wolloch, Y., Dintsman, M., and Garti, I.: Primary malignant tumors of the liver. Isr. J. Med. Sci. *9(1)*:6, 1973.

106. Yamagiwa, K.: Zur Kenntniss des primaren parenchymatosen Leberkarcinomas. Virchows Arch. [Pathol. Anat.] *206*:439, 1911.

Chapter Five

PEDIATRIC EPITHELIAL TUMORS

INTRODUCTION

Liver tumors in children are rarely seen in the U.S., although they are probably the most common primary intraperitoneal tumor of childhood. In countries where primary liver cell carcinoma in adults is most common, reports of primary carcinoma in children are very rare.[13] Most pediatric malignant tumors are made of epithelial elements that tend to show much greater variation in histologic pattern than do adult tumors. Areas within a single tumor may show histologic features suggesting fetal liver, embryonal tissue, osteoid and benign or malignant mesenchyme; other areas resemble adult liver cell cancer or liver cell adenoma. Classification was understandably difficult and delayed, but in the last 10 to 15 years a generally accepted division of the primary epithelial tumors into two groups has been made. The first type of tumor occurs largely in children under 2 years of age and is made up of fetal and embryonal elements, usually, but not always, "mixed" with mesenchymal tissue. The second group of tumors resembles liver cell carcinoma in the adult, and these tumors are likely to occur in older children. Arbitrarily we shall call these two tumors that form the basis of this chapter "hepatoblastoma" and "hepatocellular carcinoma."

Although Griffith (1918) collected from the literature 57 cases of what he considered to be primary carcinoma of the liver in infants and children, he was able to find only one report of an attempted removal

105

and this was unsuccessful.[31] Grey Turner successfully removed a 2 lb, 3 oz well-differentiated primary cancer from the liver of a 13-year-old boy in 1921,[61] and sporadic case reports continued until after World War II. As experience accumulated it became apparent that primary epithelial cancers in the pediatric group were most common in infants under 2 years of age. The tumors usually were found as mass lesions in otherwise healthy children, and occasionally were associated with other conditions such as hemihypertrophy, biliary atresia, and cysto-thioninuria. The tumors often reached enormous size without spread beyond Glisson's capsule.

During the last two decades improvements in anesthesia, fluid and blood replacement, operative technique, and perioperative support have made possible truly heroic efforts at removing up to 90 per cent of the bulk of a child's liver to control disease. More recently, the combined use of chemotherapy and radiation therapy with resection of metastatic lesions in the lung and elsewhere has resulted in a few apparent "cures," and allowed us the hope that in the future most children with primary epithelial cancer may be permanently rid of their disease by aggressive therapy.

PATHOLOGIC CLASSIFICATION OF PRIMARY EPITHELIAL MALIGNANCY IN CHILDREN

Although sporadic case reports and collected reviews of primary liver cancer in children had been published prior to 1938, the first comprehensive and critical survey of the modern era was done by Steiner.[64] Reviewing reports dating back as far as 1854, Steiner collected and studied 77 cases of primary liver cancer in children under 16 years of age (including two of his own). More than one-half of these tumors occurred in children under 2 years of age, and two-thirds occurred in males. Accepting the classification first recommended by Yamagiwa (1911), which separated primary liver cancers into those arising from the hepatocyte and those from biliary epithelium,[70] he found 52 cases of "hepatoma" and three cases of "cholangioma." Twenty-two cases were of unclassified type. Cirrhosis was an associated finding in only one child.

Bigelow and Wright updated the collected experience in 1953 by adding 21 more cases. They noted mixed epithelial and mesenchymal components in three tumors and discussed the significance of these "sarcomatous-appearing" elements.[3] Edmondson classified most carcinomas of children as liver cell carcinoma, but described a "hepatic mixed tumor" group in which was seen a wide variety of histologic patterns of liver cell, bile duct cell, and even squamous epithelium admixed with osteoid, cartilage, and other mesenchymal elements, including mesenchymal sarcoma.[13, 15]

Shorter, et al. (1960) further defined these groups as they reviewed 11 cases from the Mayo Clinic. They stressed that the presence of any osteoid, cartilage, bone, or muscle precluded the diagnosis of "liver cell cancer," and necessitated the designation of "mixed tumor."[62]

Willis, who had been among the first to recognize a group of mixed tumors distinct from liver cell carcinoma and teratomas in 1948,[68] coined the word "hepatoblastoma" and defined these tumors as distinct embryonal neoplasms arising from hepatic blastema in infants and young children (1962).[69] He classified embryonal neoplasia of the liver as: (1) embryonic hepatoma; (2) mixed hepatoblastoma; or (3) rhabdomyoblastic mixed tumors. Ishak and Glunz (1967)[35] carefully analyzed 47 epithelial tumors in children. They did not consider the rhabdomyoblastic sarcomatous tumors of children in this report. Their clinicopathologic study of 35 patients with hepatoblastoma and 12 patients with hepatocellular carcinoma forms the basis of the classification that we, and most other students of the disease, have adopted. They divided the hepatoblastomas into epithelial and mixed epithelial and mesenchymal types. Hepatocellular carcinoma in children was morphologically indistinguishable from adult liver carcinoma. Hepatoblastomas were found exclusively in children below the age of 5 years, and hepatocellular carcinoma was found in children from 5 to 15 years of age, with a single exception occurring in the 12- to 23-month age range. Others[16, 40, 58, 71] add to the experience that consistently suggests that hepatoblastomas occur in younger children and carry a better prognosis.

Misugi, et al. (1967), on the basis of histologic and ultrastructural criteria, distinguished two types of tumors.[50] The first occurred in infants and children up to 3 years of age and was characterized by a combination of embryonal liver parenchyma and mesenchyme with an ultrastructure that showed a limited number of cytoplasmic organelles. The second tumor type occurred in children older than 6 years of age and showed ultrastructural changes characterized by increased mitochondria and irregular endoplasmic reticulum. Ito and Johnson (1969) also noted ultrastructural differences between hepatoblastoma and hepatocellular carcinoma.[36] The hepatoblastoma showed few cell organelles and absence of glycogen, whereas hepatocellular carcinoma showed well-developed cytoplasmic organelles. Gonzalez-Crussi and Manz (1972) demonstrated ultrastructural differences in the organelles of fetal and embryonal areas in a purely epithelial hepatoblastoma, and suggested that these represented degrees of differentiation of cells within a hepatoblastoma.[30]

Figures 5–1 through 5–8 illustrate histologic features of hepatocellular carcinoma and hepatoblastoma.

Text continued on page 116

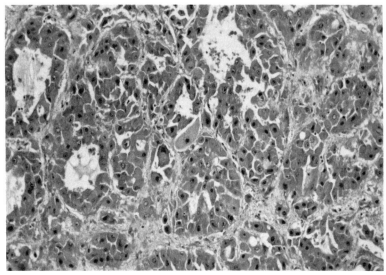

Figure 5–1. Hepatocellular carcinoma, adult type, in an eight-year-old child. The histopathology is essentially identical to adult hepatocellular carcinoma with pseudoglandular features.

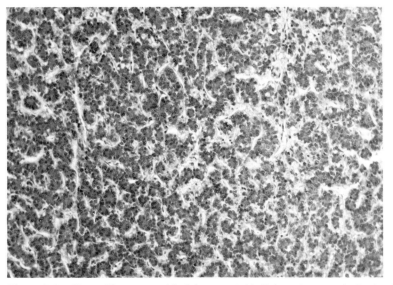

Figure 5–2. Hepatoblastoma, epithelial type. Epithelial cords comprised of cells resembling differentiated fetal hepatocytes.

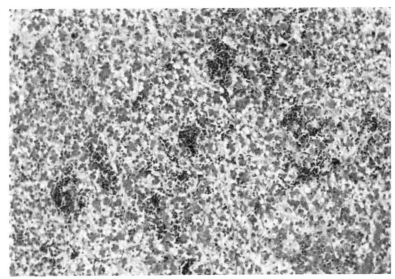

Figure 5–3. Hepatoblastoma, epithelial type. Prominent islands of hematopoietic cells in sinusoids within the tumor are a common finding in the pure epithelial type of hepatoblastoma.

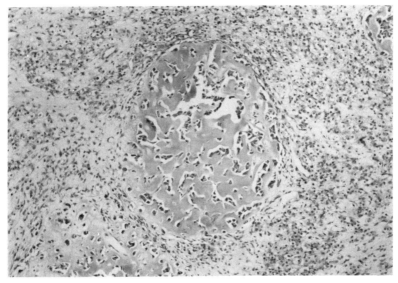

Figure 5–4. Hepatoblastoma, mixed type. A nodule of osteoid within the mesenchymal component of a hepatoblastoma with mixed features of epithelial and mesenchymal differentiation.

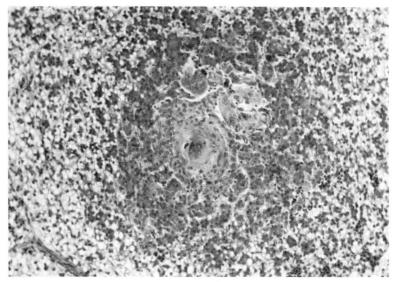

Figure 5–5. Hepatoblastoma, mixed type. A focus of squamous metaplasia occurring within the fetal epithelial component of a mixed hepatoblastoma.

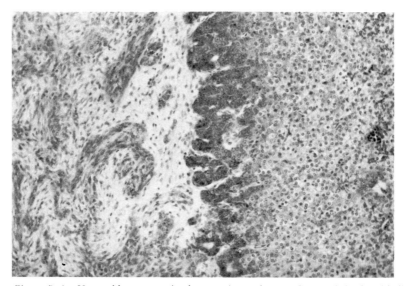

Figure 5–6. Hepatoblastoma, mixed type. A contiguous focus of fetal epithelial elements adjacent to differentiated mesenchyme showing invaginating buds of epithelium. This appearance closely approximates the embryonic differentiation of portal bile ductules by the extension of buds from the periphery of the liver lobule into the embryonic mesenchyme.

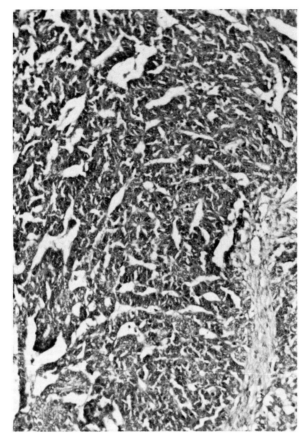

Figure 5-7. Hepatoblastoma, embryonal type. Epithelial cords of markedly de-differentiated embryonal hepatocytes arranged in a gyriform pattern.

Those pediatric patients with "mixed" tumors in which the mesenchymal malignancy is predominant (rhabdomyoblastic type, Willis,[69] or mixed mesenchymal tumor, Keeling[40]) have been grouped separately in this monograph and are discussed under the term "embryonal sarcoma" in Chapter Seven.

1974 LIVER TUMOR SURVEY

A total of 107 cases of resected primary liver tumor occurring in children less than 16 years of age were collected in the 1974 Liver Tumor Survey from six children's hospitals and 33 other general hos-

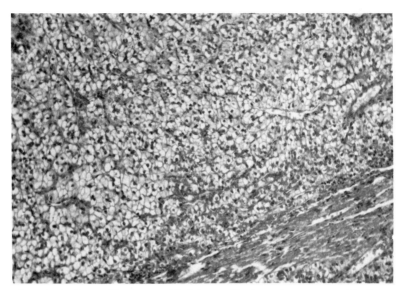

Figure 5–8. Hepatoblastoma, epithelial type. Fetal-type hepatocytes with clear cytoplasm may comprise the major histologic appearance of the fetal epithelial hepatoblastoma.

pitals. Table 5–1 outlines this experience. The 35 tumors that were classified as other than hepatoblastoma or hepatocellular cancer are discussed in Chapters Six and Seven. Of the 72 primary epithelial cancers in children found in the 1974 LTS, the histologic sections were seen by at least one of us for 20 of the 21 hepatocellular cancers, for 45 of the 47 hepatoblastomas, and for none of the four "unclassified" tumors. The written pathology report was read in every instance, and the reports for the seven patients whose slides we did not review indicate clearly that the tumors were primary in the liver and of epithelial origin. Three reports were complete enough to allow categorization of the tumors as hepatoblastoma in two instances and as a hepatocellular carcinoma in one instance. The other four tumors are listed as "unclassified" in the ensuing tabulation and discussion. Even when we were privileged to see the slides, categorization was often difficult and our initial decisions were changed after re-review in several instances. Most of the hepatocellular carcinomas were moderately well differentiated. Three patients had the unique histologic pattern which we have called polygonal cell with fibrous stroma, discussed in Chapter Four (Cases 56, 64, and 65, Appendix IV). Figure 5–1 illustrates the typical appearance of hepatocellular carcinoma in a child. These tumors are indistinguishable histologically from those of adults.

Histologic sections were sent to Dr. Berman for 35 of the 47 hepatoblastoma cases. Twenty-seven of these tumors were composed entirely of malignant epithelium which was further classified as pure fetal

Table 5–1.   Resected Pediatric Tumors —
1974 Liver Tumor Survey*

	Six Children's Hospitals	33 General Hospitals	Total
Primary Epithelial Tumors			
Hepatoblastoma	20	27	47
Hepatocellular carcinoma	11	10	21
Unclassified	0	4	4
Malignant Mesenchymal			
Angiosarcoma	1	4	5
Other sarcoma	1	10	11
Teratocarcinoma	1	0	1
Benign Tumors			
Focal nodular hyperplasia	3	6	9
Mesenchymal hamartoma	1	4	5
Miscellaneous other	4	0	4
	42	65	107

*See final footnote, Appendix V, p. 324.

(seven tumors), pure embryonal (four) and mixed fetal and embryonal (16). The remaining eight tumors showed a mesenchymal component consisting of osteoid, squamous metaplasia, or mature mesenchyme in addition to the predominant malignant epithelium. No histologic malignant mesenchymal elements were noted in the group we have classified as hepatoblastoma. Figures 5–2 to 5–8 illustrate typical features of hepatoblastoma. Appendix V lists pertinent clinical data for these 72 patients. Twenty-five of the 72 cases have been reported elsewhere. Table 5–2 demonstrates the real differences in age distribution between hepatoblastoma and liver cell cancer, but, contrary to the reports of others,[35] it does not show a striking difference in sex incidence.

Preoperative Evaluation

Most of the patients presented with a history of abdominal enlargement or an asymptomatic mass lesion found by their physician. In at least four patients this enlargement was known for more than 12 months before resection.

Jaundice was noted in one patient four months of age whose general development had been slow after an apparently normal birth. A

Table 5-2. Pediatric Epithelial Cancer — 1974 Liver Tumor Survey: 72 Resected Patients*

	47 Hepatoblastoma Patients	21 Hepatocellular Carcinoma Patients	4 Unclassified Patients	Total
AGE AND SEX				
Age				
Range	9 days–5 years	5 months–15 years	1 year–8 years	9 days–15 years
Mean	14 months	8 years	$3^{1}/_2$ years	3.2 years
Median	8 months	$8^{1}/_2$ years	$2^{1}/_4$ years	15 months
Sex				
Male	25	12	1	38
Female	22	9	3	34

*See final footnote, Appendix V, p. 324.

diagnosis of hepatitis was made and the patient was treated with pred-nisolone. Intermittent episodes of jaundice were followed by the development of pruritus at 16 months of age, and an abdominal mass was found at 2 years and resected. A large hepatoblastoma of the left lobe with direct involvement of adjacent jejunum was removed from an otherwise normal liver, but the child died with recurrent disease six months after resection (Case 37, Appendix V). Autopsy showed no evidence of hepatitis. This tumor may have been present for at least a year and eight months before resection.

Two hepatoblastomas were noted at birth, both in association with jaundice (Cases 1 and 2, Appendix V). In one child a definite tumor was palpable, but the other had only diffuse hepatomegaly. A ring of calcification that was visible on a radiograph of the abdomen and a "flush" of liver tumor seen on an intravenous pyelogram prompted exploration. Three other patients with hepatoblastomas had radiographic evidence of calcification, two with some "stippling" on a preoperative abdominal film, and the other with considerable calcification in a tumor that was excised 11 months after radiotherapy for an "unresectable" lesion.

One child with left hemihypertrophy noted since birth developed a hepatoblastoma in the right lobe of his liver that was noted at 10 months of age. Fraumeni, et al. have reported this association previously.[25] Two patients had endocrine symptoms: the first was a 15-year-old girl who was being evaluated for short stature, primary amenorrhea, and absence of development of secondary sexual characteristics when liver enlargement was noted on physical examination and the radioisotope scan showed a mass lesion. Eleven months after resection of a large solitary liver cell carcinoma she was doing well and had rapidly developed secondary sexual characteristics (Case 66, Appendix V). The other patient was a 2½-year-old male with a gonadotropin-secreting hepatoblastoma. Palliative resection of most of his tumor was done to relieve his symptoms of rapid growth, deep voice, and precocious puberty, but pulmonary and axillary metastases had developed by the tenth month after the liver resection (Case 42, Appendix V).

Two siblings four years apart in age developed identical hepatoblastomas which were diagnosed when each infant was 15 months of age (Cases 33 and 34, Appendix V). Both had enormous tumors originating in the right lobe that required extended right lobectomy for removal. Others[26, 37, 43] also have reported a familial incidence of primary epithelial carcinoma, but this must be extremely rare.

All 39 patients who were under 18 months of age presented with an abdominal mass or liver enlargement. Nineteen of these infants were healthy and without symptoms except for the mass; seven others had associated fever and pain; eleven had anorexia and weight loss; and in one patient hepatomegaly was associated with abnormal calcification on a radiograph. Adequate historical information was provided for 30 of the 33 older children (18 months of age or older), and 26 had a mass lesion. Eleven of these older children had no other symptom. The mass was associated with anorexia in five, pain in three, and pain and fever in six. Two children presented with endocrine symptoms (see above). The only instance of hemoperitoneum occurred in a 2-year-old female with abdominal pain and fever of several days' duration. A ruptured hepatoblastoma was found at emergency operation. Bleeding was temporarily controlled, allowing transfer to a larger center, but unfortunately the child died of blood loss during a second urgent attempt to resect the tumor (Case 40, Appendix V).

A 15-year-old boy was the only pediatric patient whose tumor occurred in a cirrhotic liver. A 9-cm liver cell carcinoma was noted in the left lateral segment of the liver during removal of his spleen for traumatic rupture, four years after a diagnosis of chronic active hepatitis was made and 2½ years after he had bled from esophageal varices. The tumor was successfully resected from a liver showing diffuse micronodular cirrhosis, and the patient is still alive 118 months later after two more operations to remove biopsy-proved recurrent abdominal tumor masses (Case 68, Appendix V).

Preoperative liver function tests were obtained in at least 43 patients. The SGOT proved to be the test most often abnormal, but in most cases transaminase elevation was minimal. Table 5–3 outlines the results of preoperative testing.

Radioisotope scans were done for 30 patients. Two scans failed to

Table 5–3. Pediatric Epithelial Cancer – 1974 Liver Tumor Survey: Preoperative Evaluation

	Within Normal Limits	Abnormal
Bromsulphalein retention	3	2
Alkaline phosphatase	28	15
SGOT	15	23
Bilirubin	35	10
Prothrombin time	10	2
Alpha-fetoprotein	2	6
Radioisotope scan	2	28
Angiography		
Arteriography	1	19
Venacavography	1	1
Splenoportography	1	0

reveal hepatoblastomas of the right lobe, but otherwise the scan accurately localized solitary lesions in 23 patients and predicted multiple lesions in four of five patients found to have multiple lesions at laparotomy. In one child treated with chemotherapy and radiotherapy because of an "unresectable" situation, serial scans showed a decreased size of the tumor and eventually formed the basis of an imaginative and aggressive attack on the tumor that resulted in a long survival (Case 36, Appendix V).[32]

Arteriography was done in 20 patients. Vascularity was noted in 16 reports, and was increased in 14 and decreased in two. The only patient in whom the arteriogram did not reveal the lesion had a 4-cm well-differentiated tumor along the free edge of the left lateral segment of the liver. Two patients had inferior venacavography. One had no evidence of obstruction from a tumor of the left lateral segment, and the other had complete obstruction of the inferior vena cava by extrinsic pressure from a huge tumor in the posterior one-half of the right lobe, which was resected successfully but which recurred early (Case 48, Appendix V). Obstruction of the inferior vena cava diagnosed by venography cannot be taken as absolute proof of direct involvement or unresectability, unless tumor is demonstrated at the hepatic vein–inferior vena cava junction at the diaphragm. Splenoportography was within normal limits in the one case in which it was done.

Sixteen patients had both arteriography and a radioisotope scan done preoperatively. In one case the scan showed a lesion that was not seen on arteriography, and in one the arteriogram showed a lesion that was not seen on scan. In those three patients who were proved at

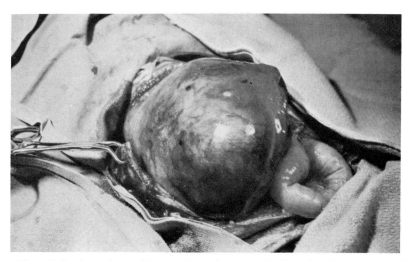

Figure 5-9. Large hepatoblastoma limited to the right lobe of an 8-month-old white girl. She died of her disease 18 months after liver resection.
  (Case 22, Appendix V).

subsequent laparotomy to have multiple tumors, and who had both scan and arteriogram done preoperatively, multiple tumors were suggested by the scan in two cases and by the arteriogram in one.

OPERATION

At operation the tumors always involved one or more surfaces of the liver and were readily distinguishable from normal liver tissue. They usually were soft and of a lighter color than surrounding normal liver tissue, with prominent surface vessels (Figs. 9, 10, 11). Umbilication was not seen. Most of the resected tumors were contained within Glisson's capsule, but one had invaded adjacent jejunum (Case 37), one was attached to the anterior abdominal wall (Case 16), and one had involved the diaphragm (Case 61). Table 5–4 outlines the site and size of these tumors and Table 5–5 lists the operations done. The details of hepatic resection for neoplasm will be discussed more thoroughly in Chapter Eleven.

MORTALITY

There were 14 deaths after liver resection for primary epithelial cancer in 72 pediatric patients (19 per cent). Three of the 14 infants under 6 months of age and nine of the 29 children from 6 to 24 months of age died during or after operation. The only two youngsters

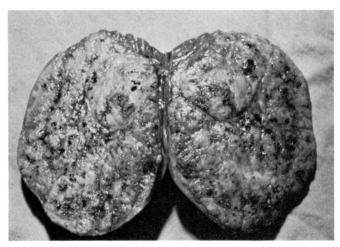

Figure 5–10. Cross-section of resected hepatoblastoma. Note soft, variegated appearance with focal necrosis.
(Case 22, Appendix V).

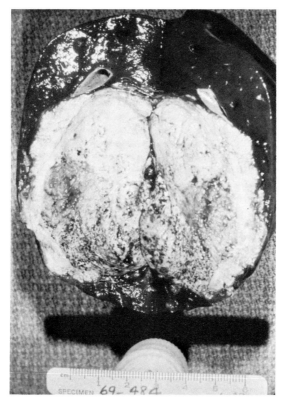

Figure 5–11. Primary hepatocellular carcinoma (clear-cell type) resected by left lobectomy from 5-year-old girl. Patient alive and well six years later.
(Case 55, Appendix V). (Photo courtesy of William Livingston, M.D. of New Britain, Connecticut.)

who died of the 29 from 2 to 15 years of age were both lost in the operating room because of failure to control hemorrhage.

Nine of the 14 deaths occurred because of technical problems with the control of hemorrhage. Eight patients died on the operating table and one survived without consciousness for 12 days after cardiac arrest during operation. In at least seven instances this fatal hemorrhage occurred in relation to the control of the junction of the major hepatic veins and the inferior vena cava.

Two patients died seven and 15 days after "90 per cent" resection with ascites and liver failure. Both of these patients were under 2 years of age and had undergone extended right lobectomy for huge hepatoblastomas. Two other deaths occurred, because of bile duct injury in one patient and because of late sepsis and liver failure in another whose liver inflow was totally occluded during resection. The last death

Table 5–4. Pediatric Epithelial Cancer – 1974 Liver Tumor Survey: Site and Size of Tumor*

	HEPATOBLASTOMA	HEPATOCELLULAR CARCINOMA	UNCLASSIFIED	OVER-ALL
Patients	47	21	4	72
Location of Tumor				
Right lobe	36	17	2	55
Left lobe	8	4	2	14
Central	2	0	0	2
Bilateral tumors	1	0	0	1
Size of Tumor (max. Diam.)				
Mean	11 cm	12 cm	13 cm	11.5 cm
Median	12 cm	12 cm	13 cm	12 cm

*See final footnote, Appendix V, p. 324.

Table 5–5. Pediatric Epithelial Cancer – 1974 Liver Tumor Survey: Operation*

	HEPATOBLASTOMA	HEPATOCELLULAR CARCINOMA	UNCLASSIFIED	TOTAL
Right lobectomy	27	13	1	41
Extended right lobectomy	7	3	1	11
Extended right lobectomy plus multiple wedge, left	1	—	—	1
Left lobectomy	2	3	1	6
Left lateral segmentectomy	5	—	1	6
Wedge, left lobe	1	1	—	2
Wedge, right lobe	3	1	—	4
Wedge, central	1	—	—	1
				72

*See final footnote, Appendix V, p. 324.

was associated with persistent tumor and sepsis in a patient who probably never should have been resected and who received chemotherapy immediately postoperatively.

Information was obtained about eight pediatric patients who came to postmortem examination in the postoperative period after liver resection for tumor. No residual cancer was found in five patients; two had small pulmonary metastases; and the last patient had a solitary 1-mm nodule of residual tumor in the liver very near to the line of transection.

Most of these pediatric patients did quite well after resection. Of the three requiring reoperation to control hemorrhage during the first 24 hours, one child died and the other two recovered rapidly.

Five patients developed subphrenic abscesses that needed drainage, and three others required reoperation to remove Ivalon and Teflon "bolsters" at one month, three months, and five and one-half years respectively after liver resection to control draining sinus tracts. Four of these patients with abscess are long-term survivors (longer than five years), and two others are alive and free of disease eight and eleven months respectively after resection. Thus perihepatic sepsis seems to have no serious adverse effects on the potential of an operation to cure cancer. Two patients required drainage of sterile bile collections, and one patient who developed progressive jaundice had repair of a compromised left hepatic duct and is still doing well 66 months later. Only two patients had significant upper gastrointestinal hemorrhage postoperatively, and both were controlled with transfusion. Transient jaundice was common, but persistent and progressive jaundice was always associated with a major bile duct injury or liver failure.

LATE SURVIVAL

The effect of operative mortality has been excluded from the following tabulations of late survival because the technical details of operation, rather than the type of disease, related more closely to operative and postoperative deaths. Over-all mortality is easily calculated from the data provided by adding the number of operative deaths to the denominator of the appropriate fraction.

Tables 5–6, 5–7, and 5–8 outline the survival data available at the time of the 1974 LTS. Thirty-three of the 57 patients surviving operation with follow-up information are alive and free of disease, 17 more than five years after resection.

All but one of the 23 children dying with recurrent cancer were dead by the end of three years, and the last child died 38 months after resection. If one makes a theoretic calculation of five-year survival on the assumption that those children who are alive and well more than 36

Table 5–6. Pediatric Epithelial Cancer—1974 Liver Tumor Survey: Survival, Tumor, and Age*

Age	Hepatoblastoma Under 2 years	Over 2 years	Hepatocellular Carcinoma Under 2 years	Over 2 years	Unclassified Under 2 years	Over 2 years
Patients	36	11	6	15	1	3
Operative deaths	9	1	3	0	0	1
Alive, N.E.D.	21	4	0	8	0	0
Mean survival	53 months	81 months	—	55 months	—	—
Dead with disease	6	4	3	7	1	2
Mean interval	10 months	25 months	6 months	16 months	5 months	4 months
Alive with recurrent disease	0	1 (10 months)	—	—	—	—
No follow-up information	—	1	—	—	—	—

*See final footnote, Appendix V, p. 324.

Table 5–7. Pediatric Epithelial Cancer — 1974 Liver Tumor Survey: Determinate Survival After Liver Resection*†

	HEPATOBLASTOMA		HEPATOCELLULAR CARCINOMA		UNCLASSIFIED	OVER-ALL	
Survival							
1-Year	29/34	(85%)	9/15	(60%)	0/3	38/52	73%
2-Year	22/30	(73%)	6/14	(43%)	0/3	28/47	60%
3-Year	17/26	(65%)	5/14	(36%)	0/3	22/43	51%
4-Year	12/22	(55%)	4/14	(29%)	0/3	16/39	41%
5-Year	9/19	(47%)	4/14	(29%)	0/3	13/36	36%

*Excludes operative deaths.
†See final footnote, Appendix V, p. 324.

months after resection will be "cured," the five-year survival rate for hepatoblastoma would be 65 per cent and the five-year survival rate for the over-all group of 58 operative survivors would be 51 per cent.

Many have said that the prognosis of an infant child who survives operation for cancer is better than that of an older child[18, 39] Table 5–8 looks at the data in this light. The differences are not impressive but are in favor of the younger child with hepatoblastoma.

The microscopic sections of the epithelial tumors in 46 patients were sent to Dr. Berman at Hartford Hospital for critical review. Table 5–9 has been organized from his final classification in an attempt to draw clinicopathologic correlations. Unfortunately, the number of patients in any single category is not large enough to provide a basis for firm conclusions. It is interesting to note, however, that, with the exception of age-incidence, there is little difference between the clinical features and course of the patients with hepatoblastoma and those with hepatocellular carcinoma.

Two patients had small satellite nodules close to the parent tumor that were totally excised. One patient died in the operating room; the other is alive and apparently free of disease 47 months after resection. Six patients had *clinically* positive lymph nodes in the liver hilum, the gastrohepatic omentum, the omentum, or along the aorta. Two whose nodes proved to be negative on histologic section are alive, one with evidence of recurrent disease ten months after resection and the other apparently free of disease at ten years. Four other patients with histologically positive lymph nodes died with recurrent disease six to 36 months after liver resection.

Five patients who had complete removal of all grossly evident tumor (two hepatocellular carcinomas, three hepatoblastomas) received "prophylactic" chemotherapy immediately after liver resection, and all five patients are alive at eight, 20, 32, 58, and 61 months after their operations. Two patients without known residual tumor received prophylactic radiotherapy; one is alive without evidence of disease at 27 months and the other died six months after resection with recurrent

Table 5–8. Pediatric Epithelial Cancer – 1974 Liver Tumor Survey: Determinate Survival – Age*

Age (years)	Hepatoblastoma		Hepatocellular Carcinoma		Over-all	
	Under 2	Over 2	Under 2	Over 2	Under 2	Over 2
1-Year survival	22/26	7/8	0/3	9/12	22/30 (73%)	16/22 (73%)
2-Year survival	16/22	6/8	0/3	6/11	16/26 (62%)	12/21 (57%)
3-Year survival	12/18	5/8	0/3	5/11	12/22 (55%)	10/21 (48%)
4-Year survival	10/16	2/6	0/3	4/11	10/20 (50%)	6/19 (32%)
5-Year survival	8/14	1/5	0/3	4/11	8/18 (44%)	5/18 (28%)

*See final footnote, Appendix V, p. 324.

Table 5-9. Primary Epithelial Cancer of Children—1974 LTS: Clinicopathologic Correlations†

		Male/Female	Mean Age	Tumor Size	46 PATIENTS* SURVIVAL**			
	Patients				Mean	Median	2-year	5-year
Hepatoblastoma	35	19/16	23 months	12 cm	39 months	26 months	16/23	5/13
Pure epithelial	27	17/10	14 months	12 cm	33 months	26 months	12/17	3/9
Fetal	7	4/3	8 months	13 cm	60 months	53 months	4/5	2/3
Embryonal	4	1/3	30 months	9 cm	25 months	32 months	2/3	0/2
Mixed fetal and embryonal	16	12/4	12 months	12 cm	29 months	24 months	6/9	1/4
Mixed	8	2/6	4.6 years	11 cm	61 months	24 months	4/6	2/4
Hepatocellular Carcinoma	11	6/5	11 years	12 cm	46 months	27 months	6/8	4/8
Polygonal cell	3	2/1	11 years	9 cm	50 months	18 months	1/1	1/1
Others	8	4/4	11 years	13 cm	44 months	31 months	5/7	3/7

*46 patients whose histologic sections were sent to Hartford Hospital for review by Dr. Berman.
**Excludes operative deaths.
†See final footnote, Appendix V, p. 324.

cancer. Aggressive combined therapy for two children deserves attention. A 15-month-old male infant with anemia, fever, and hepatomegaly was found at laparotomy to have an unresectable hepatoblastoma involving both lobes of the liver. He was treated with vincristine without effect, and then with cobalt irradiation and Cytoxan with objective regression of the tumor seen on serial radioisotope scans. When the child was 23 months of age a calcified tumor was totally resected by extended right lobectomy, and the patient is alive and free of any evidence of disease 87 months after liver resection at the time of the 74 LTS (Case 36, Appendix V).[32] Another patient, a 6-month-old male infant, had a partial right lobectomy for a multinodular hepatoblastoma with satellite nodules and adherence to the abdominal wall. Twelve months later an umbilical metastasis was resected, and, when a pulmonary metastasis did not respond to chemotherapy, it too was resected 20 months after liver resection. When last followed, the child was alive without evidence of disease 47 months after liver resection (Case 15, Appendix V).

Two other patients received radiotherapy before liver resection for hepatoblastomas thought to be unresectable. In both instances the tumor regressed, and resection was eventually done 11 and 15 months respectively after the first histologic confirmation of the diagnosis. However, both children died of recurrent disease 32 and 38 months after liver resection.

Six of 47 patients with hepatoblastomas, and four of 21 with liver-cell carcinomas, had multiple nodules of tumor. Two of these ten patients died at operation, one was lost to follow-up, and six are dead with disease from six to 38 months after liver resection. The only survivor (Case 16, Appendix V) developed abdominal wall metastases that were resected (see above). The prognosis of a child with a solitary nodule, however large, is clearly better.

Fifteen patients had significant fever as presenting symptoms (8 out of 21 with liver cell cancer and 7 out of 47 with hepatoblastoma). Four died at operation, but survival in the remaining 11 patients paralleled that of the afebrile group, suggesting that the presence of systemic symptoms does not have an adverse effect on eventual prognosis.

Can we learn anything about prognosis by looking at the patients who died with recurrent disease after hospital discharge, or at the patients who survived more than five years? Twelve female and 11 male patients died with recurrent disease from two to 38 months after liver resection (mean 13 months for liver cell cancer and 16 months for hepatoblastoma).

Table 5–6 documents that the older child with recurrent disease is more likely to live longer, although his chances for "cure" are less than those of a younger child. Tumor size at operation averaged 12 cm maximum diameter for those who died with disease, 11.6 cm for the 13 five-year survivors, and 11.5 cm for the over-all group. Thus, there was no correlation between the size of the "cured" tumors and the ones that recurred and claimed the lives of these pediatric patients. There also was no correlation between long-term survival and the type of operation done to resect the tumors. In the cases of those children whose grossly evident tumor was entirely removed, it generally was difficult to predict which one would do well after operation.

When a patient developed evidence of recurrence, was there anything that could be offered to him? Nine patients had reoperation for evaluation of recurrent disease. Four patients at laparotomy done from three to 27 months after liver resection and two patients at thoracotomy done five months after liver resection were found to have unresectable recurrent or persistent liver cancer. A single attempt at resecting recurrent disease in the liver 15 months after primary resection was followed by death with recurrent disease eight months after the second operation. Two patients had resection of metastatic disease and are alive. The first (discussed above) had resection of umbilical and pulmonary metastases (Case 16, Appendix V), and the second was the 15-year-old boy with cirrhosis who developed a liver cell carcinoma in the left lateral segment of his liver (Case 68, Appendix V). Fifty-five months after liver resection, four large nodules of biopsy-proved recurrent liver cell carcinoma were removed from the omentum, and 12 months after that a partial gastrectomy with excision of a piece of diaphragm was done to remove additional biopsy-proved recurrent disease. This patient is alive 51 months after his last operation, or 118 months after primary resection of his liver cell carcinoma.

Chemotherapy was used in at least 11 children when recurrent disease was recognized, but with the exception of Case 16, Appendix V, who also had resection of all known metastases, no child survived more than 12 months after chemotherapy was begun. Radiation therapy for recurrent disease was used in at least ten children. Seven patients died within six months of the start of radiation therapy. One is alive with diffuse metastatic disease ten months after radiotherapy was begun, and two others lived more than one year. The first is alive without evidence of disease 17 months after radiotherapy was given to a scan-diagnosed but unbiopsied recurrent nodule. The second child died 35 months after radiation to a biopsy-proved recurrence of liver cell carcinoma, which was found at laparotomy three months after an extended right lobectomy for hepatoblastoma (Case 45, Appendix V).

LITERATURE REVIEW

The subject of liver cancer in children has been a popular one with medical authors in spite of the rarity of the condition. The American

Table 5–10.   References for Pediatric Tumors

History	5, 41, 55, 64
Incidence	26, 35, 39
Epidemiology	25
Associated Conditions	25, 35
Cystothioninuria	28
Biliary atresia	21
Hemihypertrophy	25, 28
Cirrhosis	40
Familial incidence	26, 44
Endocrine symptoms	25, 58
Pathology	3, 13, 14, 15, 35, 36, 39, 40, 50, 56, 62, 64, 67, 69, 71
Symptoms	19, 35
Diagnosis	
Laboratory tests	19, 35, 44
Alpha-fetoprotein	16, 19, 26
Radiology	52, 53, 59
Scans	53
Operation—Technique	2, 47, 52
Metabolic	
Consequences	47, 65
Radiation Therapy	19, 32, 35, 39
Chemotherapy	20, 32, 39, 42
Survival	4, 19, 21, 24, 35

General reports of problem: Toronto—16, India—27, London—34, 40, Taiwan—44, Chicago—52, Barti (Italy)—56, New York—17, 18, Japan—39, Los Angeles—10, 46, Columbus—7, 8, 9, 50, Denmark—58.

Academy of Pediatrics Surgical Section Survey of 1974 was on the subject of liver tumors in children. This questionnaire survey collected data on 129 children with hepatoblastoma and 98 children with liver cell carcinoma. The resulting report of Exelby, Filler, and Grosfeld is the most comprehensive source of raw clinical data now available on these two tumors.[19] The reader is referred also to other general reviews[9, 35, 39] for a comprehensive look at the subject, and to Table 5–10 for references about specific aspects of pediatric liver carcinoma.

Rather than attempt a summary of all this material, we shall focus instead on the results of therapy as reported in the literature.

It is certain that, without resection of their tumors, all children with primary liver cancer will die. Ninety per cent of the 76 patients dying with hepatoblastoma and 80 per cent of 82 patients dying with liver cell carcinoma, as reported by Exelby, et al., were dead within 12 months of diagnosis, and little or no palliation was achieved by radiotherapy or chemotherapy.[19] How often will a primary epithelial cancer of the liver in a child be resectable for cure after the diagnosis is made? In the American Academy of Pediatric Surgery, 86 (67 per cent) of the 129 patients explored for hepatoblastoma had resection done, and this excision was felt to be curative in 78 cases. Of 92 patients undergoing laparotomy for liver cell cancer, resection was possible in only 37 and was thought to be complete in 33.[19] Lin, et al. found five of eight tumors in children under 5 years of age to be resectable, but only one of 13 over 5 years of age.[44] Nineteen of 23 children with liver tumors treated at Memorial Hospital underwent laparotomy, and resection was possible in only nine.[18]

When resection is possible, what is the risk of operation and will resection provide long-term survival? To answer these questions a review was made of the literature back to 1950. The report of Foster (1970)[24] includes the comprehensive data collected by Fish and McCary[21] and Ishak and Glunz.[35] To that report has been added information from 26 other sources about 74 patients with resected hepatoblastomas and 28 patients with resected liver cell carcinoma to compile the data tabulated in Tables 5–11, 5–12, and 5–13.

The operative mortality rate from different reports is quite consistent and remains between 20 and 25 per cent (see Table 5–11). Most of these deaths occur in younger children, and many are related to blood loss on the operating table. Postoperative liver failure, even after extended hepatic lobectomy, is rare, and, with a greater understanding of pre- and postoperative support, most children should do well if they leave the operating room in good condition. Improvements in surgical technique should lower intraoperative mortality, but technical experience is difficult to achieve because the tumors are so rare. Most general surgeons develop some competence with liver resection and hemostasis as they deal with trauma, and pediatric surgeons may well profit from similar experiences.

Late survival figures are remarkably consistent when compiled

Table 5–11. Pediatric Epithelial Cancer: Operative Mortality

	Hepatoblastoma	Hepatocellular Carcinoma	Over-all
Foster (1970)[24]	—	—	21/91
26 References*	16/74	7/28	23/102
1974 LTS	10/47	3/21	14/72
	26/121 (21%)	10/49 (20%)	58/265 (22%)

*1, 6, 11, 12, 16, 18, 23, 26, 27, 29, 33, 34, 38, 39, 45, 51, 52, 53, 54, 56, 57, 58, 60, 63, 66, 71.

Table 5–12. Pediatric Epithelial Cancer: Long-term Survival*

	FOSTER (1970)	26** REFS	1974 LTS	TOTAL	
1-Year	23/31	54/69	38/52	115/152	76%
2-Year	16/28	36/59	28/47	80/134	60%
3-Year	12/25	27/55	22/43	61/123	50%
4-Year	9/22	20/49	16/39	45/110	41%
5-Year	7/20	14/44	13/36	34/100	34%

*Excludes operative deaths.
**See Table 5–10.

from three different sources (see Table 5–12). Most patients who are not cured will die in the first year or two after resection. Of the 43 deaths due to cancer that are reported in the 26 references and the collected review of Foster,[24] 23 occurred in the first year after resection, 12 in the second, six in the third, one in the fourth, and none in the fifth year. However, Ein and Stephens report the death of a child due to pulmonary metastases from a hepatoblastoma resected 62 months previously,[16] and Exelby, et al. received reports from their questionnaire survey of deaths due to liver cell carcinoma in three patients at two, three, and 11 years respectively after the diagnosis was made.[19]

Many reports conclude that the prognosis is better for the younger child, and for the child with hepatoblastoma rather than liver cell carcinoma. Table 5–13 does not show a significant difference at five years

Table 5–13. Long-term Survival After Resection—Pediatric Patients*: Hepatoblastoma versus Hepatocellular Carcinoma

	HEPATOBLASTOMA			HEPATOCELLULAR CARCINOMA		
	26 Refs.**	1974 LTS	Total	26 Refs.	1974 LTS	Total
1-Year	39/52	29/34	79%	15/17	9/15	75%
2-Year	30/45	22/30	69%	6/14	6/14	43%
3-Year	21/41	17/26	57%	6/14	5/14	39%
4-Year	14/35	12/22	46%	6/14	4/14	36%
5-Year	9/31	9/19	36%	5/13	4/14	33%

*Excludes operative deaths.
**See Table 5–10.

Table 5-14. Pediatric Epithelial Cancer – Literature Survey:
Survival for More than Five Years After Resection

AUTHOR	AGE/SEX	TUMOR	RESECTION	RESULT	
(1) Novy, et al. (1974)[53]	1 year M	LCCa	RL	AFD	13 years
(2) Novy, et al. (1974)	9 year M	LCCa	LL	AFD	10 years
(3) Ein and Stephens (1974)[16]	Less than 3½ years	HB	—	AFD	6 years
(4) Ein and Stephens (1974)	Less than 3½ years	HB	—	AFD	7 years
(5) Ein and Stephens (1974)	Less than 3½ years	HB	—	AFD	10 years
(6) Ein and Stephens (1974)	Less than 3½ years	HB	—	AFD	13 years
(7) Ein and Stephens (1974)	Less than 3½ years	HB	—	DWD	62 months
(8) Gandhi, et al. (1973)[27]	1 year F	HB	LL	AFD	6 years
(9) Modlin, et al. (1967)[51]	6 months M	LCCa	RL	AFD	17 years
(10) Kasai and Watanabe (1970)[39]	12 months M	HB	—	AFD	72 months
(11) Honjo and Mizumoto (1974)[33]	5 months F	HB	LL	AFD	65 months
(12) Exelby, et al. (1971)[18]	1½ year M	LCCa	RL	AFD	12 years
(13) Exelby, et al. (1971)	14 year M	LCCa	RL	AFD	18 years
(14) Ochsner, et al. (1971)[54]	NS	HB	RL	AFD	8 years

Key: LCCa – Liver cell carcinoma.   AFD – Alive, free of disease.
HB – Hepatoblastoma.   DWD – Dead with disease.
N.S. – Not stated.

in the resected patients collected from the literature and from the 1974 LTS. However, resectability rates usually are lower for liver cell carcinoma, and therefore the prognosis for all children with resected *and* unresectable liver cell carcinomas probably remains worse than for hepatoblastoma. The older child with a liver cell carcinoma who is not cured by resection is more likely to live a year or two before dying with his disease than is the younger child with recurrent or persistent hepatoblastoma.

To the 21 five-year survivors of resection collected by Fish and McCary,[21] Ishak and Glunz,[35] and Foster[24] can be added 13 new cases from the 1974 LTS and 14 others that are documented in Table 5–14.

The alpha-fetoprotein was abnormal in six of eight children tested in the 1974 LTS, and in 33 of 58 children collected by Exelby, et al.[19] This test may prove to be a valuable adjunct in following patients after resection. A change from negative to positive in the alpha-fetoprotein is probably reason enough to justify a "second look" operation if diagnostic studies do not reveal the spread of disease outside the abdomen.

There are a few reports of shrinkage of nodules of primary or metastatic liver cancer after radiation therapy, but there is little evidence that the patients' lives were improved or prolonged. Chemotherapy also has been of little benefit in controlling recurrent disease after resection, or in affording palliation for patients with unresectable disease. However, in at least three instances a combination of chemotherapy and radiotherapy has transformed an unresectable situation into one allowing "curative" resection, with subsequent long-term survival.[19, 32, 60]

The adjunctive use of chemotherapy in patients after "curative" resection has been followed by survival of all five patients in the 1974 LTS who received it, and in eight of 11 patients with hepatoblastoma reported by Exelby, et al.[19] (there may be some duplication of these reports). This combination will probably be used more often in the future, although Filler, et al.[20] warn of its dangers.

SUMMARY AND RECOMMENDATIONS

Hepatoblastomas and hepatocellular carcinomas are uncommon but highly malignant diseases of insidious onset that are curable by aggressive therapy in more than one-third of the pediatric patients in whom a diagnosis is made. The neoplasms usually occur in otherwise normal livers and remain within Glisson's capsule for a prolonged period before metastasizing. Although abdominal distention or palpation of a mass are the most common presenting findings, failure to thrive, fever of undetermined etiology, unexplained anemia, and/or weight loss should bring to mind the possibility of a liver tumor in a child. The use of radioisotope scans, serum transaminase values, and alpha-feto-protein determinations will uncover most lesions. Needle biopsy is discouraged because of the vascularity of most lesions.

Although much has been made of the real differences in the pathology, incidence, and prognosis of hepatoblastoma as contrasted with liver cell carcinoma, criteria for resection are essentially the same for both.

The child with a hepatoblastoma or liver cell carcinoma confined within the capsule of the liver needs resection unless the geography of the tumor precludes this possibility. Open biopsy usually should be done, largely to rule out mesenchymal hamartoma (which need not be completely excised). Up to 85 per cent of the liver volume may be safely resected by those experienced in liver surgery. The size of the tumor, and the presence or absence of preoperative systemic symptoms such as fever, do not correlate with long-term survival and should not discourage resection. However, the presence of biopsy-proved lymph node metastasis or of multiple tumor nodules is of grave prognostic significance, and life-threatening resections probably should not be done when they are found.

Preliminary results with the use of adjunctive chemotherapy for patients after "curative" resection are favorable enough to warrant further clinical trials. Combined radiation and chemotherapy should be employed aggressively in patients with unresectable tumors within or without the liver, to ascertain whether sufficient transient regression will occur to allow subsequent "curative" resection. When recurrent but localized disease is found after resection, the possibility of re-resection should be considered.

Today, the two keys to improved therapy are early diagnosis and safe control of hemorrhage in the operating room. Tomorrow, the use of combined therapy may increase our already significant ability to provide long life to patients with these rare tumors.

REFERENCES

1. Adam, Y. G., Huvos, A. G., and Hajdu, S. I.: Malignant vascular tumors of the liver. Ann. Surg. *175(3)*:375, 1972.
2. Adson, M. A.: Major hepatic resections: elective operations. Mayo Clin. Proc. *42*:791, 1967.
3. Bigelow, N. H., and Wright, A. W.: Primary carcinoma of the liver in infancy and childhood. Cancer *6*:170, 1953.
4. Bradham, R. R., et al.: Malignant hepatoma in a child—survival following right hepa-

tectomy, right pneumonectomy, and resection of diaphragmatic and parietal recurrence. Surgery *57*:767, 1965.

5. Castle, O. L.: Primary carcinoma of the liver in childhood. Surg. Gynecol. Obstet. *18*:477, 1914.
6. Chappell, J. S.: Hepatic tumors in infancy and childhood. S. Afr. J. Surg. *10*:171, 1972.
7. Clatworthy, H. W., Jr., Boles, E. T., Jr., and Kottmeier, P. K.: Liver tumors in infancy and childhood. Ann. Surg. *154*:475, 1961.
8. Clatworthy, H. W., Jr., Boles, E. T., Jr., and Newton, W. A.: Primary tumors of the liver in infants and children. Arch. Dis. Child. *35*:22, 1960.
9. Clatworthy, H. W., Schiller, M., and Grosfeld, J. L.: Primary liver tumors in infancy and childhood. Arch. Surg. *109*:143, 1974.
10. Cleland, R. S.: Benign and malignant tumors of the liver. Pediatr. Clin. North Am. *6*:427, 1959.
11. Curutchet, H. P., et al.: Primary liver cancer. Surgery *70*:467, 1971.
12. Dean, D. L., and Bauer, H. M.: Primary cystic carcinoma of the liver. Am. J. Surg. *117*:416, 1969.
13. Edmondson, H. A.: Progress in pediatrics: differential diagnosis of tumors and tumor-like lesions of liver in infancy and childhood. A.M.A. J. Dis. Child. *91*:168, 1956.
14. Edmondson, H. A.: Tumors of the liver and intrahepatic bile ducts. Section VII, Fascicle 25, Atlas of Tumor Pathology. Armed Forces Institute of Pathology, 1958.
15. Edmondson, H. A., and Steiner, P. E.: Primary carcinoma of the liver; a study of 100 cases among 48,900 necropsies. Cancer *7*:463, 1954.
16. Ein, S. H., and Stephens, C. A.: Malignant liver tumors in children. J. Pediatr. Surg. *9(4)*:491, 1974.
17. Exelby, P. R.: Other abdominal tumors. Cancer *35*:910, 1975.
18. Exelby, P. R., et al.: Primary malignant tumors of the liver in children. J. Pediatr. Surg. *6*:272, 1971.
19. Exelby, P. R., Filler, R. M., and Grosfeld, J. L.: Liver tumors in children in the particular reference to hepatoblastomas and hepatocellular carcinoma: American Academy of Pediatrics, Surgical Section Survey – 1974. J. Pediatr. Surg. *10*:329, 1975.
20. Filler, R. M., et al.: Hepatic lobectomy in childhood: effects of x-ray and chemotherapy. J. Pediatr. Surg. *4*:31, 1969.
21. Fish, J. C., and McCary, R. G.: Primary cancer of the liver in childhood. Arch. Surg. *93*:355, 1966.
22. Fong, J. A., and Ruebner, B. H.: Primary leiomyosarcoma of the liver. Hum. Pathol. *5(1)*:115, 1974.
23. Fortner, J. G., et al.: Vascular problems in upper abdominal cancer surgery. Arch. Surg. *109*:148, 1974.
24. Foster, J. H.: Survival after liver resection for cancer. Cancer *26*:493, 1970.
25. Fraumeni, J. F., Jr., Miller, R. W., and Hill, J. A.: Primary carcinoma of the liver in childhood: an epidemiologic study. J. Natl. Cancer Inst. *40*:1087, 1968.
26. Fraumeni, J. F., Jr., et al.: Hepatoblastoma in infant sisters. Cancer *24*:1086, 1969.
27. Gandhi, R. K., Deshmukh, S. S., and Bhalerao, R. A.: Hepatoblastoma in children. Indian Pediatr. *10*:259, 1973.
28. Geiser, C. F., et al.: Epithelial hepatoblastoma associated with congenital hemihypertrophy and cystothioninuria. Pediatrics *46*:66, 1970.
29. Goldman, R. L., and Friedman, N. B.: Rhabdomyosarcohepatoma in an adult and embryonal hepatoma in a child. Am. J. Clin. Pathol. *51*:137, 1969.
30. Gonzalez-Crussi, F., and Manz, H. J.: Structure of a hepatoblastoma of pure epithelial type. Cancer *29*:1272, 1972.
31. Griffith, J. P. C.: Primary carcinoma of the liver in infancy and childhood. Am. J. Med. Sci. *155*:79, 1918.
32. Hermann, R. E., and Lonsdale, D.: Chemotherapy, radiotherapy and hepatic lobectomy for hepatoblastoma in an infant: report of a survival. Surgery *68*:383, 1970.
33. Honjo, I., and Mizumoto, R.: Primary carcinoma of the liver. Am. J. Surg. *128*:31, 1974.

34. Howat, J. M.: Major hepatic resections in infancy and childhood. Gut *12*:212, 1971.
35. Ishak, K. G., and Glunz, P. R.: Hepatoblastoma and hepatocarcinoma in infancy and childhood. Cancer *20*:396, 1967.
36. Ito, J., and Johnson, W. W.: Hepatoblastoma and hepatoma in infancy and childhood. Light and electron microscopic studies. Arch. Pathol. *87*:259, 1969.
37. Kaplan, L., and Cole, S. L.: Fraternal primary hepatocellular carcinoma in three male adult siblings. Am. J. Med. *39*:305, 1965.
38. Kappel, D. A., and Miller, D. R.: Primary hepatic carcinoma: a review of 37 patients. Am. J. Surg. *124*:798, 1972.
39. Kasai, M., and Watanabe, I.: Histologic classification of liver cell carcinoma in infancy and childhood and its clinical evaluation. Cancer *25*:551, 1970.
40. Keeling, J. W.: Liver tumors in infancy and childhood. J. Pathol. *103*:69, 1970.
41. Knox, W. G., Zintel, H., and Begg, C. F.: Portal hepatectomy for primary carcinoma of the liver in childhood. Cancer *11*:1044, 1958.
42. Lascari, A. D.: Vincristine therapy in an infant with probable hepatoblastoma. Pediatrics *45*:109, 1970.
43. Lin, T. Y.: Primary cancer of the liver. Quadrennial review. Scand. J. Gastroenterol. *6*:223, 1970.
44. Lin, T. Y., Chen, C. C., and Liu, W. P.: Primary carcinoma of the liver in infancy and childhood: report of 21 cases with resection in 6 cases. Surgery *60*:1275, 1966.
45. Longmire, W. P., Passaro, E. P., and Joseph, W. L.: The surgical treatment of hepatic lesions. Br. J. Surg. *53*:852, 1966.
46. Longmire, W. P., et al.: Elective hepatic surgery. Ann. Surg. *179*:712, 1974.
47. Martin, L. W., and Woodman, K. S.: Hepatic lobectomy for hepatoblastoma in infants and children. Arch. Surg. *98*:1, 1969.
48. Mays, E. T.: Hepatic lobectomy. Arch. Surg. *103*:216, 1971.
49. Mersheimer, W. L.: Successful right hepatolobectomy for primary neoplasm — preliminary observations. Bull. N.Y. Med. Coll. Flower & Fifth Ave. Hosp. *16*:121, 1953.
50. Misugi, K., et al.: Classification of primary malignant tumors of liver in infancy and childhood. Cancer *20*:1760, 1967.
51. Modlin, J. J., et al.: Long-term survival in carcinoma of the liver. Mo. Med. *64*:985, 1967.
52. Nikaidoh, H., Boggs, J., and Swenson, O.: Liver tumors in infants and children. Arch. Surg. *101*:245, 1970.
53. Novy, S., et al.: Angiographic evaluation of primary malignant hepatocellular tumors in children. Am. J. Roentgenol. Radium Ther. Nucl. Med. *120(2)*:353, 1974.
54. Ochsner, J. L., Meyers, B. E., and Ochsner, A.: Hepatic lobectomy. Am. J. Surg. *121*:273, 1971.
55. Packard, G. B., and Stevenson, A. W.: Hepatoma in infancy and childhood. Surgery *15*:292, 1944.
56. Pollice, L.: Primary hepatic tumors in infancy and childhood. Am. J. Clin. Pathol. *60*:512, 1973.
57. Purtilo, D. T., et al.: Alpha-fetoprotein: diagnostic and prognostic use in patients with hepatomas. Am. J. Clin. Pathol. *59*:295, 1973.
58. Schiodt, T.: Hepatoblastoma and hepatocarcinoma in infancy and childhood. Acta Pathol. Microbiol. Scand. (Suppl.) *212*:181, 1970.
59. Sorsdahl, O. A. and Gay, B. B. Jr.: Roentgenologic features of a primary carcinoma of the liver in Infants and Children. Amer. J. Roentgen. *100*:117, 1967.
60. Sharpstone, P., et al.: The diagnosis of primary malignant tumors of the liver. Findings in 48 consecutive patients. Q. J. Med. New Series. *41(161)*:99, 1972.
61. Shaw, A. F. B.: Primary liver cell adenoma (hepatoma). J. Pathol. Bacteriol. *26*:475, 1923.
62. Shorter, R. G., et al.: Primary carcinoma of the liver in infancy and childhood. Pediatrics *25*:191, 1960.
63. Stanley, R. J., Dehner, L. P., and Hesker, A. E.: Primary malignant mesenchymal tumors (mesenchymoma) of the liver in childhood. An angiographic-pathologic study of 3 cases. Cancer *32(4)*:973, 1973.
64. Steiner, M. M.: Primary carcinoma of the liver in childhood. Am. J. Dis. Child. *55*:807, 1938.

65. Stone, H. H., et al.: Physiologic considerations in major hepatic resections. Am. J. Surg. *117*:78, 1969.
66. Sugahara, K., et al.: Serum alpha-fetoprotein and resection of primary hepatic cancer. Arch. Surg. *106*:63, 1973.
67. Willis, R. A.: Pathology of Tumours. 3rd ed. Butterworth & Co., London, 1960.
68. Willis, R. A.: Embryonic Tumours of Kidney and Liver. *In* Pathology of Tumours. London, Butterworth & Co., 1948.
69. Willis, R. A.: The Pathology of the Tumors of Children. Springfield, Ill., Charles C Thomas, 1962.
70. Yamagiwa, K.: Zur Kenntniss des primaren parenchymatosen Leberkarcinoms. Virchows Arch. [Pathol. Anat.] *206*:439, 1911.
71. Yang, S. S., Brough, A. J., and Bernstein, J.: Hepatoblastoma. Mich. Med. *71*:539, 1972.

Chapter Six

THE BENIGN LESIONS: ADENOMA AND FOCAL NODULAR HYPERPLASIA

INTRODUCTION

In no area of liver tumors is there so much controversy about classification, etiology, and even prognosis as in that of the tumors to be discussed in this chapter. Minimum deviation hepatoma, adenoma, hamartoma, and a long list of other names (see Table 6–1) have been used to describe these usually solitary but occasionally multiple solid tumors that occur in the noncirrhotic liver. The tumors are quite rare and no one institution has a large experience. In the last decade, however, the number of reports about these tumors has increased dramatically from Western countries, largely as a result of the association of these benign tumors with intra-abdominal hemorrhage and because of their possible association with birth control medication. However, very few reports have come from the areas of Asia and Africa that have very high incidence rates for primary carcinoma, and the reason for this difference remains unclear.

There are several ways to approach this problem. We have chosen to begin with no particular bias about nomenclature, histologic features, or clinical correlations. We have reviewed 90 years of published reports of cases and classifications, reading the original articles whenever possible. Most of the pertinent information was published in Ger-

Table 6–1.   Terms Applied to Benign Liver Tumors

Nodular hyperplasia[67]
Adenoma, hepatocellular or liver cell[13, 22, 64, 66, 77]
Solitary adenoma[22]
Benign hepatoma[26, 32, 35]
Hepatoma, Grade I
Focal cirrhosis[5, 10]
Hamartomatous cholangiohepatoma[29]
Mixed adenoma[13, 38, 43]
Solitary hyperplastic nodule[49]
Isolated nodule of regenerative hyperplasia[8]
Hamartoma[9, 15, 24]
Focal nodular hyperplasia[22]

man before 1900, and even a few of those classic references have been reviewed.

Of the 621 cases collected in the 1974 Liver Tumor Survey, 323 were primary tumors of the liver. Of these, we have called 111 (34 per cent) benign on the basis of histologic criteria. Eleven were classified as either cystadenoma, mesenchymal hamartoma, or miscellaneous tumors, and are discussed in Chapter Seven. There remained 100 solid tumors variously classified by the pathologist in the involved hospital as hamartoma, adenoma, benign hepatoma, focal nodular hyperplasia, focal cirrhosis, and median deviation hepatoma. There were even a few tumors that were called "malignant" by the hospital pathologist but which we have called "benign." Our independent categorization was based on the gross and microscopic features of these 100 tumors, ignoring the clinical presentation and eventual course of the patient.

When we finished this review of tumor pathology we discovered what many other students of liver tumors have found, i.e., that the pathologic classification of benign tumors proposed by Edmondson in the 1958 AFIP Fascicle[22] is entirely adequate. This classification needs no alteration, but rather needs to be understood and adopted more widely. The matter of nomenclature will be discussed more fully toward the end of this chapter. When we finally correlated pathologic and clinical data, there emerged two clinical entities with a few features in common, but with distinctive characteristics that allow separation in the vast majority of cases.

The two lesions that emerge from our survey correspond with what Edmondson called "liver cell adenoma" (LCA) and "focal nodular hyperplasia" (FNH). By sheer weight of numbers, the importance of these two lesions to the clinician overwhelms the importance of all other benign primary liver tumors found in adults in the 1974 LTS.

However, 14 of 33 primary benign solid tumors of children less than 16 years of age were other than LCA or FNH, and these "other" tumors are discussed in Chapter Seven (see Table 7–1). The nine pediatric patients with focal nodular hyperplasia are discussed together with this lesion in this chapter. No pediatric patients with liver cell adenoma were found in the 1974 LTS.

A description of the gross and histologic criteria by which we made the diagnosis of LCA or FNH will be followed by an analysis of the clinical data from the 1974 LTS, in which we found 63 patients with FNH and 37 with LCA. Using that combination of pathologic definition and clinical correlation as a platform, we shall then attempt to review the reported experience of others to see if some sense can be made out of the confusion of case reports and nomenclature, which has proved so difficult to interpret in the past.

We will then discuss nomenclature anew with a view to simplification, and will finally end the chapter with some recommendations for therapy.

PATHOLOGIC CRITERIA FOR DIAGNOSIS OF FNH

FNH tumors usually are solitary, less than 5 cm in diameter, and occur in both lobes in approximate proportion to the volume of liver substance. They frequently are found near the free edge of the liver, often as incidental findings at laparotomy for other conditions. FNH tumors in children tend to be larger, and often are manifest as abdominal masses.

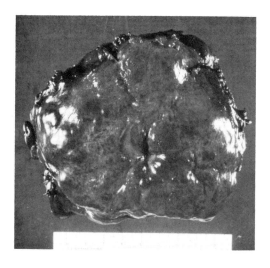

Figure 6–1. Focal nodular hyperplasia. Eleven cm tumor resected from 9-year-old girl by wedge excision. Free of recurrence at 68 months after operation. Tumor is tan, nodular, and firm, with intact capsule. (Case 5 – Appendix VI-A.)

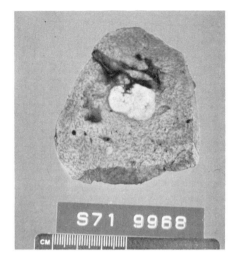

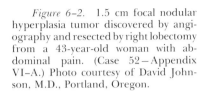

Figure 6–2. 1.5 cm focal nodular hyperplasia tumor discovered by angiography and resected by right lobectomy from a 43-year-old woman with abdominal pain. (Case 52–Appendix VI–A.) Photo courtesy of David Johnson, M.D., Portland, Oregon.

FNH tumors usually are visible on the surface of the liver (Fig. 6–1), but may be central (Fig. 6–2). They are often on a pedicle of thinned-out liver that appears to be dragged down off the free edge of the liver by the mass lesion. They are grossly nodular with surface scarring, and may be highly vascular with prominent surface vessels. They are firmer than surrounding liver tissue, dark red-brown to tan in color, and almost never white or gray. They may or may not have a thin capsule. Expanding tumor usually compresses normal liver enough to allow a plane for blunt dissection and enucleation. On cross-

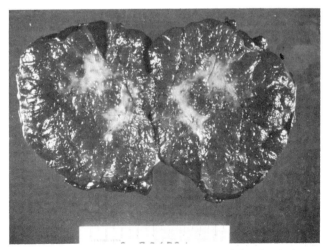

Figure 6–3. Cross-section of FNH tumor illustrated in Figure 6–1. Note stellate central scar and liver-like appearance of tumor tissue.

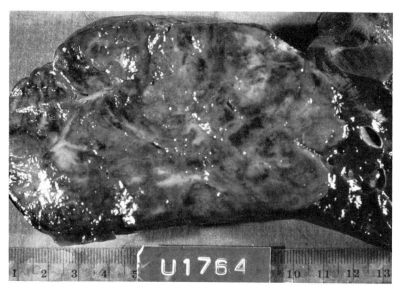

Figure 6–4. Eleven cm FNH tumor resected by right lobectomy from a 23-year-old woman 12 months after delivery of normal baby. Note diffuse scarring and soft nodularity. (Case 17–Appendix VI–A.) Photo courtesy of William Newman, M.D. of Washington, D.C.

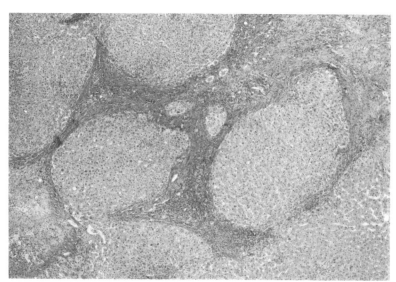

Figure 6–5. FNH. Multiple regenerative liver nodules surrounded by broad bands of investing connective tissue closely resembling the histologic appearance of a macronodular cirrhosis.

section there is nodularity laced by fibrous septa that may extend out from a broad central stellate scar (Fig. 6–3). Occasionally, instead of a large central scar, there are narrow fibrous bands criss-crossing the sectioned tumor throughout its extent (Fig. 6–4).

The histologic appearance is characterized by nodules made up of mature hepatocytes resembling the regenerating nodules of the cirrhotic liver. The nodules are outlined by bands of fibrous connective tissue (Fig. 6–5). The liver cells within the nodules are arranged in cord formation, the liver cell plates being more than one cell in thickness with intervening Kupffer cell-lined sinusoids. The nuclei show no significant anisocytosis or mitosis. The presence of intracytoplasmic glycogen is variable, and patchy fatty change is seen occasionally. The fibrous connective tissue bands show variable thickness, but generally are delicate. Foci of bile duct proliferation and occasional aggregates of lymphocytes are present within the connective tissue septa (Fig. 6–6). In most instances, the fibrous septa could be traced to a characteristic large central scar in a stellate arrangement with a prominent myxoid stroma (Fig. 6–7). Embedded within the scar are vascular structures, both venous and arterial, which often show extensive mucoid degeneration of the medial layer (Fig. 6–8). The thickness of the blood vessel walls is variable, but generally thicker vascular walls are present in the larger lesions. Elastic stains of the blood vessels show fragmentation and splitting of elastic fibers in thickened blood vessel walls.

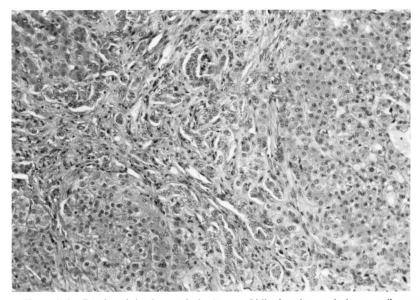

Figure 6–6.   Focal nodular hyperplasia. Focus of bile duct hyperplasia at confluence of adjacent liver nodules.

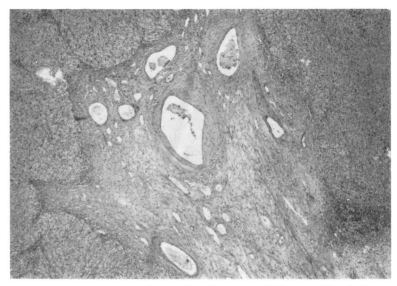

Figure 6-7. FNH. A broad central hyaline scar with large thick-walled centrally located blood vessels and radiating bands of fibrous connective tissue extending into liver parenchyma.

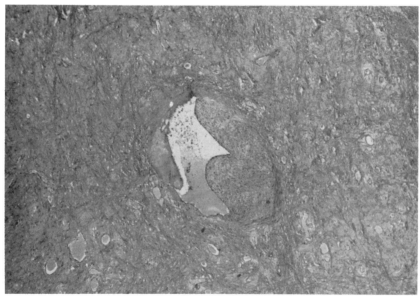

Figure 6-8. FNH. The high-power appearance of a thickened arterial vessel within a central scar. Note the proliferation of medial fibers *(right)* and the focal hyalinization of the vessel wall *(left).*

Over-all, one is left with an impression that FNH is a reaction to injury or change rather than a true neoplasm. The process seems reparative or regenerative. The blood vessel changes suggest that a primary vascular phenomenon may play a role in etiology. However, the absence of necrosis suggests that the vascular problem and the reaction thereto is a chronic one such as arteriovenous malformation, rather than an acute one such as thrombosis.

PATHOLOGIC CRITERIA FOR DIAGNOSIS OF LIVER CELL ADENOMA

LCA usually are fairly large tumors that are soft in consistency and of a lighter color than surrounding normal liver tissue. They may be tan, orange-gray, yellow, or even white. Most tumors are smooth, but surface nodularity is present occasionally. Central umbilication is not seen and pedunculation is rare. These tumors occur in both lobes of the liver, and when discovered almost always involve a liver surface. Cross-section often reveals areas of necrosis and hemorrhage (Fig. 6–9). Central scars are seen occasionally but do not have the stellate characteristics of those seen with FNH, nor is there evidence of extension into surrounding normal liver (Fig. 6–10). When the

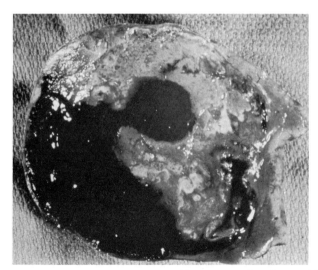

Figure 6–9. Liver cell adenoma resected with a narrow rim of normal liver from a 32-year-old woman with acute abdominal pain and hemoperitoneum. Note light color of tumor, hemorrhage, and necrosis. (Case 26 – Appendix VI–B.) Photo courtesy of Malcom Ellison, M.D., New London, Conn.

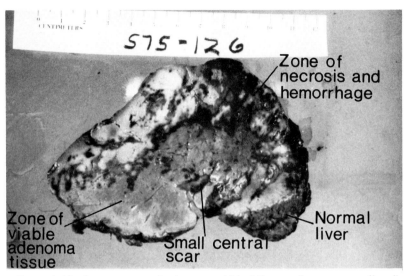

Figure 6–10. Large ruptured adenoma which fell away from surrounding liver during emergency right lobectomy (Case 18 – Appendix VI–B). Note peripheral zone of infarction and hemorrhage, sharp demarcation between adenoma and normal liver, and small non-radiating fibrous central scar.

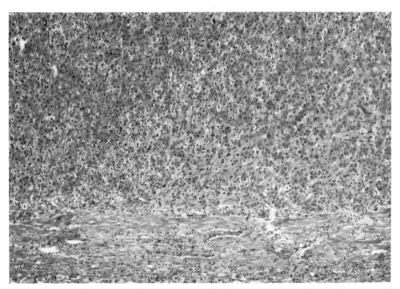

Figure 6–11. Hepatocellular adenoma. Peripheral section of an adenoma with a fibrous capsule component and a homogeneous monotonous arrangement of hepato-cyte cords without blood vessel or bile duct structures.

tumors have ruptured, a large ragged laceration usually is found in Glisson's capsule, with an underlying cavity filled with clot and lined with soft necrotic tumor. Satellite nodularity is not seen but the tumors may be multiple. Fibrous encapsulation usually is not grossly evident.

Although demarcation between LCA and normal liver tissue generally is quite evident, grossly this distinction may be more difficult to make under the microscope. The histologic appearance of liver cell adenomas is characterized by a monocellular pattern of mature hepatocytes without organization into lobules by portal areas and central veins (Fig. 6–11). The epithelial cells often have a clear or foamy cytoplasm. The presence of glycogen is variable; however, the adenoma cells appear to contain more glycogen than the surrounding normal liver parenchyma and more than the hepatocytes of focal nodular hyperplasia. Variability in nuclear size and prominence of the chromatin pattern is more pronounced than in the hepatocytes of focal nodular hyperplasia, but mitoses are not noted. Generally the liver cell adenomas are sharply demarcated at the periphery from the normal liver parenchyma by a partial or complete thin fibrous capsule or zone of compression of adjacent normal liver parenchyma. Necrosis is quite common, with a gradual fading from normal liver cell to areas of "ghost" cells without much cellular reaction (Fig. 6–13). Zones of hemorrhage are common in the necrotic areas. Bile ducts are conspicuously lacking, although there may be evidence of bile stasis.

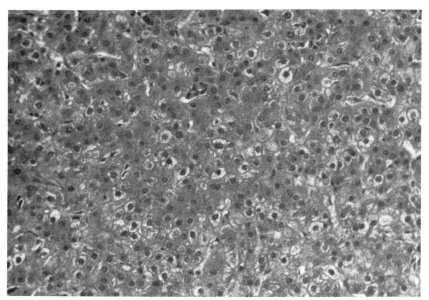

Figure 6–12. Hepatocellular adenoma. A high-power view showing the uniform pattern of liver cell cords composed of granular and clear hepatocytes arranged in a monotonous pattern.

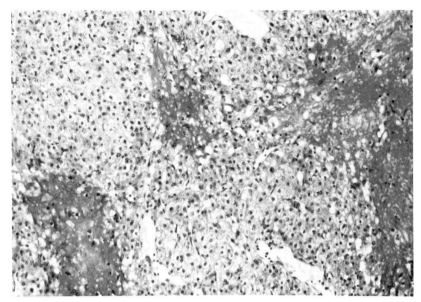

Figure 6–13. Liver cell adenoma with multiple foci of hemorrhagic zonal necrosis.

Small thin-walled blood vessels are seen, but larger vessels are uncommon, and the abnormally thickened vessels so characteristic of FNH are nowhere to be found.

Under the microscope one gets the impression of an expanding, purely epithelial process, which often has outstripped its blood supply. Although necrosis is common, there is little evidence of inflammatory reaction, fibrous scarring, or regeneration.

The histopathologic differentiation of liver cell adenomas from the well-differentiated liver cell carcinoma can be a difficult problem. Liver cell adenomas, although demonstrating nuclear variation in size and chromatin pattern, do not show significant nuclear atypia, mitoses, or the presence of intracytoplasmic bile production. Liver cell carcinomas demonstrate nuclear atypia, with irregularity of the nuclear envelope and the presence of mitoses. Most of the very well-differentiated liver cell carcinomas of borderline differentiation will demonstrate occasional more well-defined areas of malignancy if multiple sections are reviewed. However, inadequate sampling is an important source of diagnostic error. This point was underscored by one of our cases that fulfilled all the cytologic criteria for a liver cell adenoma with the exception of a microscopic malignant tumor thrombus in a single section.

FOCAL NODULAR HYPERPLASIA—1974 LIVER TUMOR SURVEY

Clinical History

From 32 hospitals, 63 cases were collected with tumors that met our criteria for focal nodular hyperplasia. In 24 patients these tumors had been labeled as "FNH" by the hospital pathologist. Other diagnoses made were "focal cirrhosis" (four patients), "benign hepatoma" (five), benign "harmartoma" (15), "liver cell adenoma" (eight), and "segmental post-necrotic cirrhosis," "portal cirrhosis," "cord cell adenoma," "hepatic pseudotumor," "Grade I hepatoma," "low grade hepatoma," and "congenital anomaly" (one patient each). As we reviewed the slides of 59 of the 63 patients, we found the typical appearance of FNH tumors in 56 cases. The three exceptions resembled liver cell adenoma or true hamartoma in some respects, but were finally classified as FNH.

Table 6–2 lists the age and sex of these patients, and Appendix VI-A outlines the details of each case. Eight female patients were Negro and all the rest were Caucasian. The youngest patient was a 10-month-old male infant and the oldest was a 70-year-old female who was the only patient over 56 years of age. Table 6–3 outlines the major symptoms with which these patients presented to their physician or surgeon. Most FNH tumors were incidental findings at laparotomy for another condition. Thirteen were found at the time of cholecystectomy, ten at a pelvic laparotomy for gynecologic disease, four at the time of exploratory laparotomy for vague abdominal symptoms or fever of undetermined etiology, and three at the time of appendectomy. Six other tumors were found incidentally at elective operations for hiatus her-

Table 6–2. Focal Nodular Hyperplasia—1974 LTS: Age and Sex

Age in Years	Female	Male
0–10	6	2
11–19	4	1
20–29	13	0
30–39	20	2
40–49	9	0
50–59	4	1
60–69	0	0
70 and over	1	0
	57	6

Table 6–3. Focal Nodular Hyperplasia — 1974 LTS:
Presenting Symptom

Incidental finding at laparotomy for other disease	36
Mass	21
Laparotomy for unexplained upper abdominal pain	3
Abnormal upper gastrointestinal radiograph	2
Positive selective arteriogram	1

nias, duodenal ulcer, umbilical hernia, colectomy for colitis, nephrec-
tomy, and aortic aneurysm.

No patient with an FNH tumor presented with shock or pain due
to an intraperitoneal rupture of the tumor. The only patient with any
evidence of bleeding from her tumor complained of two days of right
upper quadrant pain, and was operated upon with the presumptive
diagnosis of acute cholecystitis. A small nodule of FNH was found close
to the gallbladder with a "rough, inflamed" surface. There was "evidence of recent bleeding" in the area, but this patient experienced no
drop of blood pressure, she required no blood transfusion, and surface
rupture of necrotic tumor was not seen.

Adequate information about the ingestion of medications was not
obtained for 16 patients. Of the remaining 47, five were definitely taking contraceptive medication at the time their tumor was found. Three
other patients had taken birth control pills in the past (one to five years
before the diagnosis of FNH was made), two were pregnant, and two
postmenopausal females were taking Premarin. The remaining 35 had
not taken birth control pills either before, or at the time of, the diagnosis
of their FNH tumors.

We looked for clues to etiology as we studied the histories of these
63 patients. A few brief outlines are included below which may or may
not contribute to an understanding of the etiology and natural history
of the lesion.

(1) A 10-month-old male fell off his high chair three weeks prior to
the diagnosis of FNH.

(2) An 8-year-old girl had abdominal trauma as an infant. Her
epigastric mass was known for two years and had recently increased in
size prior to resection of an FNH tumor.

(3) A 47-year-old female had epigastric trauma six months before
the incidental finding of an FNH tumor at the time of elective repair of
esophageal hiatus hernia.

(4) A 7-year-old girl had two laparotomies for small bowel disease
while less than 2 years of age, and then had elective resection of an
FNH tumor at age 7 because of a newly-discovered abdominal mass.

(5) A 28-year-old female who was jaundiced at age 12 had needle

biopsy of a liver mass at age 24 which showed cirrhosis. Four years later she underwent elective resection of an 8 cm right lobe FNH tumor occurring in an otherwise noncirrhotic liver.

(6) A 53-year-old female on Premarin had an incisional biopsy of a liver tumor at the time of elective cholecystectomy at age 47. The diagnosis of a well-differentiated liver cell carcinoma was made and nothing further was done. She did well until a mass became palpable in the right upper quadrant six years later. Liver scan suggested multiple defects, but at laparotomy a solitary 8 cm FNH was found hanging off the edge of the right lobe of the liver.

(7) A 32-year-old woman had biopsy of an asymptomatic 5 cm mass on the superior surface of the left lobe of the liver at the time of cholecystectomy. A diagnosis of hepatoma was made, but because she gained 10 lbs in weight and felt well, re-exploration was done 12 months later. The tumor had shrunk to 2 cm in maximum diameter and was easily wedged out at this second operation.

(8) A celiac arteriogram showed a small vascular lesion in the right lobe of a 43-year-old woman being evaluated for two months of constant abdominal pain. No other cause for the pain was found, and right lobectomy was done to remove a 1.5 cm central FNH tumor (see Fig. 6–2).

(9) A final history deserves particular attention. The only patient in the 1974 LTS whose tumor was not resected was a 17-year-old girl who, at the time of appendectomy, was noted to have an 8 × 10 cm tumor in the right lobe of her liver near the gallbladder. Needle biopsy was inconclusive. After a liver scan showed a 7 cm tumor in the right lobe, reoperation two months after appendectomy confirmed the presence of a large tumor involving most of the right lobe. Because the tumor "could not be shelled out" and because a frozen section diagnosis of "benign" was made, the tumor was left in place. A pathologic diagnosis was made of liver cell adenoma, but to us this tumor represents focal nodular hyperplasia under the microscope. A liver scan six months later showed a marked reduction in the size of the tumor, and subsequent scans one and two years after the biopsy were entirely normal. The patient remains well 35 months after her appendectomy (Case 11, Appendix VI-A).

Seven patients had an abdominal mass that was palpable for six, 12, 14, 18, 18, 24 and 84 months respectively prior to resection of an FNH tumor.

Only six of the sixty-three patients with focal nodular hyperplasia were male. Three boys aged 10 months, 10 years, and 14 years of age presented with large tumors. The three adult males (age 32, 33, and 55) had small tumors found incidentally at laparotomy for different diseases.

Four of the five FNH tumors in female patients more than 50 years of age were discovered as incidental findings, and these patients all had small tumors. The only patient over 50 who presented with a mass lesion was mentioned above.

One gets the impression that these tumors can grow in youngsters of both sexes and in adult females in the menstrual age-groups. There was no evidence in this review to suggest that tumors will increase in size or cause serious complications in adult males or postmenopausal females.

The lesion may be related to trauma; it may be present for a long while, with increase or even decrease in size; and these tumors are seldom related to life-threatening complications.

Diagnostic Tests

Many of these tumors were incidental findings, so that liver function tests and radioisotope scans and angiograms often were not done preoperatively. However, the serum alkaline phosphatase level was measured preoperatively in 40 patients and was minimally elevated in five, three of whom had large tumors, one of whom had gallbladder disease, and the last of whom had suffered recent epigastric trauma. The serum glutamic oxalic transaminase (SGOT) was measured in 35 instances and was elevated in seven patients: three with large tumors; two with gallbladder disease; one with recent trauma; and one with a small FNH tumor and no other disease. Bromsulphalein retention was evaluated in six patients preoperatively and was elevated in four, three of whom had large tumors. Serum bilirubin was measured 36 times and was elevated only once in a 23-year-old female with a 13 cm tumor. Prothrombin time was normal in the nine instances when it was measured. Preoperative radioisotope liver scans were done in 16 patients. In those four instances when the scan showed no abnormality, two patients proved to have pedicled tumors hanging below the liver, and the other two had smaller (5 and 3 cm) intrahepatic tumors. In three instances, the radioisotope scan suggested multiple lesions and a solitary lesion was found at laparotomy. The largest FNH tumor in this series was associated with a liver scan showing only "vague abnormalities" in the right lobe. In eight patients the liver scan accurately showed the location and number of FNH tumors.

Angiography was done in 13 patients who had 11 arteriograms and two inferior venocavograms. One 12 cm tumor in the left lateral segment of the liver was missed by selective arteriography. Ten arteriograms showed vascular tumors that were well localized by this technique (five of these tumors were diagnosed radiographically as carcinoma). The two venous studies were not helpful in either diagnosis or location of the tumor (see Chapter Three and Figure 3–7) for further details about angiography of FNH tumors).

Eight patients had both radioisotope scan and angiography, and all eight proved to have solitary tumors at laparotomy. In only four did the scan agree with the arteriogram and eventually prove to be accurate. In two liver scans and one angiogram a diagnosis of multiple lesions was made, but only one tumor was found at operation. Of the other two patients one had a positive scan and a negative angiogram; the second had a negative scan and a positive angiogram.

OPERATIVE FINDINGS

Table 6–4 documents the size and location of the FNH tumors found at operation. Eight tumors were connected to the liver by a narrow stalk of normal liver tissue. Fifty-five patients had solitary tumors and eight had multiple tumors, four with nodules in both anatomic lobes of the liver. Forty-eight patients underwent wedge excision of their liver tumors. Seven patients had right lobectomy. Three had left lateral segmentectomy, and one patient each had left lobectomy, extended right lobectomy, middle lobectomy, and biopsy only. Residual tumor was left consciously in only two patients, one of whom had the spontaneous remission as discussed above. The other patient was a 7-year-old girl who had an 8 cm tumor removed from the undersurface of her left lobe, but another 6 cm tumor in her right lobe was left in place after frozen section suggested that the first tumor was benign. Unfortunately there is no follow-up on this patient.

OUTCOME

No follow-up information was available for 16 patients. There were no operative or postoperative deaths, but two patients died of

Table 6–4. FNH – 1974 LTS: Size and Location

SIZE		LOCATION	
Less than 2 cm	13	Right lobe	22
2–4.9 cm	25	Quadrate lobe	8
5–9.9 cm	10	Left lateral segment	24
10–19.9 cm	14	"Central"	5
20 cm or greater	1	Bilateral	3
		Unknown	1

other causes 39 and 73 months respectively after resection of FNH. Neither patient had evidence of recurrent liver disease before death or at autopsy. Forty-six patients were alive and well at the date of their last follow-up, which ranged from one to 256 months after liver resection. There was not a single recognized instance of persistent, recurrent, or metastatic disease in this period.

LIVER CELL ADENOMA – 1974 LIVER TUMOR SURVEY

CLINICAL HISTORY

Thirty-seven patients in the 1974 LTS had tumors that we have classified as LCA, and that were resected. We had an opportunity to review the histologic sections on all these cases, collected from 16 different hospitals. These lesions were called "carcinoma" 11 times (with a qualifying term of "grade I" in five patients), "hepatoma" seven times (well-differentiated, five; benign, two), "adenoma" 17 times, and "hamartoma" twice. Most of these LCA had typical histologic patterns of monotonous sheets of liver cells as described above. Two tumors had zones of mature mesenchymal tissue interspersed with large areas of hepatic cells. At least five of these tumors showed fatty change in hepatocytes that was often patchy in distribution, and special stains demonstrated excessive glycogen storage in several patients.

Table 6–5 outlines the age and sex of the 36 Caucasian and one Negro patients. Information about contraceptive medication was incomplete for six of the 32 female patients between 17 and 45 years of age. Of the 26 remaining, 22 were taking or had taken birth control pills and four were not, one of whom was in the third trimester of pregnancy when the mass eventually proved to be a LCA was found on physical examination. Thus, at least nine patients (four menstruating

Table 6–5.   Liver Cell Adenoma – 1974 LTS

AGE IN YEARS	FEMALE	MALE
17 – 19	3	0
20 – 29	17	1
30 – 39	10	0
40 – 49	2	0
50 and over	2	2
	34	3

females, two aged females, and three males) who had LCA were *not* on birth control pills either before or at the time their tumor was discovered.

The five patients who were not females in the menstruating age-group deserve a special look. A 29-year-old male, otherwise perfectly well, suffered an acute intraperitoneal hemorrhage and was found to have a ruptured 15 cm tumor in the right lobe of the liver. Technical problems with control of hemorrhage at operation probably contributed to a prolonged septic course, ending with death three and one-half months after resection (Case 17, Appendix VI-B). A 54-year-old male had a mass known to be present and growing for at least four years prior to resection. His tumor was dark red and had a central scar (features typical of FNH), but under the microscope the typical appearance of LCA was noted. This huge (23-cm) tumor was "scooped out" from around the inferior vena cava without a margin of normal liver, yet the patient is alive and free of disease 54 months after right lobectomy (Case 34, Appendix VI-B). The third and last male patient, aged 62, had bilateral adenomas found incidentally when his gallbladder was removed for stone disease. He remains well 43 months after removal of only one of these tumors (Case 35, Appendix VI-B). The other two patients were postmenopausal females on no hormone medication who were known to have abdominal masses for at least one year prior to resection (Cases 36 and 37, Appendix VI-B).

Table 6–6 outlines the chief symptoms that brought the 37 patients with LCA to medical attention. Of particular concern are the 11 who presented with intraperitoneal hemorrhage manifested by pain and shock. Eight of these 11 patients underwent emergency operation to control hemorrhage at a hospital other than that in which resection was eventually done. Temporary control of hemorrhage was accomplished by a variety of methods prior to transfer to the second hospital.

Table 6–6.   LCA – Presenting Symptom

	1974 LTS	LITERATURE REVIEW
Mass	23	19
Intraperitoneal hemorrhage	11	21
Upper abdominal pain without rupture	2	5
Incidental finding at laparotomy	1	2
Vague abdominal symptoms		4
Radioisotope scan		1
Unknown		3
	37	55

The only patient whose LCA was found incidentally (at the time of cholecystectomy) was the 62-year-old male mentioned above, who was found to have a 4 × 4 cm mass in his right lobe which was resected, and a 2 × 2 cm palpable mass in his left lobe which was neither resected nor biopsied after a frozen section diagnosis of adenoma was made on the right-sided tumor. Sixteen patients had been aware of an abdominal mass for at least three months prior to resection. The mass had been discovered in six patients more than a year before resection, and in two patients more than three years before resection. In several instances the mass appeared to have grown during the period of preoperative observation.

DIAGNOSTIC TESTS

Preoperative liver function tests were not available for 11 patients, in several cases because they underwent emergency operation to control hemorrhage. Of the 26 patients with laboratory evaluation of liver function before resection, 13 had results within normal limits. Bromsulphalein retention was done in only eight patients, but was elevated to the 6 to 12 per cent range in seven. SGOT was elevated in seven patients, and to very high levels in two patients with necrosis. The serum alkaline phosphatase was minimally elevated in five patients. Serum bilirubin was within normal limits in patients without bleeding. The serum alpha-fetoprotein was measured in six patients preoperatively and one patient postoperatively, and was not found in all seven instances.

A radioisotope liver scan was done preoperatively in 16 patients, and postoperatively in a 17th. Two of the preoperative scans were within normal limits, and 14 had some abnormality. In two instances patients who proved to have solitary lesions were diagnosed as having multiple lesions on isotope scan. A scan was done preoperatively in three patients proved at operation to have multiple lesions. In one who eventually was shown to have four tumors, the scan showed three, and in two patients, each proved at laparotomy to have one large and one small lesion, the scan picked out the larger lesion but not the smaller.

Tumor angiography was attempted in 19 patients before resection was successful in demonstrating a lesion in 17. This included one venous angiogram (an unsuccessful splenoportogram) and one instance in which an aortic flush did not demonstrate a 12-cm adenoma after unsuccessful attempts to cannulate the celiac axis. In the 17 patients with positive selective arteriograms, six tumors had decreased vascularity and ten had increased vascularity. Four of the vascular lesions were diagnosed as "probably malignant" on the basis of arteriographic findings. In one angiogram a huge tumor was nicely outlined, but the vascularity was not described as "increased" or "decreased" in the report. Thirteen patients had both radioisotope scan and successful angiography, and in all 13 the lesions were seen by both techniques.

Operative Findings

There was no evidence of cirrhosis of the liver in any of these patients with LCA. Usually the tumor was recognized as a discrete nodule of different color and consistency at operation. The tumors generally were orange-yellow or white in color and were soft and vascular, but clinically not as vascular as malignant liver cell cancers. A few were dark brown, and most had some surface nodularity. Many tumors had large zones of necrosis and hemorrhage, and four had a small central scar that was fibrotic but did not extend out into the peripheral areas. in the stellate fashion characteristic of FNH. When rupture had occurred it often appeared that central necrosis and hemorrhage had "blown out" a ragged hole in Glisson's capsule.

Table 6–7 outlines the size and location of these adenomas. Four tumors were on a stalk that appeared to be a thinned-out isthmus of normal liver tissue dragged down by a tumor that probably originated on the free edge of the liver. In 30 patients the tumors were solitary, and in seven they were multiple. In two patients with multiple nodules, at least one of the nodules was not removed. These two patients have had no evidence of progression of symptoms or signs in the five and 43 months respectively since their resection (Cases 8 and 35, Appendix VI-B).

Operation

In 19 patients some type of sublobar wedge resection was done. One of these patients died on the operating table and two died in the

Table 6–7.   LCA – 1974 LTS: Size and Location

Size		Location	
Less than 5 cm	2	Right lobe	22
5 – 9.9 cm	14	Left lobe	8
10 – 14.9 cm	14	Caudate lobe	1
15 – 19.9 cm	3	Quadrate lobe	1
20 cm or larger	4	Central	1
		Bilateral (multiple)	4

postoperative period, one of early unrecognized hemorrhage and the other of late septic complications. Nine right lobectomies were done, with one operating room death due to uncontrolled hemorrhage. Three extended right lobectomies, one extended left lobectomy, two left lobectomies, and two left lateral segmentectomies were done without operative death. Thus, there were four deaths: three due to failure to control hemorrhage.

LONG-TERM SURVIVAL

What happened to the 33 patients who survived resection of LCA? No follow-up information was available on three patients. One patient died of cerebrovascular disease at the age of 93 years, 89 months after resection of an adenoma (at age 86). She had no symptoms or signs of recurrent disease in her abdomen, but a postmortem examination was not carried out. The remaining 29 patients were all well and free of any evidence of disease when last examined from two to 101 months after resection. Fifteen patients have been followed for more than two years, and three for more than five years.

In seven patients either the masses were enucleated or transection was done through tumor, some of which was left at the margin of resection. One of these patients was referred to another hospital for re-exploration after enucleation of an 8 cm tumor, and at reoperation a rim of "grossly normal" liver was resected in the area of previous resection. Adenomatous tisue was found in this second operative specimen. These seven patients are alive and well at five, 12, 16, 30, 43, 54 and 84 months respectively after liver resection, without evidence of recurrent disease. Two are male, and two others may have continued to take birth control pills after liver resection.

DISCUSSION AND LITERATURE SURVEY

We have defined two clinical entities by analyzing the experience of the 1974 LTS and by emphasizing the differences between their presentation and the significance of these symptoms to the patient and to the surgeon. A retrospective look at the reported experience of others can be used to support and justify this position.

FOCAL NODULAR HYPERPLASIA — LITERATURE SURVEY

Simmonds (1889)[67] is usually credited with first defining the solitary hyperplastic nodule that we are calling "FNH," although he credits

Rokitansky (1859), Klob (1865), and Mahomed (1877) with prior descriptions. Simmonds found an isolated mass in the dome of the left lobe of an otherwise normal liver at the autopsy of a woman who died with pneumonia. On morphologic grounds he postulated that the process was reparative rather than neoplastic. Sporadic English-language reports were made[9, 13, 26, 29, 32, 35, 38, 49, 64] in the first five decades of this century, but it was not until 1953 that a detailed study was made of the pathology of this lesion and its clinical correlations. In that year Begg and Berry reported four cases of what they called isolated nodules of "regenerative hyperplasia," and collected 29 others. In seven patients, the tumor was an incidental finding at laparotomy for other disease. In two patients (both in Spanish-language reports from South America), intra-abdominal hemorrhage from ruptured surface vessels was reported. Nineteen of the 33 patients had pedunculated tumors, with evidence of twisting of the pedicles and vascular compromise in four. These authors thought that transition of these tumors to carcinoma was a distinct possibility.[8]

Also in 1953, Benz and Baggenstoss reported 34 cases found by reviewing all the autopsies at the Mayo Clinic from 1922 to 1951.[10] They excluded all nodules found in the liver of patients with generalized cirrhosis, and they called this lesion a "focal cirrhosis." There were 15 male and 19 female patients ranging from 37 to 74 years of age, who had a total of 43 nodules that measured from 0.3 to 5.5 cm in maximum diameter. No patient had antemortem symptoms attributable to the tumors, but 20.6 per cent were found also to have hemangiomas of the liver at autopsy. These authors rejected the neoplastic concept of etiology, and thought the lesion was a regenerative nodule or possibly a reaction to abnormal blood supply, trauma, or bile duct malformation.

Edmondson described this lesion in adults and children and called it "focal nodular hyperplasia."[21, 22] Because the "early" lesions observed in autopsy specimens did not show vascular change or necrosis of cells, he had trouble accepting a regenerative etiology. More recently Aronsen, et al.[5] and Whalen, et al.[80] have studied the extensive blood flow to these tumors that can be documented both by angiography and flow techniques. Is increased flow the result of increased demand by a growing tumor, or is some sort of arteriovenous malformation the cause, rather than the effect, of the isolated nodule? Whalen advances persuasive arguments in favor of the latter position.

An attempt was made to collect published reports of cases of FNH to learn more of this curious lesion. Table 6–8 outlines clinical data on 56 patients reported since 1940 whose tumors met our criteria for FNH. In addition, reports were reviewed of 35 patients who had FNH tumors found at autopsy.

Of the 56 clinical cases, nine of the 52 patients whose sex was

Text continued on page 163

Table 6–8. Focal Nodular Hyperplasia: Cases Reported from Literature

REFERENCE	YEAR OF REPORT	AGE/SEX	SYMPTOMS	OPERATION	OUTCOME
(1) 9	1942	7 months F	Mass, 5 weeks	Wedge	AFD 4 months
(2) 32	1942	38 F	Mass, 2 weeks	Wedge	NFU
(3) 13	1945	32 F	Mass, 1 week	Wedge	NFU
(4) 26	1947	23 M	Mass, weeks	Wedge	AFD 12 months
(5) 35	1949	28 F	Mass, 8 months	Enucleate	NFU
(6) 38	1950	7 months F	Mass, 1 month	Wedge	Op. death
(7) 38	1950	13 M	Nausea, mass	Biopsy	AFD 1½ years
(8) 49	1950	28 F	Vague, GI	Wedge	NFU
(9) 29	1951	8 M	Mass, 2 months	Biopsy	AFD 1 month
(10) 8	1953	59 M	Mass	Wedge	AFD 3 years
(11) 8	1953	46 F	Incidental	Multiple, wedge	AFD 2 years
(12) 8	1953	23 F	Mass	Multiple, wedge	AFD 2 years
(13) 8	1953	47 F	Mass	Biopsy	AFD 1½ years
(14) 15	1953	12 M	Mass	Wedge	AFD 9 months
(15) 15	1953	7 F	Mass, 10 days pain	Wedge	AFD 3 years
(16) 30	1956	5 F	Mass, 1 month	Wedge	AFD 47 years
(17) 30	1956	28 F	Mass and pain, 1 year	Wedge	AFD 2 years
(18) 30	1956	39 F	Incidental	Biopsy	AFD 2 years
(19) 30	1956	64 M	Incidental	Wedge	AFD 3½ years
(20) 16	1959	6½ F	Mass, 5½ years	Wedge	Op. death
(21) 16	1959	8 months F	Mass, 1 day	Biopsy	AFD 8 years
(22) 45	1966	7	Mass	Right lobe	AFD 5½ years

(23)	45	1966	34		Mass	Right lobe	AFD	33 months
(24)	45	1966	41		Incidental	Wedge	AFD	31 months
(25)	45	1966	38		—	Biopsy	AFD	2½ years
(26)	74	1968	38	F	Incidental	Wedge (2)	AFD	2 years
(27)	5	1968	23	M	Incidental	Wedge	AFD	8 months
(28)	24	1969	20	F	Mass, pregnant	Wedge	AFD	3 years
(29)	28	1969	8	M	Mass, 6 months	Wedge	NFU	
(30)	28	1969	8	F	Mass, 2 years	Wedge	NFU	
(31)	28	1969	14	F	Mass	Wedge	NFU	
(32)	28	1969	18	F	Incidental	Wedge	NFU	
(33)	82	1969	47	F	Incidental	Wedge	AFD	3 years
(34)	82	1969	38	F	Incidental	Wedge	DOD	4 months
(35)	82	1969	23	F	Incidental	Biopsy	AFD	?
(36)	82	1969	33	M	Incidental	Wedge	AFD	?
(37)	12	1969	7	F	Pain and mass	Biopsy, radiation	No change 12 mos	
(38)	65	1970	7	F	Mass	Wedge	AFD	22 years
(39)	63	1970	40	F	Incidental	L. lat. seg.	AFD	9 months
(40)	63	1970	34	F	Incidental	Wedge	AFD	5 months
(41)	54	1970	12	F	Mass	Wedge	AFD	2 years
(42)	20	1971	3½	F	Mass	L. lat. seg.	AFD	15 months
(43)	47	1972	18	F	Incidental	Wedge	NFU	
(44)	47	1972	40	F*	Incidental	Wedge	AFD	34 months
(45)	47	1972	38	F**	Incidental	Wedge	NFU	
(46)	56	1973	31	F	Mass	Wedge	AFD	1½ years
(47)	80	1973	36	F	Incidental	Wedge	AFD	2½ years
(48)	80	1973	21	F	Mass, pregnant	Left lobe	Op. death	
(49)	80	1973	7	F	Mass, 4 weeks	Left lobe	AFD	79 months
(50)	80	1973	6	F	Mass, few days	Right lobe	AFD	5 years

Table continued on following page.

Table 6-8. *Continued.*

REFERENCE	YEAR OF REPORT	AGE/SEX		SYMPTOMS	OPERATION	OUTCOME	
(51)	1973	23	F	Mass, 16 months	Left lobe	AFD	3 months
(52)	1974	34	F	Mass	Wedge	AFD	4 years
(53)	1974	35	F	Mass, 3 years	Biopsy	AFD	3 months
(54)	1974	51	F	Incidental	Wedge	AFD	2 months
(55)	1975	22	F	Incidental	Wedge	AWD	14 months
(56)	1975	27	F	Incidental	Wedge	AFD	6 months

CASES FOUND AT POSTMORTEM

Ref.	Year	Age/Sex	Symptoms	Operation
10	1953	34 patients 15 male, 19 female aged 27–74 years.		All incidental at postmortem.

*Case also included in 1974 LTS – Case 49. Appendix VI–A.
**Case also included in 1974 LTS – Case 44. Appendix VI–A.

Key: AFD – Alive, free of disease.
NFU – No follow-up available.
Op. death – Operative death.
AWD – Alive, with nodules left.
DOD – Died of other disease.

reported were male, and 43 were female. Nineteen patients were less than 16 years of age, and only nine were 40 years or older. The youngest patient was an 8-month-old boy and the oldest was a woman 64 years of age. The lesions measured less than 5 cm in maximum diameter in 15 patients, between 5 and 10 cm in 38 patients, and over 10 cm in eight patients. All of the 35 postmortem cases had lesions less than 5.5 cm in diameter.

There were multiple tumors in seven of the 56 clinical cases and in six of the 35 postmortem cases. The tumors occurred with approximately equal frequency in the right and left lobes of the liver (anatomic lobes). The tumors were incidental findings in 55 patients (20 at laparotomy for other diseases and 35 at postmortem), and in 40 patients the tumors presented as mass lesions first discovered one day to five and one-half years prior to laparotomy. It is interesting to note that at least seven of the larger tumors in the clinical series were pedunculated, yet none of the smaller autopsy-discovered tumors were on a stalk, which suggests that pedunculation is a phenomenon related to size.

Two patients had a history of trauma occurring two[5] and five years[38] prior to a diagnosis of FNH, and another had incision and drainage of a liver abscess 19 years before a diagnosis of FNH.[8] Two tumors were palpated for the first time during pregnancy.

An accurate history is not available about the use of contraceptive medication in many of these patients, but at least 66 of the 91 patients reported in the literature review could not have been taking birth control pills (19 adult female patients prior to 1960, 11 children and two adult males reported since 1960, plus 34 postmortem cases all reported in the 1950s).

None of the 56 clinical patients presented with intraperitoneal hemorrhage. The absence of rupture with bleeding for FNH tumors is an important finding in this literature review. Mays, et al. have recently reported three patients with what they called "focal nodular hyperplasia" who had massive intraperitoneal hemorrhage causing shock.[48] Because the description of their cases more closely resembles what we have called LCA, we have not included these cases in our discussion of FNH. With that exception, and the exception of the two Spanish-language cases from South America cited above, no patient in this review or in the 1974 LTS presented with intraperitoneal hemorrhage of significant degree.

What has been the surgical experience with FNH tumors? Keen, in his three papers and collection of 75 case reports, probably had no cases of focal nodular hyperplasia (see Chapter Two). Henson, et al., reporting in 1956, described a typical FNH tumor removed from a 5-year-old girl 47 years previously, in 1909.[30] The Tinkers[71] and Warvi[77, 78] in their comprehensive reviews list no tumors that can definitely be identified as focal nodular hyperplasia. Other reports[9, 13,]

[26, 32, 38, 49] describe cases resected in the 1940s or earlier. Table 6–8 lists most of the others reported in the literature review who had undergone some sort of resection for focal nodular hyperplasia. Nine patients had a major resection (three each: right lobectomy, left lobectomy, and left lateral segmentectomy). The remainder of the patients had wedge excision or enucleation of the tumors. There were three operative deaths following resection in the patients listed in Table 6–8, all due to problems with operative control of hemorrhage and their sequelae.

The tumors in nine patients were biopsied without excision, leaving the bulk of the tumor in place, and four additional patients had only one of several tumors excised. Of these 13 patients with incomplete excision, there is no follow-up information on one, and the other 12 patients were alive without symptoms referable to their tumors at the time of reporting at one, three, six, 12, 14, 18, 18, 24, 24, 24, and 40 months and eight years respectively after operation.

There was no evidence of recurrent disease or metastatic spread in the 30 patients in whom all tumor was resected and who have been followed now for periods of two months to 47 years. Eleven patients had been followed for more than three years at the time of reporting.

What can we learn about the natural history of these tumors by looking at the reported experience reviewed above and at the 1974 LTS? First, these tumors are the most common of the primary benign solid tumors occurring in the liver. They can occur at all ages, but are most common in females between 18 and 40 years of age. They are usually small and are found most often at laparotomy for other diseases or at autopsy, but occasionally they may reach large size.

A look at the larger tumors may give us a clue to etiology. In the 1974 LTS, 14 focal nodular hyperplasia tumors were 10 cm or larger in greatest diameter. Five of these large tumors occurred in children – in fact five of the nine FNH tumors in children under 16 years of age were 10 cm or greater in size, whereas only nine of 54 tumors occurring in adults were larger than 10 cm. From the literature, eight cases of tumors larger than 10 cm were found, five of which were in patients less than 16 years of age.

Of the 12 adults from the 1974 LTS and the literature with large (10 cm or larger) tumors, three had tumors first noted during pregnancy or during the first few months post partum. Of the over-all experience (63 cases from the 1974 LTS and 50 clinical cases from the literature review with known gender) only 15 of 113 patients were male, yet five of 18 large tumors occurred in males – four in boys under 15 years of age.

All the tumors discovered at post mortem were small lesions, and 15 of 35 occurred in males.[10, 63] The oldest patient in the 1974 LTS with a large tumor was a 53-year-old white female with a mass known and biopsied six years prior to eventual resection for continued growth.

She was taking Premarin and thyroid medication at the time of liver resection.

From all these data, it would seem that rapid growth of FNH tumors occurs chiefly in children or in pregnant adults. It remains to be determined whether or not contraceptive medication or the ingestion of other exogenous hormones affect this process.

Thirteen patients in the literature survey and one patient from the 1974 LTS had FNH tumor left after laparotomy, yet in no case has the tumor subsequently metastasized or caused disabling symptoms or life-threatening complications. Three patients, who eventually had resection, had a biopsy diagnosis of FNH made one, three, and six years, respectively, prior to resection. In two the tumor seemed to increase in size under observation, and in one the tumor decreased in size. Case 11, Appendix VI-A was the only nonresected patient in the 1974 LTS, and her tumor "disappeared" in the course of 18 months (see above). Clearly these lesions are benign clinically as well as pathologically, and they should not be resected, if to do so would risk the life of the patient.

Why do we rarely see necrosis in FNH tumors in spite of the fact that vascular changes are a common finding in the central scar tissue, and why is necrosis such a common finding in LCA? If FNH is a reaction to the presence of an arteriovenous malformation, the resulting changes might well occur over a prolonged period, with gradual pressure necrosis and subsequent nodular regeneration of hepatocytes at the periphery of the lesion, with replacement at the center by mature scar tissue. The thickened blood vessel walls show splitting and fragmentation of elastic tissue. Such abnormal vessels are most prominent in the center of the larger lesions, suggesting an association with larger fistulas and high intravascular pressure. The remarkable regenerative ability of the liver may explain why its reaction to chronic injury might be one of nodular regeneration, rather than replacement solely with scar tissue. The normal liver is a maze of shunts, alternate pathways, and vascular connections unique to this organ. Perhaps these vascular channels are particularly susceptible to malfunction during periods of active growth or hormonal change. The necrosis of the LCA must be related to acute vascular insufficiency which occurs as growing neoplasms outstrip their blood supply, or to endophlebitis and hepatic vein thrombosis which has been associated with birth control medication.[83]

What, then, shall we call these lesions? Edmondson avoided the term "regenerative nodule" because he saw no evidence of necrosis or vascular changes in the "early" (presumably because they were small) lesions found at postmortem examination. Could it be that the tumors found at autopsy were actually late lesions that had shrunk with time after a period of active but unrecognized growth?

Another theory of origin more in keeping with Edmondson's early observations might suggest that the FNH lesion begins from an epithelial origin and develops as an adenomatous hyperplasia.

Although Phillips, et al. beautifully distinguished between adenoma and what we have called "focal nodular hyperplasia," they prefer the term "hamartoma" for this latter lesion.[61] We agree with Edmondson that "hamartoma" is a misnomer, because it suggests a malformation with a disorganized structure. Focal nodular hyperplasia, in contrast, has a characteristic pattern with orderly and predictable organization of the several components that make up its structure.

On the basis of the above, the term "regenerative nodule" or "focal cirrhosis" would seem as appropriate as "focal nodular hyperplasia" to describe these FNH tumors. However, until we understand the process more thoroughly, perhaps we should preserve the purely descriptive, although somewhat awkward, name of "focal nodular hyperplasia."

The word "adenoma" connotes neoplasia and a possible relationship to malignant change. Whether or not the tumor we call LCA is truly a neoplasm capable of unlimited growth and possible malignant transformation will be considered further after we look at the reports and opinions of others.

Liver Cell Adenoma — Literature Survey

Liver cell adenoma was defined by Edmondson in 1958 as a "benign neoplasm, usually solitary, composed of fairly normal to atypical hepatic cells arranged in cords, occasionally forming bile, and devoid of portal tracts and central veins."[22] He thought encapsulation was nearly always present. The lesion was very rare and probably was capable of malignant change if present for a long while.

Few cases reported in the literature prior to 1965 meet our criteria for true liver cell adenomas. Although Warvi excluded nodules of regenerative hyperplasia from his encyclopedic review in 1944, he still reported a collection of 67 cases of microscopically proved "adenomas" of the liver, 38 of which apparently had been resected.[77] Neither our confidence in his diagnoses of a "true liver cell adenoma," nor our knowledge of the German literature before 1900, allows safe acceptance of that figure. Schrager (1937),[64] in a good review, nicely illustrates the confusion of solid, cystic, and probably regenerative lesions termed "adenoma" by contemporary authors. Before 1950 only a few cases[15, 39, 44, 72, 76, 81] seem acceptable by our retrospective criteria.

Table 6–9 lists some clinical data about the 55 case reports that satisfied our criteria as true LCA tumors. Five of these reported cases are also included in the 1974 LTS, bringing the total experience to 87 cases. Edmondson, et al. studied 42 patients with LCA, but data on individual cases were not given.[23] There may be overlap with Edmondson's cases and with the present literature survey and the 1974 LTS in this group of 87 cases. A case previously reported by one of us as a

Text continued on page 170.

Table 6-9. Liver Cell Adenoma: Cases Reported from Literature

REFERENCE	YEAR OF REPORT	AGE/SEX	SYMPTOM	OPERATION	OUTCOME
(1) 72	1923	29 F	Rupture	Wedge	Op. death
(2) 39	1923	57 F	Pain, 12 days	Wedge	NFU
(3) 81	1938	8 months M	Mass, 2 weeks	Biopsy	Op. death
(4) 76	1941	23 F	Mass, 4 years	Wedge	AFD 5 years
(5) 46	1948	27 F	Mass, 5 years	Wedge	AFD 18½ years
(6) 15	1953	13 months F	Mass, 1 month	Wedge	Died of other causes, 25 years
(7) 11	1959	71 F	Vague abd. pain 6 weeks	Wedge × 2	AFD 80 months
(8) 14	1964	2½ F	Mass, 2 months	Wedge	AFD 5 years
(9)* 51	1964	21 F	Mass, 5 months	Ext. right lobe	AFD 7 years
(10) 50	1967	29 F	Mass, 2 years	Left lobe (mult.)	NFU
(11) 25	1967	20 F	Pain, fever, 1 week	Right lobe	AFD 7 years
(12)** 58	1967	23 F	Incidental (angio)	Wedge (mult.)	AFD 5 months
(13) 84	1969	20 F	Rupture	Right lobe	AFD 5½ years
(14) 54	1970	2½ M	Mass	Wedge	AFD 3 years
(15) 54	1970	3½ F	Mass	Left lat. seg.	AFD 5 years
(16)*** 47	1970	27 F	Postpartum pain and mass	Left lat. seg.	AFD 93 months
(17)**** 47	1970	29 F	Rupture	Right lobe	Op. death
(18) 37	1971	23 F	Recurrent mass	Wedge × 2	AFD 43 months
(19) 53	1972	23 F	Mass, 2 months	Left lobe	AFD 56 months
(20) 53	1972	30 F	Acute pain	Left lobe	AFD 3 years
(21) 53	1972	20 F	Postpartum mass	Right lobe	AFD 27 months

Table continued on the following page.

Table 6–9. *Continued.*

REFERENCE	YEAR OF REPORT	AGE/SEX	SYMPTOM	OPERATION	OUTCOME
(22)	53	1972	40 F	Mass, 2 months	Wedge	AFD 25 months
(23)	53	1972	38 F	Incidental	Left lat. seg.	AFD 5 months
(24)	34	1972	28 F	Pain. mass	Wedge	NFU
(25)	19	1973	36 F	Rupture	Right lobe	AFD 3 years
(26)	19	1973	24 F	Rupture	Right wedge	AFD 11 months
(27)	19	1973	15 F	Acute pain	Left lobe	AFD 9 years
(28)	6	1973	26 F	Rupture	Left lobe	AFD 4 years
(29)	6	1973	27 F	Rupture	Right lobe	Op. death
(30)	6	1973	25 F	Mass, 1 month	Wedge	NFU
(31)	6	1973	25 F	Pain, anemia	Right lobe	AFD 2 months
(32)	6	1973	29 F	Mass	Right wedge	AFD 3½ years
(33)	6	1973	30 F	Rupture	Right lobe	AFD 15 months
(34)	6	1973	39 F	Rupture	60% resection	In-hospital 2 months postop.
(35)	17	1973	30 F	Mass, 4 months	Right lobe	AFD 2 years
(36)	62	1973	10 M	Mass, 3 months	Left wedge	AFD 9 years
(37)	31	1973	29 F	Rupture	Right lobe	AFD 1½ years
(38)	31	1973	20 F	Rupture	Left lobe	AFD 4 years
(39)	42	1973	24 F	Mass, 6 months	Right lobe	AFD 4 years
(40)	3	1974	22 F	Diarrhea, 6 months	Right lobe	AFD 15 months
(41)	3	1974	43 F	Incidental, 2 years	Left lat. seg.	AFD 1 year

(42)	3	1974	25	F	Rupture	Right lobe	AFD	1½ years
(43)	3	1974	41	F	Pain, fever	Bilat. wedge	AFD	16 months
(44)	75	1974	34	F	Rupture	Multiple wedge	Op. death	
(45)	48	1974	42	F	Pain	Right lobe	AFD	2 years
(46)	48	1974	26	F	Rupture	Right lobe	AFD	1 year
(47)	48	1974	25	F	Rupture	Left lobe	AFD	5 years
(48)	73	1974	40	F	Rupture	Right lobe	AFD	6 months
(49)	40	1974	55	F	Rupture	V segment	AFD	6 months
(50)	57	1974	37	F	Rupture	Right lobe	Op. death	
(51)	57	1974	33	F	Rupture	Right lobe	Op. death	
(52)	57	1974	36	F	Rupture	"Large"	Op. death	
(53)*****	69	1975	25	F	Postpartum mass	Left wedge	NFU	
(54)	69	1975	29	F	Mass, 2 months	Left wedge	AFD	3 months
(55)	55	1975	27	F	Rupture	Partial wedge	AWD	8 months

Key: AFD – Alive, free of disease.
      AWD – Alive with disease.
      Op. death – Operative death.
      NFU – No follow-up information.
*Cases also included in 1974 Liver Tumor Survey:
    *Case 4, Appendix VI-B.
   **Case 12, Appendix VI-B.
  ***Case 15, Appendix VI-B.
 ****Case 17, Appendix VI-B.
*****Case 10, Appendix VI-B.

post-traumatic central hematoma of the liver has been reconsidered in the light of new knowledge and a review of the pathology, and is almost certainly a classic liver cell adenoma.[25] The case cited by Frederick, et al. may be a similar instance, but is not included because the history could not be reviewed.[27] Forty-six of the 55 acceptable cases in the literature have been reported since 1965, reflecting either an increased awareness, a greater interest, or an increased incidence of these tumors in the last decade. We have included with the LCAs three cases reported by Mays, et al.[48] and two by Stauffer, et al.[69] which they called "focal nodular hyperplasia." The clinical presentation with rupture, the size of the lesions, the absence of nodularity or of a well-defined central scar with fibrous septa, and the absence of bile duct proliferation in these five cases seem to correlate more closely with the entity we are calling "liver cell adenoma." To alter their classification is presumptuous, but the opportunity of retrospective review may afford some advantage.

Table 6–10 outlines the age and sex incidences of the 55 cases for which this information is available. There were multiple LCAs in eight patients and solitary lesions in 47, without a predilection for any particular area of the liver. Stumpf, et al. report a unique case of diffuse multiple adenomatosis in a young male dying of renal failure, but this case is not included in our tabulation.[70] Thirty-eight of the included tumors were more than 10 cm in diameter, 12 were less than 10 cm, and size was not clearly defined for five other patients.

The most remarkable thing about patients with LCA, and the factor that probably is most different from FNH, is the way in which the patients presented to their physician. Twenty-one patients had massive intraperitoneal hemorrhage due to rupture of their tumor, 19 were

Table 6–10.   Liver Cell Adenoma: Literature Survey

| | | PATIENTS |
AGE IN YEARS	*Males*	*Females*
Under 20	3*	4**
20 – 29	None	30
30 – 39	None	10
40 – 49	None	5
Over 50	None	3***
	3	52

*Males age 8 months, 2½ years, and 10 years.
**Females age 13 months, 2½, 3½, and 15 years.
***Females age 55, 57, and 71 years.

found to have a mass occasionally associated with vague abdominal symptoms, five had acute abdominal pain which in retrospect was probably due to hemorrhage into the adenoma, and four had vague abdominal complaints unassociated with a palpable mass. The adenomas were incidental findings in only three patients, two at laparotomy for other problems and one in which a liver scan picked up a "cold" lesion. The presenting symptom was not clearly documented for the remaining three patients in this collected series. The palpable mass was known to be present for two weeks to five years prior to laparotomy but this interval was a short one in most patients (see Table 6–6).

Of those patients who presented with rupture and intraperitoneal hemorrhage, all but two were females between ages 19 and 40. The two exceptions were a 29-year-old male[47] (already included in and discussed with the 1974 LTS) and a 55-year-old female reported by Krajka in 1974.[40] Most of the 42 women recently reported by Edmondson, et al. presented with a mass (18 patients), pain (12), or rupture with intra-abdominal hemorrhage (10). Only two had their adenomas found incidentally.[23]

One patient found in this literature survey of LCA did not undergo resection and died shortly after exploratory laparotomy.[81] Therapy was not discussed in four other patients with liver cell adenoma.[61] Five others were included in the 1974 LTS, leaving 49 from whose follow-up review some information about prognosis may be derived. Six of these patients, all of whom presented with massive intraperitoneal hemorrhage, died either during or after operation. One patient was still in the hospital two months after resection,[6] and another was dead 35 years after resection of an LCA without signs or symptoms of recurrent liver tumor.[15] No follow-up information was available for four patients, leaving 36 who were living at the time of the published report.

Thirty-four of these 36 patients were alive and well without a sign of recurrent disease two months to 18 and one-half years after resection of LCA, in spite of the fact that in three patients grossly evident tumor had been left at the time of resection.[3] Eighteen of these patients had been followed for more than three years, and nine for a period of more than five years after liver resection.

Two other patients had evidence of recurrent liver tumor. The first, a 71-year-old white female, had wedge resection of an 11 cm LCA from the right lobe, and then six years later underwent reoperation with resection of recurrent tumor from the right lobe, together with resection of another nodule from the left lateral segment of the liver. Both nodules were histologically similar to the original adenoma, and the patient is well eight months after her second operation.[11] The other patient was a woman who at the age of 23 had resection of a large adenoma from the right lobe.[37] Three years later a liver scan showed evidence of recurrent disease, although no mass was palpable. At reoperation an orange-sized mass was found in the right lobe, which on frozen section proved to be a recurrent LCA. No resection was done, and she was asymptomatic in the ensuing seven months before the last report.

No evidence of metastatic disease was found in any report, nor in any case examined in the 1974 LTS. There is also no clear-cut report of malignant transformation of LCA in either series.

What, then, is this disease? Is it becoming more common, perhaps in relation to the increasing use of oral contraceptive agents, or is the increasing number of reports related to a better recognition and definition of the lesion? Is it a true neoplasm with a propensity toward progressive growth?

No conclusive answer can be given to any of the above questions, but it is tempting to speculate about them.

The question that has received the most attention in the lay press, as well as in scientific journals, is whether the lesion we are calling LCA is caused by, or at least related to, the use of oral contraceptive medication.

Davies, as early as 1948, raised the question about the relationship of high estrogen levels to an increased incidence of hepatic tumors in Africans.[18] However, it was not until 1973, when Baum et al. reported seven cases of "benign hepatomas" in young women taking birth control pills, that what had been considered a theoretic possibility in man became instead a probable association.[6] As we have seen, the preponderance of patients developing LCA tumors are, and have been, in the child-bearing age-group. The use of oral contraception became widespread in the early 1960s, and the incidence and recognition of LCA has increased markedly since that time. Both true facts, but are they related? With so many using "the pill," any phenomenon occurring largely in young females would necessarily have a strong association with, if not relation to, that use. The basis for our suspicion lies on the solid evidence that exogenous hormone therapy does produce injury to some human livers, and on animal experimentation which has demonstrated an increased incidence of hepatic tumors in mammals fed oral contraceptive agents.

In 1950 Werner, et al. described liver damage during androgen therapy.[79] Jaundice was associated with norethindrone therapy in 1962,[60] and Adlercreutz and Ikonen discussed the liver damage associated with oral contraceptives in 1964.[1] A comprehensive 1970 review of the relationship of natural and synthetic female sex hormones and the liver concluded that the use of oral contraceptives usually produced ultrastructural changes in the liver cells of human subjects even if liver function tests were normal.[2] Bromsulphalein excretion is delayed in most patients if measured carefully, but increases in SGOT and SGPT levels are more often transient, suggesting the possibility of enzyme induction by medication. The synthetic progesterones, particularly the 19-norprogesterones, have a more pronounced effect on the liver, resembling that of the androgens.[2] The relationship between sex hormone therapy and liver injury seems dose-related, yet from human work the suspicion also arises that individuals vary in their ability to metabolize and/or adapt to exogenous hormones. Perhaps the patient who develops an adenoma lacks a specific enzyme, or develops an extra one.

The ultrastructural changes in the hepatocytes of women taking oral contraceptives are minimal for the first six months of therapy, and are limited to an increased amount of smooth endoplasmic reticulum. However, striking changes in mitochondria are seen with therapy that is continued for 12 to 30 months.[59]

In 1972 Horvath, et al. noted similar mitochondrial changes in the cells of an adenoma removed from a 28-year-old woman on contraceptive medication, and questioned a possible relationship.[34] In the same year the British Committee on the Safety of Medicine showed an increased frequency of liver tumors in rats fed norethynodrel,[7] and Johnson, et al. reported four hepatocellular carcinomas occurring in patients receiving androgenic-anabolic steroid therapy for aplastic anemia.[36] This last report must be viewed cautiously since (1) one of the liver "cancers" regressed with cessation of steroid therapy; (2) the tumors were all confined to the liver; (3) they were described as "well-differentiated" microscopically; and (4) autopsy evidence was lacking in two of the four cases.

In any case, however, the background was well set for the 1973 report of Baum, et al.,[6] and subsequently there has been an extraordinary proliferation of case reports describing an association of birth control medication and other endocrine phenomena with liver cell adenomas and/or "hamartomas." Focal nodular hyperplasia also has been related to the use of oral contraceptive by Mays, et al.[48] and Stauffer, et al.,[69] but they may have been discussing the lesion we are calling "adenoma" (see above).

Frederick, et al. related spontaneous rupture of the liver to the venous thrombotic potential of contraceptive medication, and cited multiple reports of Budd-Chiari syndrome in women on "the pill."[27] Mosonyi reported multiple benign hepatomas in a 62-year-old woman who also had an adrenal adenoma and was eventually found to have a virilizing Leydig-cell adenoma of the ovary.[52] O'Sullivan and Wilding noted the association of a liver hamartoma with adrenal carcinoma,[57] and Mays, et al. remind us of the relationship of clear cell tumors of the cervix and vagina to intrauterine exposure to estrogen therapy[48] — a relationship even more interesting when one remembers that many of the hepatocytes in liver cell adenomas resemble clear cells. Hooghe states that estrogen therapy may stimulate the production of estrogen-binding proteins such as alpha-1-fetoprotein, and tries to relate that theory to the growth of benign hepatomas.[33]

A recent report by Edmondson begins what must eventually supplant circumstantial and anecdotal evidence about the possible relationship between the use of contraceptive medication and liver cell adenomas in humans. Forty-two women with documented adenomas were found, 34 of whom were paired with normal controls to examine the effect of contraceptive medication. The patients with adenomas were taking birth control pills for a longer time than the controls, and those taking mestranol-containing pills were at increased risk.[23] Finally, peliosis hepatitis, a condition in which vascular lakes may be found throughout the liver substance, has been seen after administration of steroids,[69] and also has been described as a feature of a few liver cell adenomas.

One is left with a strong impression that exogenous sex hormone therapy is certainly related to liver injury and possibly to liver tumor formation, but the relationship remains obscure. Most patients with focal nodular hyperplasia, and many patients with liver cell adenoma, have never taken oral contraceptive medication. Pregnancy, too, may be related to the incidence or at least to the rapid growth of benign liver tumors. Does the avoidance of pregnancy by oral contraception increase or decrease the risk of liver disease in a young woman? There simply are not yet sufficient data to answer that vital question.

In the meantime, it seems prudent to measure liver function tests in all women taking oral birth control medication, and to be suspicious of those with elevated BSP and transaminase values in their sera. Liver scanning should detect most large adenomas before they are palpable or symptomatic. Certainly one could not advise a woman with a proved benign liver tumor to continue oral contraception. Horvath states that the patient with a recurrent adenoma reported by Kay and Schatski[37] was taking oral contraceptive medication,[34] but there are precious few other reports of recurrent problems in women who had adenomas diagnosed before the possible association of liver tumors and oral contraception was recognized, and who presumably continued their medication.

Is the lesion we are calling LCA really an adenoma, i.e., a neoplasm capable of growth and possible malignant change? For the present that name will probably have to suffice for want of a better one, because the weight of available evidence suggests that the growth of this tumor is purely epithelial—connoting neoplasia or hyperplasia rather than repair. Necrosis, however, could be due to the outstripping of blood supply by epithelial neoplasia in excess of angiogenesis, or to acute thrombosis related in some as yet undefined, but almost certainly existent, propensity toward thrombosis in patients taking oral contraceptive medication.

Malignant transformation may be seen when our experience with the lesion increases, but, theoretic considerations aside, no such transformation has yet been documented. However, in contrast with FNH, no LCA has decreased in size while under observation. With the rapidly accumulating evidence about etiologic association with contraceptive medication, a trial of observation, off medication and with careful follow-up with liver scans or angiography, may soon provide us with better information about the natural history of these lesions upon which decisions about therapy may more rationally be based.

If, indeed, the epithelial proliferation proves to be due to medication and is reversible by abstinence from that medication, we shall need a new word to name it—if not adenoma, perhaps "iatrogenoma." It seems fitting that what could be the prototype for drug-dependent growths in other organs should be first recognized as a new "feature" of the pluripotential hepatocyte.

RECOMMENDATIONS FOR THERAPY OF FNH AND LCA

Most patients with FNH or LCA tumors will present to a physician or surgeon in one of three ways: (1) with a mass; (2) with abdominal pain—either acute or chronic; or (3) with an asymptomatic, nonpalpable lesion found incidentally at laparotomy for another disease or by angiography or liver scan done for investigation of some other problem. Patients with vague abdominal symptoms, fever of undertermined origin, or symptoms of gallbladder disease associated with normal oral cholecystograms should have liver function tests and radioisotope liver scans looking for either benign or malignant tumors. The Bromsulphalein and SGOT tests are probably most sensitive for FNH and LCA, although both frequently are normal even in the presence of the larger tumors.

A palpable mass lesion or a "cold" defect on a liver scan should be investigated at any age. A prolonged period of observation may not harm the patient with a benign lesion, but a "curable" cancer may be missed.

There is no way short of biopsy that can safely establish a certain diagnosis of LCA, FNH, or carcinoma of the liver. Because the biopsy should be a generous one to allow adequate differentiation, and because most such tumors are quite vascular, percutaneous needle biopsy is discouraged. Open evaluation at laparotomy, done with the patient and surgeon prepared for resection, is indicated whenever a primary liver tumor is suspected.

If the lesion is small and peripheral and can be resected safely, excision biopsy should be done. In all other cases a large wedge biopsy should form the basis for further therapy, even though the tumor's gross characteristic strongly suggests a specific diagnosis. If a rapid section diagnosis of carcinoma, adenoma, or "normal" liver is returned by the pathologist from wedge biopsy of an obvious tumor, resection with a margin of normal liver tissue is recommended. If the lesion is FNH, it should be left in place if resection would significantly endanger the patient's life. If the patient's condition, the tumor anatomy, and the surgeon's skill allow safe resection, an FNH tumor may be enucleated or removed by more formal liver resection.

REFERENCES

1. Adlercreutz, H., and Ikonen, E.: Oral contraceptives and liver damage. Br. Med. J. *2*:1133, 1964.
2. Adlercreutz, H., and Tenhunen, R.: Natural and synthetic female sex hormones and the liver. Am. J. Med. *49*:630, 1970.
3. Albritton, D. R., Tompkins, R. K., and Longmire, W. P.: Hepatic cell adenoma. Ann. Surg. *180*:14, 1974.
4. Amerson, J. R., and Stone, H. H.: Experiences in the management of hepatic trauma. Arch. Surg. *100*:150, 1970.
5. Aronsen, K. F., et al.: A case of operated focal nodular cirrhosis of the liver. Scand. J. Gastroenterol. *3*:58, 1968.
6. Baum, J. K., et al.: Possible association between benign hepatomas and oral contraceptives. Lancet *2*:926, 1973.
7. Beaconsfield, P.: Liver tumors and steroid hormones. Letter to ed. Lancet *1*:516, 1974.
8. Begg, C. F., and Berry, W. H.: Isolated nodules of regenerative hyperplasia of the liver. Am. J. Clin. Pathol. *23*:447, 1953.
9. Benson, C. D., and Penberthy, G. C.: Surgical excision of primary tumor of liver (hamartoma) in infant seven months old, with recovery. Surgery *12*:881, 1942.
10. Benz, E. J., and Baggenstoss, A. H.: Focal cirrhosis of the liver: its relation to the so-called hamartoma (adenoma, benign hepatoma). Cancer *6*:743, 1953.
11. Berkheiser, S. W.: Recurrent liver cell adenoma. Gastroenterology *37*:760, 1959.
12. Bienayme, J., and Prawerman, A.: L'hamartome de foie chez l'enfant à l'exclusion des angiomes. Ann. Chir. Infant. *10*:399, 1969.
13. Branch, A., Tonning, D. J., and Skinner, G. E.: Adenoma of the liver. Can. Med. Assoc. J. *53*:53, 1945.
14. Chandler, E. M., and Walters, W. D.: Solitary liver tumors in childhood: report of two cases. Ann. Surg. *160*:986, 1964.
15. Christopherson, W. M., and Collier, H. S.: Primary benign liver cell tumors in infancy and childhood. Cancer *6*:853, 1953.
16. Cleland, R. S.: Benign and malignant tumors of the liver. Pediatr. Clin. North Am. *6*:427, 1959.
17. Danais, S., et al.: Radiopertechnetate flow study and liver scan in a case of benign hepatoma (liver cell adenoma). Am. J. Roentgenol. Radium Ther. Nucl. Med. *118(4)*:836, 1973.
18. Davies, J. N. P.: Liver tumors and steroid hormones. Letter to ed. Lancet *1*:516, 1974.
19. Davis, J. B., Schenken, J. R., and Zimmerman, O.: Massive hemoperitoneum from rupture of benign hepatocellular adenoma. Surgery *73(2)*:181, 1973.
20. Denis, R., et al.: Hamartoma versus multiple nodular hyperplasia of the liver. Pathol. Eur. *6*:396, 1971.

21. Edmondson, H. A.: Progress in pediatrics: differential diagnosis of tumors and tumor-like lesions of liver in infancy and childhood. A.M.A. J. Dis. Child. *91*:168, 1956.

22. Edmondson, H. A.: Tumors of the liver and intra-hepatic bile ducts. Section VII-Fascicle 25, Atlas of Tumor Pathology. Armed Forces Institute of Pathology, 1958.

23. Edmondson, H. A., Henderson, B., and Benton, B.: Liver cell adenomas associated with use of oral contraceptives. N. Engl. J. Med. *294*:470, 1976.

24. Field, C. A.: Hamartoma of the liver in a pregnant woman. Minn. Med. *52*:639, 1969.

25. Foster, J. H., and Chandler, J. J.: Central rupture of the liver with lobar infarction. J. Trauma *7*:3, 1967.

26. Franklin, R. G., and Downing, C. F.: Primary liver tumors. Am. J. Surg. *73*:390, 1947.

27. Frederick, W. C., Howard, R. G., and Spatola, S.: Spontaneous rupture of the liver in patient using contraceptive pills. Arch. Surg. *108*:93, 1974.

28. Garancis, J. C., et al.: Hepatic adenoma: biochemical and electron microscopic study. Cancer *24*:560, 1969.

29. Gerding, W. J., Popp, M. F., and Martineau, P. C.: Hamartomatous cholangiohepatoma. J.A.M.A. *145*:821, 1951.

30. Henson, S. W., Gray, H. K., and Dockerty, M. B.: Benign tumors of the liver. Surg. Gynecol. Obstet. *103*:23, 1956.

31. Hermann, R. E., and David, T. E.: Spontaneous rupture of the liver caused by hepatomas. Surgery *74*:715, 1973.

32. Hoffman, H. S.: Benign hepatoma: review of the literature and report of a case. Ann. Intern. Med. *17*:130, 1942.

33. Hooghe, R.: Benign hepatomas and oral contraceptives. Letter to ed. Lancet *1*:630, 1974.

34. Horvath, E., Kovacs, K., and Ross, R. C.: Ultrastructural findings in a well-differentiated hepatoma. Digestion *7*:74, 1972.

35. Hunter, W. R.: A case of benign hepatoma. Br. J. Surg. *36*:425, 1949.

36. Johnson, F. L., et al.: Association of androgenic anabolic steroid therapy with development of hepatocellular carcinoma. Lancet *2*:1273, 1972.

37. Kay, S., and Schatzki, P. F.: Ultrastructure of a benign liver cell adenoma. Cancer *28*:755, 1971.

38. Kay, S., and Talbert, P. C.: Adenoma of the liver, mixed type (hamartoma). Cancer *3*:307, 1950.

39. Kidd, F.: Case of primary tumor of the liver removed by operation. Proc. R. Soc. Med. *16*:61, 1923.

40. Krajka, V. K., Dybicki, J., and Jankav, O.: Hämoperitoneum durch die Ruptur eines hepatozellulären Adenoms. Zentralbl. Chir. *99*:606, 1974.

41. Lawrence, G. H., et al.: Primary carcinoma of the liver. Am. J. Surg. *112*:200, 1966.

42. Leger, L., et al.: Hamartomes hépatocytaires du foie. Nouv. Presse Med. *2(6)*:353, 1973.

43. Levenson, R. M., and Mason, D. G.: Mixed adenoma (hamartoma) of the liver. Ann. Intern. Med. *38*:136, 1953.

44. Longmire, W. P., Jr., and Marable, S. A.: Clinical experiences with major hepatic resections. Ann. Surg. *154*:460, 1961.

45. Longmire, W. P., Passaro, E. P., and Joseph, W. L.: The surgical treatment of hepatic lesions. Br. J. Surg. *53*:852, 1966.

46. Longmire, W. P., Jr., and Scott, H. W., Jr.: Benign adenoma of the liver. Surgery *24*:983, 1948.

47. Malt, R. A., Hershberg, R. A., and Miller, W. L.: Experience with benign tumors of the liver. Surg. Gynecol. Obstet. *130*:285, 1970.

48. Mays, E. T., Christopherson, W. M., and Barrow, G. H.: Focal nodular hyperplasia of the liver; possible relationship to oral contraceptives. Am. J. Clin. Pathol. *61*:735, 1974.

49. McBurney, R. P., Woolner, L. B., and Wollaeger, E. E.: Solitary hyperplastic nodule of the liver simulating a neoplasm. Mayo Clin. Staff Meetings *25*:606, 1950.

50. Mercadier, M., et al.: Observation exceptionnelle d'adenomatose hépatique multinodulaire et multicentrique. Presse Med. *75*:1129, 1967.

51. Monaco, A. P., Hallgrimsson, J., and McDermott, W. V.: Multiple adenoma (hamartoma) of the liver treated by subtotal (90 per cent) resection. Ann. Surg. 159:513, 1964.

52. Mosonyi, L.: Multiple benign hepatomas and virilisation by ovarian tumor. Letter. Lancet 2:1263, 1973.

53. Motsay, G. J., and Gamble, W. G.: Clinical experience with hepatic adenomas. Surg. Gynecol. Obstet. 134:415, 1972.

54. Nikaidoh, H., Boggs, J., and Swenson, O.: Liver tumors in infants and children. Arch. Surg. 101:245, 1970.

55. Nissen, E. D., and Kent, D. R. F.: Liver tumors and oral contraceptives. Obstet. Gynecol. 46:460, 1975.

56. Orda, R., et al.: Large solitary hepatic hamartoma. Am. Surg. 39:592, 1973.

57. O'Sullivan, J. P., and Wilding, R. P.: Liver hamartomas in patients on oral contraceptives. Br. Med. J. 3:7, 1974.

58. Palubinskas, A. J., Baldwin, J., and McCormack, K. R.: Liver cell adenoma. Radiology 89:444, 1967.

59. Perez, V., et al.: Oral contraceptives: long-term use produces fine structural changes in liver mitochondria. Science 165:805, 1969.

60. Perez-Mera, R. A., and Shields, C. E.: Jaundice associated with norethindrone acetate therapy. N. Engl. J. Med. 267:1137, 1962.

61. Phillips, M. J., et al.: Benign liver cell tumors. Classification and ultrastructural pathology. Cancer 32(2):463, 1973.

62. Pollice, L.: Primary hepatic tumors in infancy and childhood. Am. J. Clin. Pathol. 60:512, 1973.

63. Ramchand, S., Suh, H. S., and Gonzalez-Crussi, F.: Focal nodular hyperplasia of the liver. Can. J. Surg. 13:22, 1970.

64. Schrager, V. L.: Surgical aspects of adenoma of the liver. Ann. Surg. 105:33, 1937.

65. Shah, J. P., Goldsmith, H. S., and Huvos, A. G.: Hamartomas of the liver. Surgery 68:778, 1970.

66. Shaw, A. F. B.: Primary liver cell adenoma (hepatoma). J. Pathol. Bacteriol. 26:475, 1923.

67. Simmonds, M.: Die knotige Hyperplasie und das Adenom der Leber. Dtsch. Arch. Klin. Med. 34:388, 1884.

68. Starzl, T. E., et al.: Alopecia, ascites and incomplete regeneration after 85 to 90 per cent liver resection. Am. J. Surg. 129:587, 1975.

69. Stauffer, J. Q., et al.: Focal nodular hyperplasia of the liver and intrahepatic hemorrhage in young women on oral contraceptives. Ann. Intern. Med. 83:301, 1975.

70. Stumpf, H. H.: Hepatocellular adenomatosis. Am. J. Med. 17:887, 1954.

71. Tinker, M. B., and Tinker, M. B., Jr.: Resection of the liver. J.A.M.A. 112:2006, 1939.

72. Turner, P.: Case of excision of an adenoma of the liver, which had ruptured spontaneously, causing internal hemorrhage. Proc. R. Soc. Med. 16:60, 1923.

73. Veyriéres, M., and Flabeau, F.: Hépatectomie droite pour adénome rompu du foie. Nouv. Presse Med. 3:517, 1974.

74. Von Sydow, C.: Multipel fokal nodulär hyperplasi i levern. Nord. Med. 80:1278, 1968.

75. Vosnides, G., et al.: Liver hamartomas in patients on oral contraceptives. Br. Med. J. 3:580, 1974.

76. Wallace, R. H.: Resection of the liver for hepatoma. Arch. Surg. 43:14, 1941.

77. Warvi, W. N.: Primary neoplasms of the liver. Arch. Pathol. 37:367, 1944.

78. Warvi, W. N.: Primary tumors of the liver. Surg. Gynecol. Obstet. 80:643, 1945.

79. Werner, S. C., Hanger, F. M., and Kritzler, R. A.: Jaundice during methyltestosterone therapy. Am. J. Med. 8:325, 1950.

80. Whelan, T. V., Jr., Baugh, J. H., and Chandor, S.: Focal nodular hyperplasia of the liver. Ann. Surg. 177(2):150, 1973.

81. Wilens, G.: Adenoma of the liver. Am. J. Dis. Child. 55:792, 1938.

82. Wilson, T. S., and MacGregor, J. W.: Focal nodular hyperplasia of the liver. Can. Med. Assoc. J. 100:567, 1969.

83. Sterup, K., and Mosbeck, J.: Budd-Chiari syndrome after taking oral contraceptives. Br. Med. J. 4:660, 1967.

84. Scorer, C. G.: Spontaneous rupture of a hepatic adenoma: a possible hazard of flying. Br. J. Surg. 56:633, 1969.

Chapter Seven

CYSTIC, VASCULAR, MESENCHYMAL, AND MISCELLANEOUS TUMORS

INTRODUCTION

Ninety per cent (317 of 353) of the resected primary tumors of the liver found in the 1974 Liver Tumor Survey could be classified as solid epithelial cancer, focal nodular hyperplasia or hepatocellular adenoma. There remained, however, an additional 36 tumors that could not be so classified and, with the exception of the cystadenomas and cystadeno-carcinomas, most occurred in pediatric patients. A few very rare types of sarcoma have been reported by others but were not encountered in this survey. These will be discussed briefly.

This chapter will attempt to tie up loose ends by briefly reviewing these other categories of primary liver tumors that are rarely seen, but which present problems and solutions clearly different from those already considered. Table 7–1 arbitrarily divides this experience into several major categories. We shall discuss our own review in the light of the reported experience of others by considering these major categories separately.

Table 7–1. Miscellaneous Tumors – 1974 Liver Tumor Survey

	PATIENTS	
	Adult	*Pediatric*
Cystadenoma	2	0
Cystadenocarcinoma	6	0
Vascular tumors	1	5
Mesenchymal hamartoma	0	5
Embryonal sarcomas	1	11
Miscellaneous benign tumors	0	4
Teratocarcinoma	0	1

CYSTADENOMA AND CYSTADENOCARCINOMA

The famous tumor removed by Keen from a 31-year-old woman (see Chapter 2) was a cystadenoma.[33] Ewing confirmed this diagnosis when he reviewed the slides in 1919.[20] Liver cysts are fairly common, but most are either solitary or multiple simple non-neoplastic, non-parasitic cysts that usually are unilocular and lined with low cuboidal epithelium. They normally contain clear serous fluid and are associated with little fibrous stroma or cellular reaction. For a comprehensive review of the historical and clinical aspects of cystic disease of the liver, the reader is referred to the encyclopedic report of Jones[30] and the more recent collected reviews of Martin, et al.[44] and Longmire, et al.[36]

Edmondson characterized the neoplastic cystadenomas as usually containing mucinous fluid, multilocular, and lined with tall columnar epithelium with papillary infoldings.[18] These neoplastic cysts have a dense cellular connective tissue stroma (Figs. 7–1 and 7–2). These features are seen also in pancreatic cystadenomas, but are lacking in simple cystic disease. Although simple hepatic cysts often are associated with polycystic disease that may involve kidney, liver, pancreas, and lung, no such relationship has been described with hepatic cystadenomas. One case of pancreatic cystadenoma has been reported in a patient with an hepatic cystadenoma.[31] Perhaps one can relate this association to the common embryologic origin of both these organs.

Moore, et al.,[49] Gerber,[22] and more recently Short, et al.[54] have described cystadenomas related to papillomas of the bile ducts. In each instance the papillary bile duct tumor probably represented an outgrowth in-continuity with the wall of the neoplastic cyst—a dragging down stream, if you will, of part of the more solid lining of the tumor. Such biliary papillomas may produce jaundice.[49] The "hamartoma" recently reported by Ansari, et al. may be another example.[6]

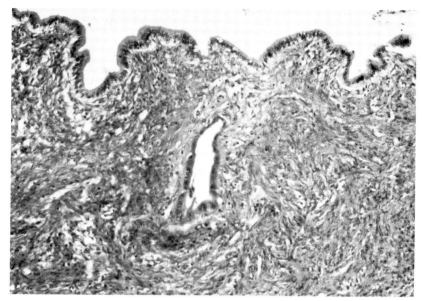

Figure 7–1. Cystadenoma demonstrating a portion of the cyst wall lined by mature, well differentiated columnar epithelium and adjacent fibrous stroma.

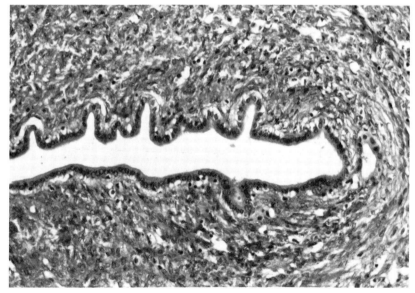

Figure 7–2. Cystadenoma (high power) showing rich cellularity of fibrous stroma and regular, mature character of the epithelial lining of a cyst.

Cystadenomas are very rare and malignant transformation is even rarer. Short, et al. in 1971 could find reports of only 30 cases of benign cystadenomas and a single case of cystadenocarcinoma in their collected review.[54] Other cases of cystadenoma or adenocarcinoma surely must be included in the voluminously documented collection of Jones (1923), but it is difficult to separate the neoplastic from the non-neoplastic in this review.[30] Marsh, et al.[43] and Martin, et al.[44] have added cases of resected benign cystadenomas since 1971. Greenwood and Orr reported epidermoid carcinoma in the lining of the wall of a simple cyst,[24] and Ameriks, et al. described a sarcomatous change in the wall of an 18 cm unilocular cyst in the right lobe of a 21-year-old woman.[5]

Two-thirds of the 32 collected benign cystadenomas are reported with adequate data about sex and age. All but one occurred in women who ranged from 14 to 69 years of age. Most of the women were between 35 and 60 years of age, and the single man was 69 years old.[43] The cystadenomas were intrahepatic in 24 instances, in the gallbladder in two instances, and involved an extrahepatic bile duct in the remaining six patients. The tumors were 1.5 to 30 cm in diameter, and usually presented with vague symptoms and/or an abdominal mass. Calcification was rarely present.[54]

Of 31 patients operated upon, 17 had an initial drainage procedure or only partial excision of the tumor. All seven patients with less than complete excision who were followed for more than three years have had recurrence of their tumor. Cattell, et al. reported recurrence ten years after partial excision of a cystadenoma, and the patient remained well six years after re-resection.[11]

The 1974 LTS found two patients who had resection of a benign cystadenoma. The first was a 20-year-old white female who had a clinical syndrome diagnosed as hepatitis. When needle biopsy yielded fluid, a laparotomy was done and a cystic structure of the liver hilum was noted and excised. This tumor was considered by the pathologist to be either a biliary cyst or a cystadenoma. Six months later the patient had itching and jaundice. At reoperation a soft mass was palpated within the dilated common hepatic duct, and a dumbbell-shaped tumor was teased out of the common hepatic duct and the left hepatic duct (Fig. 7–3). The left lateral segment of the liver was finally removed because of compromised biliary drainage. This patient was alive and well 61 months after her second operation.

The other patient was a 32-year-old white female who was known to have had an epigastric mass for one year prior to excision of a "grapefruit-sized" cystic mass in the left lobe of her liver. Several firm areas in the wall of this 10 cm cyst showed the typical histologic features of a benign cystadenoma. The patient has done well for 8½ years after resection.

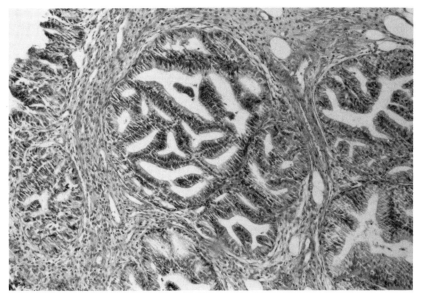

Figure 7–3. Cystadenocarcinoma. There is obvious malignant change in the lining of the cyst wall *(upper left)* and foci of carcinoma *(center)* in the fibrous stroma adjacent to the cyst wall.

Malignant transformation of a cystadenoma had not been encountered by Edmondson (1958), but Willis reported a papillary adenocarcinoma arising in a multilocular cyst in 1943,[60] and others[2, 15, 19, 43, 50] have reported individual cases of malignant cystadenocarcinoma since that time. Mersheimer resected an enormous tumor from a 54-year-old man by right lobectomy in 1954 which, in retrospect, was almost certainly a cystadenocarcinoma.[47]

Table 7–2 outlines the course of four patients reported in the literature who underwent resection for malignant cystadenoma and six other patients with cystadenocarcinoma encountered during the 1974 LTS (including three cases previously reported).[2, 14, 47] There were seven females and three males from 44 to 77 years of age. All patients presented with huge abdominal masses. In at least three instances, many liters of what was assumed to be ascitic fluid were aspirated before an accurate diagnosis of a liver tumor was made. Carcinomatous change was usually found in a solid mural plaque in a cyst wall in which the rest of the lining was made up of benign columnar epithelium (Fig. 7–4). Five of these patients are alive from 4 to 150 months after resection of their tumors, and five were dead of disease at 10 to 35 months. Extrahepatic metastases from cystadenocarcinoma of the liver have not been reported previously, although these tumors can reach enormous proportions within the capsule of the liver. However, Case 6, Table 7–2 had biopsy-proved peritoneal spread at reoperation prior to death. Of

Table 7–2.   Cystadenocarcinoma

Reported Cases

1. *53, Female.*   Left lobectomy done for 18 cm cystadenoma with foci of malignant change after 11-year history of abdominal swelling. Recurrence in omentum resected six months later but dead with persistent disease 11½ months after first operation.[59]

2. *52, W. Male.*   Cystojejunostomy done after 24 months of abdominal distention treated by multiple paracenteses. At reoperation three months later, right hepatic lobectomy done for 12 cm cystadenocarcinoma. Living and well almost three years after last operation.[15]

3. *48, Female.*   Wedge resection of cholangiocystic carcinoma. Alive more than five years after operation.[19]

4. *66, Female.*   One year of abdominal mass calcified on x-ray. Left lobectomy to remove large cyst with 3 cm mural focus of malignant alteration in biliary cystadenoma. Well four months after operation.[43]

1974 LTS Cases

5. *56, W. Female.*   Incision and drainage liver "abscess" in jaundiced patient. Repeat I. and D. seven months later when biopsy positive. Marsupialized and then partial left lobectomy after radiation therapy. Dead with recurrent disease 12 months after resection. Path.: Papillary cystadenocarcinoma.[14]

6. *53, W. Female.*   Left lobectomy for cystic tumor known to be present for at least two years. Microscopic foci of cystadenocarcinoma in wall of unilocular cyst. At laparotomy six months later had peritoneal metastases. Died ten months after liver resection.

7. *54, W. Male.*   Right lobectomy for enormous cystic liver tumor filling whole abdomen known to be present 17 months before operation. Died 11 months later after progressive decline.[47]

8. *77, W. Male.*   Aspiration of bilateral cysts, 14 months prior to partial excision. Died with recurrent abdominal tumor 35 months later. Path.: Papillary cystadenocarcinoma.

9. *53, W. Female.*   Left lobectomy for 20 cm cystadenocarcinoma and aspiration of 1000 cc of mucinous peritoneal fluid probably spilled by needle biopsy. Living and well 12½ years later.[3]

10. *44, W. Female.*   Cystogastrostomy and biopsy one month before left lobectomy for papillary cystadenocarcinoma. Alive and well 49 months later.

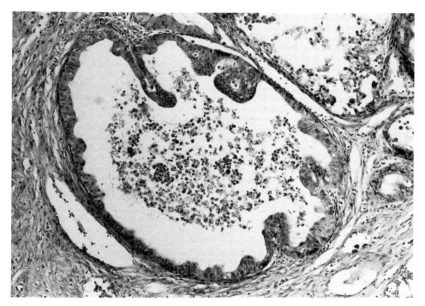

Figure 7–4. Cystadenocarcinoma (high power) with characteristic dilated duct appearance with intraductal papillary projections. Note the dedifferentiation of the epithelial cells lining the wall of the cystic space.

course, this may have represented iatrogenic spread rather than spontaneous metastasis.

The lessons seem clear. The wall of any cystic tumor of the liver should be searched carefully for suspicious mural plaques of papillary outgrowths, which should be biopsied when found. Particularly suspect are multilocular cysts, cysts that contain mucinous fluid or other than clear serous fluid, and cysts in association with jaundice. When possible, all cysts lined with tall columnar epithelium should be excised, rather than drained or marsupialized. When cystadenoma or cystadenocarcinoma is diagnosed, operative cholangiography should be performed to rule out the presence of an associated biliary polyp. These tumors are slow-growing and are quite similar clinically, histologically, and prognostically to pancreatic cystadenomas and cystadenocarcinomas.

VASCULAR TUMORS

Benign hemangiomas are quite common in the livers of pediatric and adult patients, but have been excluded from this review. The terms Kupffer cell sarcoma, hemangioendothelioma, angiosarcoma, angiomatous mesenchymoma, and hemangioblastoma have all been used to

186   SOLID LIVER TUMORS

describe neoplastic vascular tumors originating in the human liver. "Spindle cell" change has been considered as a variant of epithelial cancer by Stewart[57] and as a synonym for Kupffer cell sarcoma by others. Angiosarcoma in the adult has been closely related to Thorotrast injection[10] and vinyl chloride exposure.[8, 39, 53]

The reader is referred to the classic references of Edmondson[17, 18] and the more recent articles of Blumenfeld, et al.,[9] Dehner and Ishak,[16] and Pollice[52] for a more thorough exposition of the prevailing (although not necessarily uniform) classification of the various histologic patterns of vascular tumors, and for a comprehensive review of clinical correlations. In most reported series, vascular tumors that occur in infants appear to behave differently from those in adults, and therefore are considered separately.

PEDIATRIC VASCULAR TUMORS

Infantile hemangioendothelioma of the liver is a rare tumor (about 60 cases reported so far) that often occurs in premature babies with other congenital malformations. It usually is found within the first few months of life. It may be associated with congestive heart failure (attributed to arteriovenous fistulas in the tumor) or with cutaneous angiomas, which do not represent metastases but rather another manifestation of what is probably a common dysembryogenetic problem. The patient with this tumor may have multiple nodules spread

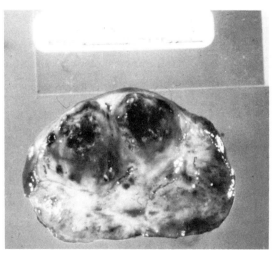

Figure 7-5. Six cm solitary infantile hemangioendothelioma wedged out from the lower aspect of the right lobe of a 1-month-old asymptomatic female (Case 4, Table 7-3). Photo provided courtesy of E. Orfei, M.D., Loyola University of Chicago.

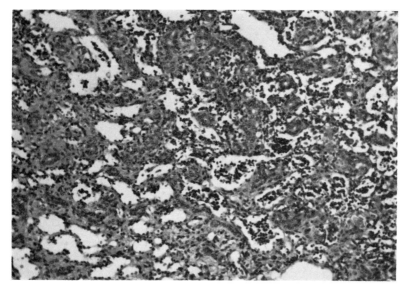

Figure 7–6.   Infantile hemangioendothelioma. The neoplasm is composed of a multitude of dilated vascular channels containing prominent groups of hematopoietic cells. Bile duct structures compressed by the dilated vascular channels are present.

throughout both lobes of the liver, or may have only a solitary nodule (Fig. 7–5). Individual nodules usually appear gray-white on the periphery with a red, blue, or purple center. Necrosis and hemorrhage into the tumor or into the peritoneal cavity are fairly common. Extrahepatic metastases do occur.[16]

Infantile hemangioendotheliomas show a variety of patterns under the microscope. They are composed of large and small endothelium-lined channels within a reticular framework. The endothelial cells range from a thin and flattened appearance (Fig. 7–6) to rather large plump cells that may narrow the lumen of the vessel (Fig. 7–7). Rare mitoses may be present, but no significant atypical nuclear changes are noted. Dilated sinusoidal channels may show large numbers of nucleated red blood cells. Occasional areas of vascular thrombosis may be present with associated foci of active proliferation of fibroblasts. The margins of the lesions are not well demarcated and there may be infiltration of surrounding liver.

Dehner and Ishak found seven of 12 hemangioendotheliomas to be solitary,[16] but Blumenfeld, et al. in a review of the literature found 32 of 37 hemangioendotheliomas in infants to be multiple. Of the five remaining patients with solitary tumors, one newborn infant died in congestive heart failure with no therapy directed at his abdominal mass. At postmortem examination his heart showed no congenital defect, and his liver showed a large solitary infantile hemangioendothelioma. The other four solitary tumors were treated with resection and the patients were all alive at the time of this report.

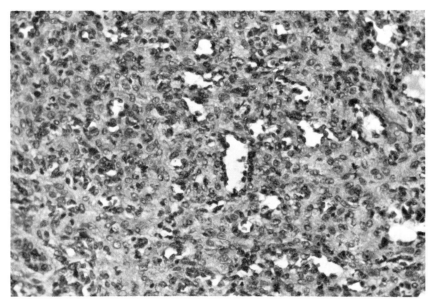

Figure 7–7. Hemangioendothelioma. A high-power view showing a focus of prominent thick-walled vascular channels lined by plump endothelial cells.

Two patients were male and two were female. Two of these tumors occurred in the right lobe and two in the left.[9]

Although some authors consider these tumors to be benign because they usually remain within the liver capsule, most regard them as malignant with an expected fatal outcome if untreated. There have been three reports of spontaneous remission in children who had biopsy-proved evidence of hemangioendothelioma diagnosed at laparotomy, and who were alive and well 4½, five, and 25 years later respectively without subsequent therapy.[17, 46] Radiotherapy may have a place in the treatment of these vascular tumors, but experience to date has not been sufficient to permit conclusions to be drawn about this.

The diagnosis of hemangioendothelioma should be considered whenever congestive heart failure occurs in a young infant with an abdominal mass. Angiography is helpful in demonstrating multifocal disease. Needle biopsy is to be avoided because of the vascularity of this tumor. Resection, when feasible, is the treatment of choice. If the tumors are multiple, a trial of radiation therapy may be given, and the child should be supported vigorously because of the possibility of a remission or involution of the vascular tumor as he matures. However, most patients with untreated infantile hemangioendotheliomas go on to a rapidly progressive course and death. When the tumor can be resected, the prognosis is good.[9] Prednisone[29] and hepatic artery ligation[3] have been advocated as symptomatic treatment in patients with nonresectable tumors.

Adult Vascular Tumors

Angiosarcoma in adults is a rare but invariably fatal disease unless treated and is characterized by a very rapid progressive downhill course, hemorrhagic ascites and cachexia leading to death within six months. Adam, et al. collected from the literature 39 cases of angiosarcoma unrelated to Thorotrast in adult patients, to which they added four additional adult cases.[1] Although angiosarcoma in adults may occur in cirrhotic livers, none of Adam's cases had an associated cirrhosis.

Thorotrast, a colloidal suspension of 232-thorium dioxide, was used extensively in diagnostic radiology for pyelography and angiography from the time of its introduction in 1928 until MacMahon, et al. (1947) reported a case of angiosarcoma of the liver associated with Thorotrast administration.[40] The liver takes up about 70 to 75 per cent of the retained Thorotrast, and the extremely long half-life of the alpha-particle emitting isotope ensures prolonged liver injury. Liver tumors may occur up to 33 years after Thorotrast injection. Two-thirds of 115 reported Thorotrast-induced liver tumors were hemangioendotheliomas,[10] although this proportion may be changing.[53] Hemoperitoneum due to rupture is common, and bloody ascites occurs preterminally in many patients. We were unable to find a report of long-term survival in a patient with resection of a Thorotrast-induced angiosarcoma.

At least 26 cases of angiosarcoma have been found in association with vinyl chloride exposure.[8] All seven vinyl chloride workers at the Louisville B. F. Goodrich plant who developed angiosarcoma of the liver had some form of nonalcoholic cirrhosis. The mean latent period of vinyl chloride exposure before development of an angiosarcoma was 17 years.[8] Makk, et al. recently have studied 15 of these cases, none of which came to resection. Seven of eight patients coming to autopsy had tumor spread outside of the liver capsule.[37, 39]

1974 Liver Tumor Survey

The 1974 LTS included six patients with malignant tumors classified as of vascular origin. Five occurred in infants less than 2 months of age, and one was found in a 79-year-old white female. Table 7–3 presents the details and the results achieved by resectional therapy. Figures 7–8 and 7–9 illustrate the gross and microscopic features of angiosarcoma.

Resection will rarely be possible in adult patients with Thorotrast- or vinyl chloride-associated tumors because of the associated liver fibrosis. However, when angiosarcoma is found in an otherwise normal liver in an adult, or when a solitary or unilobar multinodular

Table 7-3. Vascular Neoplasms – 1974 Liver Tumor Survey: Clinical Data

	AGE/SEX	SYMPTOMS	TUMOR	DIAGNOSIS	OPERATION	RESULT
(1)	3 days WM	Mass alpha-fetoprotein pos.	Solitary 18 cm right lobe	Infantile hemangio-endothelioma	Wedge	AFD 27 months
(2)	9 days WM	Mass and lethargy	Solitary 8 cm l. lat. seg.	"	Wedge	AFD 117 months
(3)	3 weeks WM	Mass	Solitary 12 cm left lobe	"	Left lobectomy	AFD 169 months
(4)	1 month WF	Mass	Solitary 6 cm right lobe	"	Wedge	NFU
(5)	2 months WM	Mass and heart failure	Solitary 6 cm right lobe	"	Right lobectomy	AFD 44 months
(6)	79 years WF	Mass	Solitary 10 cm l. lat. seg.	Angiosarcoma	L. lat. seg.	AFD 4 months

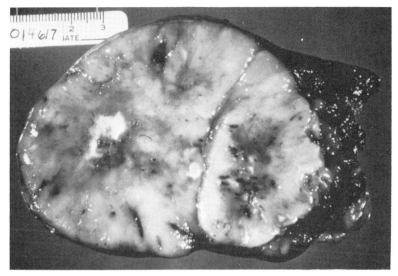

Figure 7–8. Cross-section of 10 cm angiosarcoma resected by left lateral segmentectomy from a 79-year-old female (Case 6, Table 7–3). Photo courtesy of E. Orfei, M.D., Loyola University of Chicago.

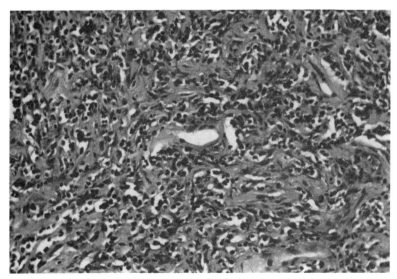

Figure 7–9. Angiosarcoma. A malignant vascular neoplasm composed of spindly endothelial cells forming fine vascular slit channels.

hemangioendothelioma is found in a child, resection should always be attempted.

MESENCHYMAL HAMARTOMA

Mesenchymal hamartoma of infancy is the only primary liver tumor that we have recognized as a "true" hamartoma. Under the microscope the tumor is characterized by an abundant highly cellular embryonal mesenchyme, throughout which are found random groups of hepatic cells and bile ducts. This largely myxoid background usually encloses multiple cysts lined by flattened cells that probably are mesodermal. The cysts are always multiple and may produce a honeycomb appearance. Because the cystic components may be the most impressive feature of these tumors, they have been called "lymphangiomas" by some authors (Figs. 7–10 and 7–11).

Maresch (1903)[42] reported a patient with such a lesion, which he called "lymphangioma of the liver." In 1958 Edmondson attached the term "mesenchymal hamartoma" to this rare lesion, which he considered to be the result of a failure in the normal development of the embryonic and fetal liver, or a degenerative change. He cited eight

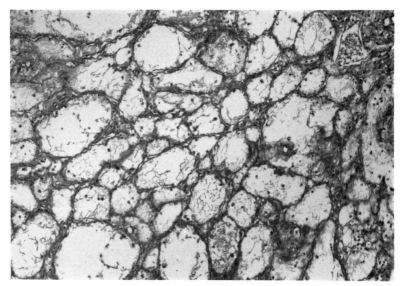

Figure 7–10. Mesenchymal harmartoma. Multiple cystic channels arising from degeneration of mesenchymal connective tissue. The cystic spaces resemble vascular channels, and this pattern may be confused with cystic lymphangioma.

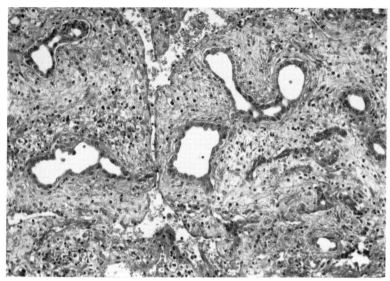

Figure 7–11. Mesenchymal hamartoma. Characteristic epithelial lined cystic structures surrounded by loose differentiated mesenchyme.

reported cases, including that of Maresch, and added four more.[18] Ishida, et al. found five additional published cases, added another one, and tabulated the reported world experience up to 1965.[28]

To that summary can be added 15 additional cases[7, 25, 26, 41, 51, 56, 58] (Table 7–4). Two other cases are described by Lannon[34] as hamartomas; one occurred in a 6-month-old female whose breasts stopped lactating after removal of the tumor, but the details of this report are not complete enough to be sure that these tumors were truly mesenchymal hamartomas as defined by Edmondson, and therefore they have not been included.

There are 10 female and 18 male patients in this collected experience. Three patients were more than 2 years old (3, 3, and 5 years) and the youngest was 3 months of age. In almost every instance, a healthy youngster developed a mass as the first, and usually the only, sign of trouble. Rapid enlargement often occurred, probably because of fluid accumulation in the cystic component of the tumor. Liver function tests were within normal limits in these patients. When preoperative angiography was done, the tumors were usually avascular. Ultrasonography was used by Ishida, et al. to differentiate cystic and solid areas within the tumors.[28]

At operation the tumors originated in the right lobe in 19 patients, in the left lobe in five, from the area of the central plane along the free edge of the liver in three, and the location was not indicated for one patient. Nine tumors were attached to the lower surface of the liver by

Table 7–4. Mesenchymal Hamartoma: Collected Experience (added to Ishida, et al.[28])

REFERENCE/YEAR	AGE/SEX	SYMPTOM	TUMOR	OPERATION	RESULT
1. Henson, et al. 1956[26]	14 months M	Mass	Mostly solid 15 cm right lobe	Excised	Op. death
2. Henson, et al. 1956[26]	10 months M	Mass	Multicystic 20 cm right lobe	Aspirated, then excised	AFD 1½ years
3. Stephens and Jenevein 1965[56]	13 months M	Mass, diarrhea	Multicystic 16 cm left lobe	Enucleated	NFU
4. Stephens and Jenevein 1965[56]	24 months M	Mass	Multicystic 22 cm right lobe	Wedge	NFU
5. Sutton and Eller 1968[58]	9 months F	Mass	Pedunculated 18 cm right lobe	Wedge	NFU
6. Sutton and Eller 1968[58]	10 months M	Mass	Multicystic 20 cm right lobe	Right lobectomy	Op. death
7. Sutton and Eller 1968[58]	13 months M	Mass	Multicystic 16 cm central	Extended right lobectomy	Op. death

8. Sutton and Eller 1968[58]	15 months F	Mass	Multicystic pedunculated 23 cm right lobe	Wedge	NFU
9. Bienaymé and Prawerman 1969[7]	18 months M	Mass	Multicystic left lobe	Wedge	AFD 1 year
10. Bienaymé and Prawerman 1969[7]	3 years M	Mass	Multicystic 15 cm right lobe	Enucleated	NFU
11. Bienaymé and Prawerman 1969[7]	3 years M	Mass	Multicystic 2100 gm left lobe	Enucleated	NFU
12. Hartemann, et al. 1969[25]	13 months M	Mass, malaise	Multicystic 17 cm central	Right lobectomy	AFD 7 months
13. Hartemann, et al. 1969[25]	27 months M	Mass	Multicystic 850 gm right lobe	Right lobectomy	AFD 9 years
14. Malt, et al. 1970[41]	5 months M	Mass	9.5 cm cystic falciform lig. plane	Enucleated	NFU
15. Nikaidoh, et al. 1970[51]	13 months F	Mass	14 cm pedunculated left lobe	Wedge	AFD 8 months

Table 7–5.   Mesenchymal Hamartoma—1974 Liver Tumor Survey

AGE/SEX	SYMPTOMS	TUMOR	OPERATION	RESULT
1. 8 months WM	Mass	Solitary, nodular 16 cm right lobe	Enucleation	Op. death
2. 12 months NM	Mass 5 months	Multicystic 18 cm right lobe	Wedge	AFD 9 months
3. 18 months WF	Mass	Multicystic 16 cm right lobe	Right lobectomy	NFU
4. 2 years WM	Mass 1 year	Jelly-like 12 cm tumor right lobe	Right lobectomy	AFD 124 months
5. 5 years WF	Mass 4 months	Multicystic 22 cm right lobe	Extended right lobectomy	AFD 47 months

a narrow margin of normal tissue through which excision could be accomplished easily. The tumors were all very large, averaging more than 16 cm in diameter at operation.

Twenty seven of the 28 tumors were enucleated or excised with a narrow margin of normal tissue. In a few instances a portion of the wall of the tumor was left for technical reasons, without subsequent morbidity. The unresected patient was a 3-month-old female who succumbed to rapid growth of the tumor.[28] There were six operative deaths, but there was no evidence of recurrence in the 18 patients who survived operation and were followed for periods of up to nine years.

Five patients with mesenchymal hamartomas were found in the 1974 LTS. Table 7–5 outlines the details of their histories. The presentation was typical in each case, with the discovery of an enlarging abdominal mass in an otherwise healthy child. At operation these five tumors were all solitary and showed multilocular cystic change; they averaged 17 cm in size. Preoperative differential diagnoses included neurogenic and renal tumors, as well as primary liver carcinoma.

There was no evidence in the literature, nor in these collected patients, of intrahepatic metastasis or extrahepatic spread. It would be reasonable to assume that all multilocular cystic lesions in young children are probably mesenchymal hamartomas, although an occasional embryonal sarcoma may have a cystic component. Frozen section should easily differentiate between these two lesions. Operative excision is recommended in every case. Two unoperated patients have apparently succumbed to the mass effects of rapidly enlarging lesions.[28] The collected experience suggests that enucleation of the tumor may be sufficient, and probably is preferable when excision through normal liver might jeopardize the life of an infant patient.

SARCOMAS

Primary malignant tumors of the liver originating in mesenchymal elements are quite rare. Various combinations of malignant and/or benign epithelium with malignant and/or benign mesenchyme have been called "mixed tumors," "hepatoblastoma," etc. by Edmondson,[17] Ishak and Glunz,[27] and others who have studied this problem and pioneered in its elucidation. Goldman and Friedman[23] and Lorimer[37] have reported large tumors in three females (aged 8, 15, and 65 years) in which definitely malignant mesenchymal elements were found together with either benign or malignant epithelial components. The two younger patients probably fit into the category that we have called "embryonal sarcoma," but the 65-year-old represents a unique experience in our review, and the relationship of her lesion to hepatoblastoma or adult sarcomas is obscure.

The tumors that we have termed "hepatoblastoma" in Chapter Five always contained malignant epithelial elements, although they often also had areas of cellular, immature mesenchyme which, on a few occasions, exhibited nuclear variation that might suggest malignancy. However, whenever the mesenchyme was clearly malignant and when it dominated the histologic features of the tumor, we have chosen to categorize the tumor as a sarcoma. The presentation and course of these patients with "sarcoma" was sufficiently different from the "hepatoblastoma" cases to justify this distinction.

The tumors we shall call "sarcoma" have been termed by others malignant mesenchymoma, rhabdomyosarcoma, embryonal sarcoma, mixed tumors, spindle cell tumors, or even a variant of hepatoblastoma. Malignant mesenchymal tumors in children may be more difficult to categorize on histologic grounds than those in adults, which tend to show more differentiation, although Mattila[45] recently reported the occurrence of a ruptured, bleeding, huge, but solitary undifferentiated sarcoma in a 68-year-old female patient. Longmire, et al. also reported a malignant mesenchymoma in a 20-year-old female patient who survived only four months after right lobectomy.[35]

There have been a few reports of differentiated sarcomas in adults, and these are outlined below.

Fibrosarcoma of the Liver

Alrenga collected 11 cases of fibrosarcoma and added a 12th.[4] These tumors occurred in eight male and two female patients (sex not mentioned in two) ranging from 30 to 66 years of age, three of whom had cirrhosis of the liver. All but two of these patients were dead within 12 months of diagnosis of their disease. A patient who died five years after diagnosis and radiation therapy for a fibrosarcoma was found at postmortem examination to have a 12,150 gm tumor in his liver and lung metastases. The other survivor was alive one year after resection of a 2780 gm tumor. These tumors obviously can reach enormous size within Glisson's capsule and probably metastasize late.

No tumors classified as fibrosarcoma were found in the 1974 LTS.

LEIOMYOSARCOMA OF THE LIVER

Malignant and benign smooth muscle tumors probably originate in walls of blood vessels when they are primary in the liver. Wilson[61] and Fong and Ruebner[21] have recently discussed primary smooth muscle tumors of the liver. Of the collected eight cases, six were malignant and two were benign. Four patients underwent resection; there were three survivors for up to two years at the time of publication, and one was dead with metastatic disease $1\frac{1}{2}$ years after resection. The tumors can reach enormous size, and metastases apparently occur late.[21] No cases of leiomyosarcoma were found in the 1974 LTS.

ANGIOSARCOMA

These tumors are discussed under a separate heading of "vascular tumors" (see above).

LIPOSARCOMA

We could not find a single clear-cut case of liposarcoma in our literature review, and none were found in the 1974 LTS. Wolloch, et al. mention a 22-year-old female who died after resection of a "lipomyxosarcoma" of the right lobe of the liver.[62] No histologic sections were presented in this report, and it is difficult to know whether this tumor should be classified separately or put into the category of undifferentiated sarcomas.

SARCOMAS IN CHILDREN

Primary sarcomas in children often are difficult to categorize into the standard histologic patterns of adult sarcomas. The tumors may not show the pathognomonic features of fibrosarcoma, liposarcoma, leiomyosarcoma, etc. In some instances, the histologic pattern of a single tumor may vary from field to field and include typical elements of several types of sarcoma. We have chosen to categorize all sarcomas in children in the 1974 LTS as "embryonal sarcoma"—first because the 11 malignant primary mesenchymal tumors we found in pediatric patients all had many histologic features in common, and second because the presentation and progress of these patients was fairly uniform.

In 1973 Stanley, et al. reported three boys, ages 6, 10, and 10 years, with malignant mesenchymal tumors. Two had resection but none were cured. He collected nine other cases from the literature, several of which have been cited by Edmondson.[55] Keeling reported three cases of highly malignant pure rhabdomyosarcomas of the liver in children more than 6 years of age,[32] but such tumors are extremely rare.

The 11 tumors found in children in the 1974 LTS and a single adult tumor had a unique histologic appearance, illustrated in Figures 7–12 and 7–13, that was characterized predominantly by a loose myxoid connective tissue background containing spindle- and stellate-shaped fibroblast-like cells with large folded nuclei, prominent nucleoli, and fine delicate filamentous cytoplasmic processes. Occasional bizarre mitoses were seen. Embedded within this tissue were both solid and ductular epithelial structures. The ductules, composed of cuboidal-shaped cells with large, slightly irregular, folded nuclei and abundant finely granular eosinophilic cytoplasm, usually were arranged in a single layer, although an occasional double layer was noted. Well-defined lumens

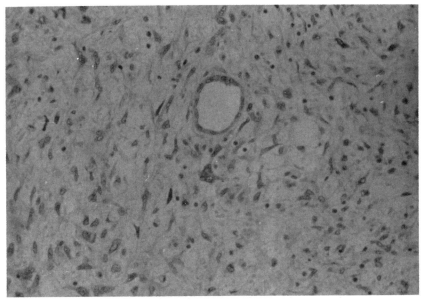

Figure 7–12. Embryonal sarcoma. A characteristic field showing a centrally embedded epithelial structure surrounded by atypical stellate mesenchymal cells.

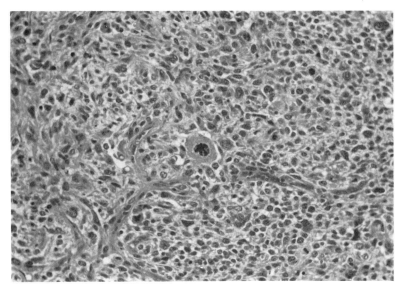

Figure 7–13. Embryonal sarcoma. Large bizarre undifferentiated mesenchymal cells with a spindle-shaped configuration and large central bizarre mitosis.

or solid nests of cells were present. The ductular structures showed an associated basement membrane, which was less evident with the solid groups of epithelial cells. Endothelial lined vascular channels were present in the connective tissue background. The presence of a basement membrane in association with the ductular and some of the solid epithelial structures suggested an abortive attempt to form bile ducts. No specific features of mesenchymal differentiation, such as rhabdomyoblasts, were found. The predominant embryonal mesenchymal background of this neoplasm, with its associated epithelial duct-like structures, was strongly reminiscent of the appearance of vitelline ducts and surrounding mesenchyme in the early stages of embryonic development. Table 7–6 outlines the clinical data on these 12 patients.

The 11 pediatric cases were all over 6 years of age except Case 1. Five patients were female and six were male. The tumors averaged 18 cm in diameter, and one tumor exhibited some cystic areas. Rare foci of ductular epithelial structures were found in at least seven tumors. In two patients the malignant mesenchymal component dominated, but epithelial elements showed significant histologic atypia. These tumors had been called "hepatoblastoma," "undifferentiated mesenchymal sarcoma," "rhabdomyosarcoma," "carcinosarcoma," "malignant mesenchymoma," "malignant mixed tumor," and "spindle cell sarcoma" by the hospital pathologists.

Case 6 had a particularly interesting presentation. A right atriotomy was done in an 8-year-old boy after five months of severe cardiac

Table 7-6. Embryonal Sarcoma—1974 Liver Tumor Survey

Age/Sex	Symptoms	Tumor	Operation	Result	Comment
1. 17 months WM	Mass, malaise	Solitary 11 cm left lobe	Left lobectomy	DWD 7 months	
2. 6½ years M	Anorexia, fatigue, fever	Solitary 15 cm left lobe	Left lat. segmentectomy	DWD 36 months	Pulmonary metastases also excised
3. 7 years WF	1 month pain and mass	Solitary 10 cm central	Extended right lobectomy	DWD 23 months	Bone metastasis
4. 7 years WM	Mass, preop. radiotherapy	Solitary 15 cm central	Extended right lobectomy	DWD 2 months	Called rhabdomyosarcoma
5. 7½ years WF	Pain and mass, 9 months	Solitary 26 cm right lobe	Right lobectomy	DWD 4 months	
6. 8 years WM	Cardiac myxoma excised, now fever and malaise	Solitary left lobe, IVC block	Left lobectomy	Operative death	See text for more history
7. 8 years WM	4–5 weeks pain	Bilobed 15 cm right lobe	Wedge	DWD 25 months	Retroperitoneal recurrence
8. 10 years WF	5 months weight loss 2 months pain	Solitary 35 cm central	Extended right lobectomy	Operative death	Desperation operation
9. 10 years NF	3 weeks fever, malaise	Solitary 25 cm right lobe	Right lobectomy	AFD 26 months	
10. 12 years	Mass, 2 weeks	Solitary 10 cm left lat. segment	Left lateral segmentectomy	DWD 8 months	
11. 14 years F	—	Solitary cystic 16 cm right lobe	Right lobectomy	DWD 17 months	
12. 47 WF	Pain and mass	Solitary right lobe	Wedge	DWD 16 months	Re-excised 7 months after first operation

symptoms. An intracardiac "myxoma" was resected that appeared to arise from the inferior vena cava. Three months later the child had fever, malaise, and evidence of obstruction of the inferior vena cava at the level of the diaphragm. A "cold" area was seen in the left lobe of the liver on radioisotope scan. At reoperation he was found to have a large solitary nodular mass that replaced the left liver lobe, and that had grown into and occluded the inferior vena cava at the level of the dia-phragm. When excision was attempted the tumor shelled out easily from the inferior vena cava and the right hepatic veins, but the patient did not survive the operation. The tumor had the typical histologic ap-pearance of an embryonal sarcoma.

There were two operative deaths, and eight other patients died from two to 36 months after resection in this small series. Local recur-rence was the rule after resection, and metastases to the lung, bone, and peritoneum were present at the time of death in most patients. The sole survivor was a 10-year-old black girl whose 35 cm solitary tumor showed definite malignant change of the mesenchyme, with areas suggesting fibrosarcoma, myxosarcoma, and possible angiosar-coma, and some areas of benign epithelium. She is alive more than two years after right lobectomy without evidence of recurrence (Case 9, Table 7–6).

The sole adult patient with a primary liver sarcoma found in the 1974 LTS was a 47-year-old white woman who had initial excision of her tumor by wedge resection. Seven months later a discrete solitary 10 cm recurrence was excised from the lower edge of the right lobe of the liver by enucleation. Six months later a cystic recurrence was found in the retroperitoneum, and she died with recurrent disease 16 months after the initial resection. The tumor had all the typical histologic fea-tures of the 11 pediatric embryonal sarcomas categorized above.

Embryonal sarcomas occur in older children and in an occasional adult. The lack of liver cell epithelial elements, the presence of a pre-dominantly malignant mesenchymal component, and the unfortunate clinical outcome for most patients clearly distinguish this lesion from the hepatoblastomas and liver cell carcinomas of childhood. Cystic areas may occur in these largely solid tumors, which may reach enor-mous size before extrahepatic spread. No relationship with cirrhosis has been established. The tumors should be resected when possible, al-though the prognosis is worse than with epithelial tumors. Radiother-apy has not proved to be of benefit in three patients with embryonal sarcoma.[55]

MISCELLANEOUS TUMORS

The 1974 LTS included four other benign solid tumors removed from pediatric patients, the case histories of whom are outlined in

Table 7-7. Miscellaneous Benign Tumors

	Age/Sex	Symptoms	Tumor	Operation	Outcome
Benign mesenchymal tumor	7 years NF	Anorexia, mass, distention 1 week	8 cm solitary right lobe.	Wedge	AFD 18 months
Myxoma	6 years WF	Asymptomatic mass	16 cm solitary left lobe	Wedge	AFD 67 months
Myxoma	7 years WM	Abdominal mass, known since birth with recent increase.	Large solitary, with invasion of diaphragm and abdominal wall.	Left lobectomy	AFD 61 months
Bile duct fibroadenoma	10 weeks WM	Asymptomatic mass	10 cm solitary right lobe	Right lobectomy	AFD 191 months

Table 7–7. There was a single benign mesenchymal tumor composed of round and vesicular fibroblast-like cells that were associated with fine fibrillary reticular processes and embedded in a loose areolar backgound. Occasional atypical mitoses were present, and there were other histologic features that suggested malignancy. However, the over-all histologic picture and the patient's course after resection supported the pathologist's impression of benign morphology in this purely mesodermal tumor.

Two myxomas were removed from 6- and 7-year-old children. The tumors were described as solitary, white, and shiny. Only a narrow rim of normal liver was excised with each tumor, but both patients have done well subsequently without evidence of recurrent disease. Although histologically benign, one of these tumors had extended into the surrounding structures and required excision of portions of the anterior abdominal wall, the diaphragm, and a small patch of pericardium (Fig. 7–14). Edmondson reported a single case of myxoma in a 58-year-old white male, but the clinical and histologic features of that case suggested a more malignant process.[18]

The "bile duct fibroadenoma" was a 13 cm tumor that occupied an estimated 80 per cent of the right lobe of this infant's liver. Its histologic appearance is perhaps best described by the term we have chosen (although it is a new term), since it consisted of irregular but mature bile ducts surrounded by dense fibrous tissue quite reminiscent of the pattern of a benign fibroadenoma of the breast. Case 5 of Bienaymé and

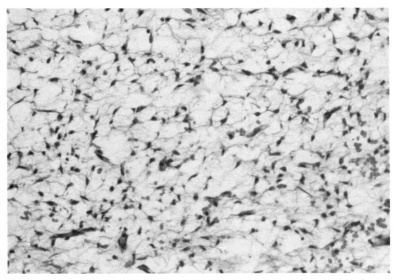

Figure 7–14. Embryonal myxoma. A characteristic field of stellate-shaped fibrillar fibroblast-like cells embedded in a loose areolar mucopolysaccharide stroma.

Prawerman may represent a similar tumor, which was treated with radiation therapy after biopsy.[7]

The microscopic pattern exhibited by this "bile duct fibroadenoma" is similar to the small subcapsular nodules occurring in adults and variously called "bile duct adenoma" or "hamartoma." Although these tumors were excluded from the 1974 LTS and are always small and of little clinical significance, they deserve a brief discussion here because the unwary may confuse them histologically with carcinoma.

Edmondson defined a bile duct adenoma as an innocuous subcapsular gray circumscribed tumor that might be either solitary or multiple. These lesions were first described by von Meyenburg in 1898.[64] Usually less than 1 cm in diameter, the nodules show mature bile duct cells embedded in dense collagen.[18] Bile-stained proteinaceous material is seen occasionally within the lumen of the ducts. Henson, et al. found seven such lesions in a 47-year review of the files of the Mayo Clinic. Their lesions were always incidental findings at laparotomy or postmortem examination, and the largest was 1.5 cm in diameter.[26] More recently Chung has reviewed the subject and emphasized the possible relationship of multiple bile duct adenomas to polycystic disease of the liver.[12] "Hamartoma" may be a more appropriate term than adenoma

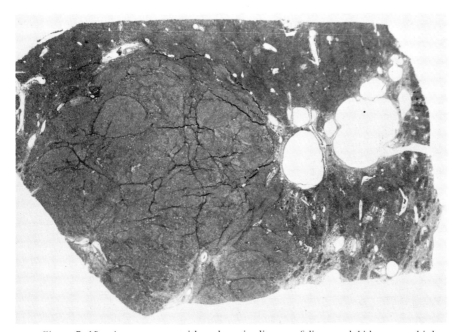

Figure 7–15. Autopsy case with polycystic disease of liver and kidneys, multiple tiny bile duct adenomas, and several nodules of focal nodular hyperplasia. Low power view illustrates a single nodule of hyperplasia, epithelium lined cystic spaces, and normal surrounding liver parenchyma.

for these rare and probably insignificant lesions, since no potential for progressive growth or malignant transformation has yet been clearly demonstrated. Perhaps the greatest importance of these small tumors to the clinician lies in the danger of interpreting such nodules as metastatic tumor. Frozen section diagnosis by pathologists unfamiliar with this lesion may be misleading in this regard.

We have recently seen at autopsy, in the liver of a woman with polycystic renal disease, four FNH tumors up to 4 cm in diameter associated with multiple hepatic cysts and many tiny bile duct adenomas (hamartomas) (Fig. 7–15). Although a solitary case, this raises the most interesting questions about etiology.

TERATOMAS

A solitary instance of teratoma was encountered in the 1974 LTS, and this case has been reported previously by Clatworthy, et al.[13] and Misugi, et al.[48] An otherwise healthy 2½-year-old white male child was noted to have a large right upper quadrant mass that showed calcification in a radiogram. Although multiple small pulmonary metastases were found after liver dissection was well under way, a 14 cm multinodular tumor was resected by right hepatic lobectomy. The child died ten days later with multiple complications. Histologic elements of all three germinal layers were represented in the tumor with areas of nerve, kidney, adrenal, cartilage, and ameloblastoma. There were also epithelial and mesenchymal elements more characteristic of hepatoblastoma.

Misugi, et al. collected the previously reported five cases in addition to discussing the case mentioned above, which is apparently the only malignant "true" teratoma so far reported in children. Its occurrence raises interesting questions about the relationship of hepatoblastoma and teratoma to the embryology of the liver. Pollice reports an additional case of a benign teratoma.[52] The benign tumors usually are encapsulated, often are cystic, and have been easily resectable. Long-term survival of 14 years has been reported by Yarborough.[63]

REFERENCES

1. Adam, Y. G., Huvos, A. G., and Hajdu, S. I.: Malignant vascular tumors of liver. Ann Surg. 175(3):375, 1972.
2. Adson, M. A., and Jones, R. R.: Hepatic lobectomy. Arch. Surg. 92:631, 1966.
3. Adlercreutz, H., and Tenhunen, R.: Some aspects of the interaction between natural and synthetic female sex hormones and the liver. Am. J. Med. 49:630, 1970.

4. Alrenga, D. P.: Primary fibrosarcoma of the liver. Cancer *36*:446, 1975.
5. Ameriks, J., Appleman, H., and Frey, C.: Malignant non-parasitic cyst of the liver: case report. Ann. Surg. *176*:713, 1972.
6. Ansari, A., et al.: Cystic hamartoma of the left hepatic bile duct. J.A.M.A. *235*:630, 1976.
7. Bienaymé, J., and Prawerman, A.: L'hamartome du foie chez l'enfant à l'exclusion des angiomes. Ann. Chir. Infant. *10*:399, 1969.
8. Block, J. B.: Vinyl chloride and angiosarcoma. J. Ky. Med. Assoc. *72*:483, 1974.
9. Blumenfeld, T. A., Fleming, I. D., and Johnson, W. W.: Hemangioendothelioma of the liver. Report of a case and review of the literature. Cancer *24*:853, 1969.
10. Campbell, I. N., and Webb, J. N.: Haemoperitoneum complicating thorotrast-induced haemangioendothelioma of the liver. J. Coll. Surg. Edin. *19*:233, 1974.
11. Cattell, R. B., Braasch, J. W., and Kahr, F.: Polypoid epithelial tumors of the bile ducts. N. Engl. J. Med. *266*:57, 1962.
12. Chung, E. B.: Multiple bile duct hamartomas. Cancer *26*:278, 1970.
13. Clatworthy, H. W., Schiller, M., and Grosfeld, J. L.: Primary liver tumors in infancy and childhood. Arch. Surg. *109*:143, 1974.
14. Curutchet, H. P., et al.: Primary liver cancer. Surgery *70*:467, 1971.
15. Dean, D. L., and Bauer, H. M.: Primary cystic carcinoma of the liver. Am. J. Surg. *117*:416, 1969.
16. Dehner, L. P., and Ishak, K. G.: Vascular tumors of the liver in infants and children. Arch. Pathol. *92*:101, 1971.
17. Edmondson, H. A.: Progress in pediatrics: differential diagnosis of tumors and tumor-like lesions of liver in infancy and childhood. A.M.A. J. Dis. Child. *91*:168, 1956.
18. Edmondson, H. A.: Tumors of the liver and intrahepatic bile ducts. Section VII - Fascicle 25, Atlas of Tumor Pathology, Armed Forces Institute of Pathology, 1958.
19. El-Domeiri, A. A., et al.: Primary malignant tumors of the liver. Cancer *27*:7, 1971.
20. Ewing, J.: Neoplastic Diseases. 1st Ed. Philadelphia, W. B. Saunders Co., 1919.
21. Fong, J. A., and Ruebner, B. H.: Primary leiomyosarcoma of the liver. Hum. Pathol. *5(1)*:115, 1974.
22. Gerber, A.: Retention cyst of the liver due to a bile duct polyp. Ann. Surg. *140*:906, 1954.
23. Goldman, R. L., and Friedman, N. B.: Rhabdomyosarcohepatoma in an adult and embryonal hepatoma in a child. Am. J. Clin. Pathol. *51*:137, 1969.
24. Greenwood, N., and Orr, W. McN.: Primary squamous cell carcinoma arising in a solitary non-parasitic cyst of the liver. J. Pathol. *107*:145, 1972.
25. Hartemann, E., et al.: Hamartoma hépatique du nournisson. Rev. Lyon. Med. 18 June, 1969.
26. Henson, S. W., Gray, H. K., and Dockerty, M. B.: Benign tumors of the liver. Surg. Gynecol. Obstet. *103*:23, 1956.
27. Ishak, K. G., and Glunz, P. R.: Hepatoblastoma and hepatocarcinoma in infancy and childhood. Cancer *20*:396, 1967.
28. Ishida, M., et al.: Mesenchymal hamartoma of the liver. Ann. Surg. *164*:175, 1966.
29. Johnson, F. L., et al.: Association of androgenic anabolic steroid therapy with development of hepatocellular carcinoma. Lancet *2*:1273, 1972.
30. Jones, J. F. X.: Removal of a retention cyst from the liver. Ann. Surg. *77*:68, 1923.
31. Keech, M. K.: Cystadenomata of the pancreas and intrahepatic bile ducts. Gastroenterology *19*:568, 1951.
32. Keeling, J. W.: Liver tumors in infancy and childhood. J. Pathol. *103*:69, 1970.
33. Keen, W. W.: On resection of the liver, especially for hepatic tumors. Boston Med. Surg. J. *126*:405, 1892.
34. Lannon, J.: Seventeen cases of hepatectomy. S. Afr. J. Surg. *12*:227, 1974.
35. Longmire, W. P., Passaro, E. P., and Joseph, W. L.: The surgical treatment of hepatic lesions. Br. J. Surg. *53*:852, 1966.
36. Longmire, W. P., et al.: Elective hepatic surgery. Ann. Surg. *179*:712, 1974.
37. Lorimer, W. S.: Right hepatolobectomy for primary mesenchymoma of the liver. Ann. Surg. *141*:246, 1955.
38. Makk, L., et al.: Liver damage and angiosarcoma in vinyl chloride workers. J.A.M.A., *230*:64, 1974.

39. Makk, L., et al.: Clinical and morphologic features of hepatic angiosarcoma in vinyl chloride workers. Cancer *37*:149, 1976.
40. MacMahon, H. E., Murphy, A. S., and Bates, M. I.: Sarcoma of the liver. Rev. Gastroenterol. *14*:155, 1947.
41. Malt, R. A., Hershberg, R. A., and Miller, W. L.: Experience with benign tumors of the liver. Surg. Gynecol. Obstet. *130*:285, 1970.
42. Maresch, R.: Ueber ein Lymphangiom der Leber. Z. Heilkd. *24*:39, 1903.
43. Marsh, J. L., Dahms, B., and Longmire, W. P.: Cystadenoma and cystadenocarcinoma of the biliary system. Arch. Surg. *109*:41, 1974.
44. Martin, A. G., et al.: Cystadenoma of the liver; a rare tumor. Wis. Med. J. *72*:220, 1973.
45. Mattila, S., Keskitalo, E., and Makinen, J.: Primary nondifferentiated sarcoma of the liver. Acta Chir. Scand. *140*:303, 1974.
46. McSweeney, W. J., Bove, K. E., and McAdams, A. J.: Spontaneous regression of a putative childhood hepatoma. A reappraisal. Am. J. Dis. Child. *125*:596, 1973.
47. Mersheimer, W. L.: Successful right hepatolobectomy for primary neoplasm — preliminary observations. Bull. N.Y. Med. Coll. Flower & Fifth Ave. Hospitals *16*:121, 1953.
48. Misugi, K., and Reiner, C. B.: A malignant true teratoma of liver in childhood. Arch. Pathol. *80*:409, 1965.
49. Moore, S. W., McElwee, R. S., and Romiti, C.: Benign tumors of the biliary tract. J.A.M.A. *150*:999, 1952.
50. More, J. R. S.: Cystadenocarcinoma of the liver. J. Clin. Pathol. *19*:470, 1966.
51. Nikaidoh, H., Boggs, J., and Swenson, O.: Liver tumors in infants and children. Arch. Surg. *101*:245, 1970.
52. Pollice, L.: Primary hepatic tumors in infancy and childhood. Am. J. Clin. Pathol. *60*:512, 1973.
53. Selinger, M., and Koff, R. S.: Thorotrast and the liver: a reminder. Gastroenterology *68*:799, 1975.
54. Short, W. F., et al.: Biliary cystadenoma. Arch. Surg. *102*:78, 1971.
55. Stanley, R. J., Dehner, L. P., and Hesker, A. E.: Primary malignant mesenchymal tumors (mesenchymoma) of the liver in childhood. An angiographic-pathologic study of three cases. Cancer *32(4)*:973, 1973.
56. Stephens, C. L., and Jenevein, E. P., Jr.: Mesenchymal hamartoma of the liver. Arch. Pathol. *80*:413, 1965.
57. Stewart, F. W.: Personal communication.
58. Sutton, C. A., and Eller, J. L.: Mesenchymal hamartoma of the liver. Cancer *22*:29, 1968.
59. Thompson, J. E., and Wolff, M.: Intra-hepatic cystadenoma of bile duct origin with malignant alteration. Milit. Med. *130*:218, 1965.
60. Willis, R. A.: Carcinoma arising in congenital cyst of the liver. J. Pathol. Bacteriol. *55*:492, 1943.
61. Wilson, J. E., et al.: Primary leiomyosarcoma of the liver. Ann. Surg. *174*:232, 1971.
62. Wolloch, Y., Dintsman, M., and Garti, I.: Primary malignant tumors of the liver. Isr. J. Med. Sci. *9(1)*:6, 1973.
63. Yarborough, S. M., and Evashwick, G.: Case of teratoma of the liver with 14 years postoperative survival. Cancer *4*:848, 1956.
64. Willis, R. A.: The Borderland of Embryology and Pathology. London, Butterworth and Co., 1958.

Chapter Eight

RESECTION OF
METASTATIC TUMORS

The discovery of embolic metastatic deposits in the liver means to most clinicians that cancer has spread beyond a hope of cure. Although there have been staunch advocates of resection of pulmonary and even cerebral metastatic disease, few have championed liver resection for the same purpose. In 1888, Garrè reported the resection by his chief, von Bruns, of a hazel nut-sized metastatic cancer from the right lobe of the liver, but the primary abdominal tumor was not resected.[16] Keen listed this case twice (as number 4 and 51) in his famous list of 76 liver resections (see Chapter 2). Cattell resected an apparently solitary liver metastasis from a rectal carcinoma in 1939, and the patient was doing well 12 months later.[9] In 1943 Owen Wangensteen proposed second laparotomy for liver resection two or three months after removal of a gastrointestinal primary cancer when liver metastasis had been found at the first operation. He admitted, however, that at the date of his report no patient had yet accepted the proposal.[45]

As experience with liver resection increased after World War II, more attempts were made to excise liver secondaries. Pack suggested that liver resection for metastatic cancer should be done when the primary growth was controlled, and when there had been a long interval between resection of the primary disease and discovery of the liver metastasis.[33, 34] Quattlebaum advocated lobectomy for any and all metastatic deposits unless the patient was obviously incurable.[37]

These opinions by pioneers in the field deserve our close attention, but are they justified by the results achieved? What is the natural his-

209

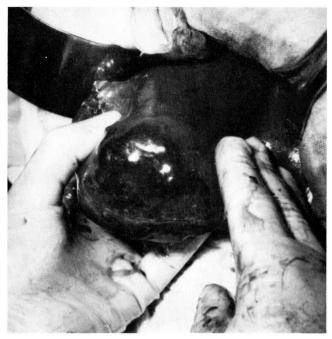

Figure 8–1. Metastatic adenocarcinoma of left kidney resected by wedge excision from left lateral segment of the liver of a 65-year-old man. Patient died with disseminated disease 7 months later. (Case 148 – Appendix VII–B.)

tory of patients with metastatic liver disease? Can the true extent of liver involvement be assayed preoperatively or even at laparotomy? Does the length of the interval between resection of the primary cancer and the discovery and resection of the metastasis truly correlate with subsequent survival? Do the number and size of the metastatic deposits influence "curability" by resection? How does the risk of resection compare with the benefits that might be achieved? How often will a situation suitable for resection be found? These questions need answers before we can put the concept of liver resection for secondary disease into perspective.

WHAT IS THE NATURAL HISTORY OF PATIENTS WITH METASTATIC DISEASE WHO DO NOT UNDERGO RESECTION?

Pestana, et al. reported a mean survival of nine months after the diagnosis of liver metastasis in 353 patients with liver secondaries from primary cancers of the colon and rectum.[36] Galante, et al. found liver metastases in 74 of 975 patients (7.6 per cent) with cancer of the colon;[14] 11.5 per cent of the 74 lived three years and four patients lived five years, but there was no histologic documentation of the liver metastasis, nor any autopsy information for the long-term survivors. Swinton, et al. found liver metastases at the time of bowel surgery in 41 of 334 patients (12 per cent) with carcinoma of the sigmoid and/or rectum. Seven of the 41 patients lived two years, but none survived as long as four years.[44] Bengmark and Hafström found liver metastasis in 38 of 156 patients undergoing laparotomy for primary carcinoma of the colon and rectum. These patients survived an average of 5.7 months after diagnosis, and the longest survivor died one year and eight months after bowel surgery.[4] Flanagan and Foster reported 43 cases of liver metastasis from primary carcinoma of the colon, with a mean survival of eight months and a median survival of six months after diagnosis. Four patients lived as long as two years, but none survived five years.[11]

Jaffe, et al. studied 390 patients with liver metastasis from multiple primary sites. The median survival in this group was 75 days, and only 7 per cent lived more than one year. The 56 patients with a solitary liver nodule had a median survival of 136 days, about twice that of patients with bilateral nodules. The 177 patients with primary carcinoma in the colon and rectum had a median survival of 146 days, considerably better than the over-all group.[20] Bengmark, et al. reported a mean survival of six months for 54 patients with liver metastasis from primary cancer of the breast. Only one patient lived more than 21 months, and she died 45 months after the diagnosis of liver metastasis was made.[6] Survival averaged only 2.4 months from the date of diagnosis in patients with liver metastasis from pancreatic cancer.[8]

There are isolated reports of long-term survivals after the discovery of liver metastasis, but in most instances further investigation reveals either that these cases do not have histologic documentation or that the metastasis is from a carcinoid or islet cell tumor. We have found no report of a patient with a histologically confirmed liver tumor secondary to a primary adenocarcinoma of bowel, breast, stomach, pancreas, or lung in which the patient has survived as long as five years after liver biopsy without treatment aimed at the liver metastasis.

CAN THE PRESENCE AND EXTENT OF LIVER INVOLVEMENT BE ACCURATELY DETERMINED BEFORE OR DURING LAPAROTOMY?

Preoperative evaluation is discussed in Chapter Three. Liver scanning, angiography, and liver function tests are quite useful in determining the presence of liver metastasis, but these tests are less reliable in defining the exact location and number of metastatic lesions. Kim, et al. remark that 28 per cent of liver tumors judged resectable at laparotomy were deemed unresectable preoperatively.[21] Most surgeons have had the opposite experience of finding at laparotomy more extensive tumor involvement than had been suggested by preoperative tests.

When the belly is open wide enough to allow careful palpation of the liver, will clinical evaluation detect the true extent of liver disease? Pack and Ariel studied 100 patients with carcinoma of the gastrointestinal tract who died of various causes while still hospitalized after resection of their primary tumors.[32] The liver of all these patients had been judged by the surgeon to be free of metastasis at the time of bowel resection. Only five patients had metastatic disease at autopsy, and only two of these unrecognized metastases were evident macroscopically.

Goligher found clinical evidence of liver metastasis in 103 patients (11.5 per cent) during 893 operations for carcinoma of the rectum. Thirty-one of the 790 patients with clinically negative livers died and came to postmortem examination in the postoperative period. Five were found to have liver metastasis.[17] Ozarda and Pickren studied at autopsy 150 livers with secondaries from a wide variety of extrahepatic primary cancers. In 134 (90 per cent) the nodules were evident on the surface of the liver.[31] Five patients in the 1974 Liver Tumor Survey who died after "curative" resection of liver metastasis came to postmortem examination, and in four there was no evidence of tumor in the liver or elsewhere. The fifth patient was found to have a previously unrecognized 2.5 cm "posterior" metastasis when she died of a myocardial infarction on the first day after combined resection of a sigmoid cancer and synchronous wedge resection of a 4 cm clinically solitary liver metastasis.

These studies suggest that, in a very high percentage of cases, the sensitive fingers of an experienced surgeon will discover the true extent of liver involvement more accurately than any scan, angiogram, or other noninvasive test. They also indicate that decisions made on the basis of careful palpation will usually be accurate.

HOW OFTEN WILL A "RESECTABLE" METASTATIC TUMOR IN THE LIVER BE FOUND?

The answer to this question will be shaded by one's definition of "resectable," but here it is taken to mean solitary and/or unilobar disease not involving major vascular trunks. Raven studied 818 patients from the Royal Marsden Hospital undergoing operation for cancer of the stomach, colon, or rectum. Of these, 186 (23 per cent) had hepatic metastases, and 42 (5 per cent) had metastases that were judged to be resectable on the basis of a solitary metastasis or multiple metastases confined to one lobe. He concluded that about one in every 20 patients operated on for cancer of the gastrointestinal tract will have technically resectable hepatic metastases.[38] Galante, et al. found liver metastasis in 7.6 per cent of 975 patients with colon carcinoma, but these authors do not discuss whether they were "resectable."[14] Bengmark and Hafström found liver metastases in 24.5 per cent of 156 patients undergoing laparotomy for primary cancer of the colon and rectum, and in nine patients the disease was quite limited.[4] Goligher found clinically evident metastases in 11.5 per cent of 893 patients with cancer of the rectum.[17] Jaffe studied 390 patients with liver metastases, and in those 173 patients for whom the location and number of the metastatic lesions were stated, he found 56 with solitary nodules and 45 additional patients with multiple nodules confined to one lobe.[20] Ozarda and Pickren found only four instances of solitary liver metastasis in 150 autopsies of patients who all had liver involvement with secondary carcinoma. However, in an additional 30 patients, multiple nodules were confined to

Table 8–1. Liver Resection for Metastatic Cancer: Location of Primary Tumor

	COLLECTED* REVIEW	1974 LIVER TUMOR SURVEY	TOTAL
Colon and rectum	109	126†	231
Stomach	17	3	20
Melanoma	4	9	13
Wilms' tumor	12	3	15
Breast	1	4	5
Leiomyosarcoma	3	7	10
Pancreas	5	1	6
Uterus and cervix	4	3	7
Ovary	2	4	6
Renal	3	3	6
Others	4**	13***	17
	164	176	336

*Foster (1970)[13] plus 19 references;[1, 2, 5, 9, 10, 12, 18, 19, 22–28, 30, 40, 42, 46] operative survivors only.

**Includes omentum 1, lung 1, adrenal 1, "sarcoma" 1.

***Includes paraganglioma 1, pericytoma 1, lung 1, neuroblastoma 1, adrenal 1, esophagus 1, miscellaneous sarcomata 3, primary unknown 4.

†Three cases reported by Adson[49] and one by Peden and Blalock[35] included in both collected review and 1974 Liver Tumor Survey.

---

one lobe of the liver. Metastatic cancer was confined to the liver in only 11 patients, but these were autopsied cases and therefore it was very late in the course of the disease.[31]

One could generalize and estimate that 10 to 30 per cent of patients with primary cancer of the gastrointestinal tract will be found to have liver metastases at laparotomy for treatment of their primary disease. Perhaps one-quarter of these patients will have solitary nodules or disease limited to one lobe or segment of the liver. Thus, any surgeon who treats patients with primary gastrointestinal tract cancer will probably encounter "resectable" liver metastases several times during his career.

The questions about interval, size, number, operative risk, and survival are not well answered by any published report—largely because few studies report enough experience from which firm conclusions might be drawn. An attempt at answering these questions will be made by collecting the reported experience of others, and by looking at the information available from the 1974 LTS. Table 8–1 outlines this experience.

LITERATURE SURVEY

To the 123 patients collected in 1970[13] can be added 41 others who survived liver resection for metastatic cancer. The additional cases include 32 patients with primary colon and rectum cancer,[2, 9, 12, 18, 22-28, 30, 42, 46] and 18 with other primary cancers.[1, 5, 10, 19, 23, 24, 30, 40] Nine of these 50 patients died during or after liver resection, leaving 41 for whom survival information is available.

Table 8–2. Liver Resection for Metastatic Cancer—Collected Review: Survival After Operation*

	ALL CASES	COLON AND RECTUM PRIMARY
Number of patients	164	109
Alive 2 years after liver resection	67/133 – 50%	39/82 – 48%
Alive 5 years after liver resection	26/110–24%	15/68 – 22%

*Excludes operative deaths.

Table 8–3. Survival After Resection of Hepatic
Metastases*—Collected Review

INTERVAL BETWEEN PRIMARY AND LIVER OPERATIONS

	Synchronous	Metachronous	
		Less than 2 years	More than 2 years
Patients	54	35	38
Mean survival	24 months	29 months	35 months
2-Year survival	18/40 — 45%	16/30 — 53%	15/31 — 48%
5-Year survival	6/36–17%	7/28 — 25%	8/27 — 30%

*Excludes operative deaths.

The risk of operation to remove liver metastases has been calculated by collecting the experience of reported series and excluding reports of individual cases. Twenty-six of 152 patients in 17 series[13, 22, 24, 25, 27, 30, 46] died after operation (17 per cent), but if the somewhat more lethal experience of two series is excluded,[8, 15] 10 of the remaining 101 patients (10 per cent) died after liver resection for embolic metastasis.

Table 8–2 documents survival in the over-all group and the more homogeneous group of patients whose tumors were primary in the colon and rectum.

Table 8–3 attempts to answer the question whether the interval between resection of the primary tumor and resection of the liver metastasis has any effect on long-term survival or "cure." The numbers are too small to be of statistical significance, but they do suggest that Pack's opinion of the favorable effect of a long interval may have merit.

Table 8–4 adds four cases to those already reported[11, 13] of patients who lived more than five years after resection of liver metastasis from colon and rectum cancers, bringing the total reported in the literature to 15 cases. Table 8–12 lists five-year survivors after liver resection for "other" cancers. There were no long-term survivors after resection of liver metastases from primary carcinomas of the breast, lung, and stomach, or from adenocarcinoma of the pancreas. Although there were two five-year survivors after liver resection for metastatic melanoma, both patients succumbed to the disease shortly after the five-year mark was reached.[11]

Fourteen patients had liver resection for metastatic Wilms' tumor,[10, 13, 19, 24, 40] often as part of an aggressive program of combined chemotherapy and radiotherapy during which several patients also had resection of pulmonary metastases. At least three of the ten who survived the operation are alive more than five years after liver resection,

Table 8–4. Patients Surviving 5 Years After Resection of Liver Metastases from Colon and Rectum Primary—Collected Review (to be added to 11 cases previously tabulated)[11, 13]

Authors	Age/Sex	Primary Tumor Site	Interval Between Tumor and Liver Resection	Liver Metastasis	Resection	Outcome
McKenzie and Wilson (1970)[28]	25 F	Rectum	3 months	Multiple small	Right lobe	AFD 6½ years
Macphee (1965)[25]	N.S.	Left colon	N.S.	Multiple	Left wedge	AFD 5½ years
Manheimer (1965)[26]	62 F	Sigmoid polyp	Synchronous	Solitary 2cm	Wedge	AFD 7 years
Bowden (1974)*[24]	N.S.	Colon	N.S.	N.S.	N.S.	DWD shortly after 5 years

*In discussion of Longmire, et al. (1974).[24]
N.S. = not stated.
AFD = alive free of disease.
DWD = dead with disease.

and four others are alive without evidence of recurrent tumor at less than five years.

Of the 15 five-year survivors reported in the literature whose primary tumor was in the colon and rectum, 14 were apparently cured of their disease. The resected liver tumors in this group of 15 were solitary in 12 patients and multiple in three; they ranged from 1 to 20 cm in size, and were resected by a variety of operations ranging from small wedge excision to extended right lobectomy. Four were resected synchronously, and nine metachronously, after an interval ranging from three months to four years (the interval was not stated for two patients).

1974 LIVER TUMOR SURVEY – RESECTION OF METASTATIC TUMOR

The records of 288 patients undergoing liver resection for carcinoma that originated outside of the liver were reviewed in the 1974 LTS. Patients with carcinoid, islet cell, or other endocrine-like metastatic tumors were placed arbitrarily in a separate category, and will be discussed in Chapter Nine. Patients with liver invasion by adjacent carcinomas who underwent liver resection to satisfy the "en bloc" principle are discussed in Chapter Ten. There remained 176 cases in which embolic metastases were resected (Table 8–1). Appendices VIII–A and VIII–B outline the clinical data on these patients, four of whom have been reported elsewhere.

METHODS

In at least ten instances, grossly visible tumor was left in the liver or elsewhere in the abdomen, and these cases are classified as "palliative" resections. When the metastatic liver disease was recognized at the time of operation for removal of the primary lesion, and when the liver metastases were resected at either the same operation or within a few weeks thereafter, the liver resection is classified as "synchronous." "Metachronous" resection refers either to the resection of liver metastases after a prolonged period of observation of limited liver disease noted at the time of resection of primary cancer, or, more often, to subsequent recognition of metastatic liver disease in a patient whose liver was judged free of disease at the laparotomy for resection of the primary tumor. The "interval" listed for metachronous resection relates to the months between resection of the primary disease and resection of the liver metastasis. When more than one operation for resection of liver metastatic disease was done, the interval refers to the first liver resection. Once again, wedge resection refers to any less than lobar resection except for left lateral segmentectomy.

Because operative deaths relate so closely to technical or "surgeon" factors, long-term survival has been calculated and reported by considering only those patients who survived operation. Over-all five-year survival can be quickly calculated from the figures given by simply adding the number of operative deaths to the denominator of the five-year fractions. Seventy-two per cent of the patients with resected liver metastases had primary tumors of the colon and rectum, and this large group will be discussed separately and first.

METASTATIC TUMORS FROM COLON AND RECTAL CARCINOMA

RESULTS

Table 8–5 defines the more homogeneous group of colonic and rectal cancers and relates the location of the primary tumor to survival after resection of liver metastasis.

Among the 62 patients undergoing synchronous resection of metastatic liver cancer, the liver problem was recognized preoperatively by physical examination in six, by abnormal liver function tests in two, and by liver scan in four. In all the other patients undergoing synchronous resection the liver metastasis was discovered as an incidental finding at laparotomy. What has been labeled as a "synchronous" resection was carried out at the same time as bowel resection in 45 patients, and was delayed one to nine weeks in 16 patients (interval not known in one case).

Liver metastases were discovered in 64 patients undergoing metachronous resection: (1) as an incidental finding at laparotomy for some other disease in 12; (2) because of a palpable abdominal mass found on routine follow-up examination in 15; (3) because of abnormal liver function tests or liver scan during routine follow-up in five; and (4) because pain and/or fever, weight loss, malaise, and other systemic symptoms had prompted further evaluation in 15. Nine other patients undergoing metachronous resection had their liver metastases discovered at the operation to remove the primary tumor, and were followed for three to 17 months before a decision for resection was finally made. No patient who had resection of metastatic tumor from a colon or rectum primary presented with rupture and/or intraperitoneal hemorrhage.

Table 8–5. Resection of Metastatic Cancer – 1974 LTS: Primary Colon and Rectum

LOCATION OF PRIMARY TUMOR	PATIENTS	OPERATIVE DEATHS	SURVIVAL* MEAN	SURVIVAL* MEDIAN	5-YEAR
Cecum and right colon	24	1	38 months	14 months	4/15
Transverse colon	11	1	33 months	16 months	2/7
Left colon	10	1	32 months	24 months	1/7
Sigmoid colon	53	3	22 months	14 months	4/40
Rectum	26	2	27 months	23 months	4/17
Unspecified	2	0	90 months	—	1/2
Over-all	126	8	29 months	16 months	16/88

*Excludes operative deaths.

Information about liver function tests was available in 96 of the 126 patients with colon and rectum secondaries (see Chapter 3). They were entirely within normal limits for 40 per cent of the patients who eventually were proved to have liver metastasis. The serum alkaline phosphatase was most frequently abnormal, being elevated in 38 patients. The SGOT was elevated in 17 patients, but was often within normal limits when the alkaline phosphatase was increased. Bromsulphalein retention was done in only 20 patients, but was elevated in 12. Serum bilirubin was elevated in only one patient, and the carcinoembryonic antigen (CEA) was positive in the single instance in which it was measured (in a patient who subsequently underwent synchronous resection of a small liver metastasis and a large sigmoid carcinoma).

Thirty-four of the 104 patients for whom information is available underwent liver scans preoperatively. The scan showed the lesion in 26 patients, was negative in seven, and was equivocal in a single patient. Selective arteriography was done in 21 patients and accurately located one or more lesions in 19. Both scan and angiogram were done in 13 patients, and both were positive in 12. The 13th patient had a positive angiogram and a negative liver scan. Of the four patients whose angiograms suggested multiple lesions, three had only a solitary metastasis at laparotomy. In five patients with multiple metastases, the angiogram showed only one lesion. There was a comment about the vascularity of the metastatic lesions in 14 patients undergoing angiography: in two the vascularity was increased and in 12 it was reduced.

There were eight deaths after operation for metastatic colon and rectal cancer.

(1) A 65-year-old woman died of cardiac failure, one day after a low anterior resection of a "Duke's C" adenocarcinoma of the sigmoid and synchronous wedge resection of an apparently solitary 4 cm metastatic nodule of the liver. Autopsy revealed acute thrombosis of the right coronary artery and an unrecognized 2.5 cm liver metastasis deep in the liver (Case 92, Appendix VIII-A).

(2) A 29-year-old woman had symptoms characteristic of cholecystitis for nine months before a laparotomy revealed large and multiple right lobe metastases from a primary carcinoma of the cecum. She died of exsanguination from a "stress" ulcer, ascites, and combined hepatic and renal failure 17 days after an "heroic" right liver lobectomy and right colectomy. Postmortem examination revealed residual tumor in the left lobe of the liver and in bone (Case 12, Appendix VIII-A).

(3) A 63-year-old white male had evaluation of three small liver metastases at the time of colostomy closure, three months after resection of an adenocarcinoma of the transverse colon. Wedge resection of two small right-sided nodules confirmed the impression of metastatic disease, but then a right lobectomy was done to remove a third small right-sided nodule and "any other hidden disease." Death followed five

days later with fever, jaundice, and hepatic and renal failure. Autopsy showed ligation of the main hepatic artery, a question of "drug-induced" hepatocellular necrosis, and no residual tumor. The grossly evident 0.3 cm subcapsular nodule of the right lobe was the only tumor found in the resected lobe. Retrospective analysis suggests that simple wedge-resection of the third small nodule, rather than lobectomy, would have removed all grossly evident tumor (Case 26–Appendix VIII-A).

(4) A 66-year-old man had high fever and positive liver scan five years after a sigmoid resection for cancer. Laparotomy revealed a woody left-sided liver mass from which pus was drained. Frozen section report was "benign," as was the repeat frozen section one month later, when re-exploration, biopsy, and then excision of the left lateral segment of the liver was accomplished to control continuing fever. At that time multiple nodules were noted, but the suspicion of recurrent carcinoma was not raised until permanent sections of the resected specimen revealed this diagnosis. The patient died in fulminant hepatic, renal, and pulmonary failure five days after operation, and an autopsy showed multinodular residual liver metastases with purulent necrosis (Case 50–Appendix VIII-A)

(5) A 55-year-old woman died of gradual liver failure nine weeks after a right lobectomy was done for two large metastases from a sigmoid carcinoma resected 17 months earlier. Autopsy revealed no tumor and an occlusion of the common hepatic duct, which had remained uncorrected in spite of a second operation (Case 98, Appendix VIII–A).

(6), (7), (8) The three other patients had bilateral multinodular metastatic disease. In two, an extended right hepatectomy resulted in removal of all grossly visible disease (confirmed at autopsy), but death in liver failure followed in 12 days and six weeks respectively. The third patient had disease left after bilateral wedge excisions, and died several weeks later without leaving the hospital (Cases 45, 102 and 116, Appendix VIII–A).

Limited resection of small nodules, denial of resection to those with bilateral disease, and more careful treatment of the bile duct in one case might well have averted seven of these eight operative deaths.

LONG-TERM SURVIVAL; COLON AND RECTUM METASTASIS

Eight of the 126 patients with liver resection for metastatic colonic and rectal cancer died after operation, and follow-up information is inadequate for five others. Of the remaining 113 patients, 25 are alive less than five years after liver resection. This leaves 88 patients available for five-year survival figures and, of these, 16 (18 per cent) were alive 60 months after liver resection. However, six of these 60 month survivors have subsequently developed evidence of recurrent cancer at the date of their last follow-up in this survey, and four of the six have died. Thus, ten of the 83 determinate cases seemed "cured."

Which patients will do well? It seemed reasonable to believe that the patient with a small, solitary metastasis, resected by major lobectomy at a long interval after resection of the primary colon cancer, would be a prime candidate for long survival after liver resection. But, is that true?—and how can we select the patient who is most likely to benefit from the resection of liver metastases? Numerous correlations were made to search for an answer to these questions, but very few clear guidelines emerged.

We first looked at the 16 who survived five years. Nine of these fortunate patients had synchronous resection and seven had metachronous resection; three patients had lobectomy, three left lateral segmentectomy, and ten had only wedge excisions—four of which were wedge excisions of multiple nodules. Nine patients had solitary tumors 0.5 to 5 cm in maximum diameter, but seven had multiple tumors, 7.5 to 14 cm in diameter.

Table 8–5 relates survival to the location of the primary lesion. In contrast to the experience of Macphee,[25] patients in this series with liver metastasis from rectal carcinoma seemed to fare better than those with lesions primary in the descending or sigmoid colon, but the differences are not significant.

Does the presence or absence of mesenteric node involvement by primary cancer correlate with the result achieved by resection of liver metastasis? Table 8–6 demonstrates that the status of the colonic lymph nodes does not help in the selection of patients for liver resection. In those 86 patients who survived liver resection and about whom it is

Table 8–6. Resection of Metastatic Cancer – 1974 LTS: Primary Colon and Rectum: Colon Lymph Node Status Versus Survival

	LYMPH NODES NEGATIVE	LYMPH NODES POSITIVE
Patients	35	51
2-Year survival* after liver resection	12/26 – 46%	15/38 – 39%
5-Year survival* after liver resection	3/23 – 13%	8/37 – 22%

*Excludes operative deaths.

Table 8–7. Resection of Metastatic Cancer – 1974 LTS:
Primary Colon and Rectum: Operation versus Survival

OPERATION	PATIENTS	OPERATIVE DEATHS	SURVIVAL* Mean	SURVIVAL* 5-Year
Extended right lobectomy	4	1	70 months	1/2
Right lobectomy	25	4	29 months	2/16
Left lobectomy	10	0	9 months	0/8
Left lateral segmentectomy	20	0	24 months	3/12
Wedge	67	3	31 months	10/50

*Excludes operative deaths.

known whether or not the colonic lymph nodes contained metastatic cancer, any advantage is in favor of those with involved nodes.

Table 8–7 relates the extent of the operation to survival, and there is no clear correlation between longevity and the amount of liver removed. Table 8–8 looks at the correlation between the maximum diameter of the largest nodule of metastatic tumor and survival in those 117 patients for whom accurate information was available. Although 12 of the 44 patients with tumors 5 cm or less in diameter lived five years (27 per cent), only three of 40 patients with tumors larger than 5 cm lived that long (8 per cent). However, the two longest survivors in the whole group of 126 patients were among the 27 patients with tumors greater than 10 cm in diameter. These two patients (one previously reported)[35] were living 13 and 16½ years after liver resection (Cases 20 and 126, Appendix VIII-A), and they skew the mean survival of this group of larger tumors. If they are excluded from the calculations making up Table 8–8, the mean survival of the other 22 survivors of operation who had very large tumors was only 12 months. Size was the one factor that correlated well with long-term survival.

Twenty per cent of the 45 patients at risk with solitary metastasis, and 16 per cent of the 43 with multiple metastases from colon and rectum cancer lived five years – a difference that has no statistical significance. Table 8–9 reviews this factor, and it would seem that unless multiple metastases involved both anatomic lobes, the prognosis was not altered significantly by more than one tumor nodule. The single five-year survivor with bilobar metastases died with recurrent disease 73 months after resection.

Table 8–10 summarizes the data on the time interval between resection of the primary cancer of the colon and rectum and resection

Table 8–8. Resection of Metastatic Cancer – 1974 LTS: Primary Colon and Rectum: Tumor Size versus Survival

MAXIMUM TUMOR DIAMETER	OPERATIVE PATIENTS	DEATHS	SURVIVAL* Mean	Median	2-Year	5-Year
Less than 2 cm	19	0	33 months	30 months	12/16	2/15
2–5 cm	39	2	37 months	22 months	16/32	10/29
6–10 cm	32	2	14 months	14 months	3/22	1/22
Greater than 10 cm	27	3	26 months	10 months	5/19	2/18

*Excludes operative deaths.

Table 8–9.   Resection of Metastatic Cancer – 1974 LTS:
Primary Colon and Rectum: Solitary or
Multiple Lesions versus Survival

		METASTASIS	
	Solitary	Multiple	
		Unilobar	Bilobar
Patients	81	30	15
Operative deaths	1	3	4
Mean survival*	29 months	40 months	19 months
Median survival*	16 months	16 months	14 months
5-Year survival	9/45 – 20%	6/19 – 31%	1/10 – 10%

*Excludes operative deaths.

of the liver metastasis. The 57 patients whose liver tumors were removed during the same operation as the bowel resection, or shortly thereafter, are compared with 56 whose liver tumors were removed after a prolonged interval. In contrast to the collected experience reported in Table 8–3, the results of the 1974 LTS indicate that a lengthy "disease-free interval" has little or no beneficial effect on the prognosis after liver resection for secondary cancer and that, therefore, a period of watching and waiting to see if anything else develops is not warranted. In fact, if one adds together the experience reported in the literature and that of the 1974 LTS, survival after synchronous resection is almost exactly the same as that after metachronous resection with an interval greater than two years.

Nine patients had liver metastases noted at the time of resection of the primary colon or rectal tumor that were watched for three to 17 months prior to liver resection. In three, rapid growth of the liver was

Table 8–10.   Resection of Metastatic Cancer – 1974 LTS: Primary Colon and Rectum: Interval Between Bowel and Liver Resection

	SYNCHRONOUS	METACHRONOUS	
	(None)	Less than 2 Years	More than 2 Years
Patients	57	25	31
Mean survival*	30 months	22 months	33 months
2-year survival*	25/48 – 52%	9/20 – 45%	4/25 – 16%
5-year survival*	9/45 – 20%	5/19 – 26%	2/24 – 8%

*Excludes operative deaths.

noted during the seven-, 12-, and 18-month intervals between operations, and all were dead with disease within one year after liver resection. Six other patients, two of whom received 5-fluorouracil during the interval, had slow growth of their metastatic tumors and no sign or symptom of systemic manifestations. All four of this latter group who survived liver resection are alive—three without evidence of disease at 6, 32, and 116 months respectively after liver resection, and one with evidence of recurrent disease at five months. This small experience suggests that a delay of a few weeks or months prior to elective resection of apparently solitary liver metastases found during colon or rectum excision probably will not affect adversely the "curability" of the metastatic cancer. The choice of such a treatment plan may be very sound for those situations in which neither the patient nor the surgeon is adequately prepared for liver resection at the time of bowel resection.

There were no long-term "cures" in those six patients who had palpable liver masses prior to synchronous colon and liver resections. In those patients who underwent metachronous resection of liver metastasis, survival did seem to vary with the way in which the metastatic disease presented itself. Four of the 11 operative survivors whose metastatic disease was discovered incidentally at laparotomy for some other problem (such as bowel obstruction, aneurysm, cholecystitis, etc). lived at least five years, and a fifth is alive without evidence of disease 12 months after resection. Only one of the 15 patients whose liver involvement presented as an asymptomatic mass is alive and free of disease after metachronous resection, and she has been followed for only five months.

Fifteen other patients undergoing metachronous liver resection presented with pain and/or fever, and 11 of these also had a palpable mass. Most are dead, but it is interesting to note again that the two longest survivors in the whole series not only had very large tumors, but also had pain and fever associated with a palpable liver metastasis.

One of the most remarkable aspects of this late follow-up information is the look it has given us at the natural history of colon cancer. In nine patients the liver metastasis was diagnosed from 66 to 101 months after resection of the primary tumor of the colon or rectum. Seven other patients had metachronous liver resection at an interval less than five years after colon surgery, but then went on to succumb to recurrent or persistent bowel cancer at an interval more than 60 months after the resection of the bowel.

The statement made above is true that no case or report of a patient with a histologically proved liver metastasis from a colon and rectum cancer could be found in which the patient lived five years after liver biopsy without therapy to the liver metastasis. However, if one can accept the premise that a liver metastasis that eventually is discovered

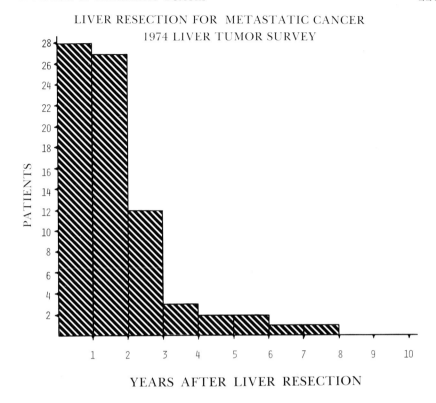

LIVER RESECTION FOR METASTATIC CANCER
1974 LIVER TUMOR SURVEY

YEARS AFTER LIVER RESECTION

TIME OF DEATH WITH RECURRENT CANCER AFTER LIVER
RESECTION FOR METASTATIC DISEASE FROM COLON & RECTUM

Figure 8–2

long after treatment of a bowel cancer must have been present in the
liver at the time of bowel resection, then the 16 cases cited above are acceptable as clearly documented examples of survival for more than five
years of patients who had colon cancer metastatic to the liver. Four
other patients died with carcinoma more than 60 months after liver
resection of metastases and can be added to the above evidence. This,
when combined with the data on interval between liver resection and
death in those 76 patients not cured by liver resection (Fig. 8–2), gives
us a picture of the natural history of patients with liver metastasis considerably different from that developed on page 211 of this chapter.

How can we reconcile these differences? It may not be possible to
do so, but perhaps the most probable explanation is that the patients
who are selected for resection of liver metastases represent a more favorable group, with localized disease and host defenses that have at
least partially "controlled" the spread of cancer.

RE-RESECTION

Three patients had a "second" liver resection for metastatic disease. A 71-year-old female had synchronous resection of a 5 cm metastasis from the left lobe of the liver at the time of resection of a sigmoid cancer that was metastatic to five of 13 mesenteric lymph nodes. Nineteen months later a right upper quadrant mass was palpable, and another apparently solitary 5.5 cm metastasis was wedged out of the free edge of the right lobe of the liver. She survives 62 months after the first liver resection and 43 months after the second (Case 57, Appendix VIII–A). The other two patients each had two metachronous resections for metastatic cancer of the rectum, but they succumbed to widespread disease, 25 and 26 months respectively after the first liver resection (Cases 115 and 118, Appendix VIII–A). Re-resection of localized liver disease would seem to make as much sense as initial resection so long as disseminated disease was carefully ruled out in each instance.

PALLIATIVE RESECTION

Thirteen patients had liver resection in which some tumor was left, either in the liver (six patients) or elsewhere in the abdomen and chest (seven patients). Three patients died after operation; seven are dead with disease at four, five, seven, 18, 19, 22, and 33 months after liver resection; and three are alive with evidence of spread of disease at 11, 14, and 26 months after liver resection. "Noncurative" liver resections were elected for several reasons. The surgeon abandoned attempts at curative resection after finding tumor on the inferior vena cava during right lobectomy in one case, and after excessive blood loss followed excision of some but not all of multiple metastases in two other cases. In at least four other instances a peripheral liver tumor was resected because it was "easy to do" and would eliminate a "mass." One tumor was about to block the duodenum, and another had purulent breakdown with fever and persistent drainage.

"Palliation" is a relative term. We should not forget Hoerr's rule, which states that "it is difficult to make the asymptomatic patient feel better."[51] However, there may be rare circumstances in which noncurative liver resection might be justified if it can be done with little threat to life and if the patient's discomfort is sufficient to limit useful survival at home without resection.

RESECTION OF LIVER METASTASES FROM PRIMARY TUMORS OTHER THAN COLON AND RECTUM

Fifty patients collected in the 1974 LTS had resection of liver metastases from cancers primary in organs other than colon and rectum, but even when these are added to the reported experience of others (Table 8–1) there are not enough cases of any one type to justify firm conclusions. However, there were important differences between these "other" tumors and metastatic colon and rectum cancers. Two-thirds of the liver resections were done metachronously (33 patients), and only ten were done synchronously. Seven were done "precociously"—i.e., before an extrahepatic primary focus was evident. In three patients it eventually became apparent that the liver tumors had originated in lung, pancreas, and ovary, but in four patients the exact site of origin was never discovered, although the liver lesions were clearly not of bile duct or liver cell origin.

Fifteen of the 33 patients undergoing metachronous resection had an interval between the primary resection and liver resection of more than five years, suggesting that the natural history of the tumor was that of slow growth, yet only four of these 15 with a long disease-free interval are alive, and three of those four have evidence of recurrent or persistent cancer. Only two of the 44 patients who survived operation lived as long as five years, and they both died with recurrent cancer 105 months after liver resection (Cases 140 and 172, Appendix VIII–B). Two-year survival in this miscellaneous group was 8/36 (22 per cent), and five-year survival was 2/32 (6 per cent), both considerably lower than that after resection of metastases from colon and rectum. Twelve of the 13 patients with multiple nodules of metastatic tumor in the liver are dead, and the 13th had evidence of recurrent disease 32 months after liver resection. Only five of the 37 patients with solitary nodules are alive without evidence of disease at five to 26 months after liver resection.

Appendix VIII–B lists the clinical data on these 50 patients. Table 8–11 relates survival to the type of operation in the 1974 LTS cases,

Table 8–11. Liver Resection for Metastatic Cancer from Primary Tumors Other than Colon and Rectum — 1974 LTS: Operation versus Survival

	PATIENTS	OPERATIVE DEATHS	SURVIVAL* Mean	SURVIVAL* Median	5-Years
Extended right lobectomy	2	0	21 months	—	0/1
Right lobectomy	11	2	19 months	9 months	1/9
Left lobectomy	2	0	6 months	—	0/2
Left lateral segmentectomy	9	3	13 months	8 months	0/4
Wedge	26	1	17 months	10 months	1/16
	50	6	17 months	9 months	2/32**

*Excludes operative deaths.
**Both 5-year survivors dead with disease at 105 months after liver resection.

Table 8–12.   Survival for More than 5 Years After Liver Resection for Cancer Metastatic from Primary Lesions Other than Colon and Rectum

REF.	AGE/SEX	PRIMARY TUMOR SITE	INTERVAL	METASTASIS	RESECTION	OUTCOME
(1) Woodington and Waugh (1963)[48]	46 M	Pancreas, islet cell	4 years		RL	DWD 5.5 years
(2) Woodington and Waugh (1963)[48]	60 F	Melanoma	Synchronous		Wedge	DWD 5 years
(3) Pack and Brasfield (1955)[33]		Melanoma, eye	13 years	Solitary 7 cm	Wedge	DWD 6 years
(4) Straus and Scanlon (1956)[43]	62 F	Kidney	5 years	Solitary 1500 gm	LLS	DOD 12 years
(5) Möller (1936)[29]	29 F	Granulosa cell, ovary	10 years	Solitary	Wedge	AFD 6 years
(6) Smrcka, et al. (1967)[41]	28 M	Pancreas, insulinoma	32 months	2 nodules	RL	AFD 5 years
(7) Gans, et al. (1966)[15] and Wedemeyer, et al. (1968)[47]	6 M	Wilms' tumor	13 months	Solitary 3 cm	Wedge	AFD 5½ years
(8) Brasfield, et al. (1972)[7]	N.S. F	Gastric leiomyosarcoma	N.S.	N.S.	RL	DWD 64 months
(9) Smith, et al. (1974)*	4 M	Wilms' tumor	9 months	Solitary 10 cm	Wedge	AFD 5 years
(10) Martin, R.G. (1974)*	N.S.	Wilms' tumor	N.S.	N.S.	N.S.	AFD 6 years
(11) Martin, R.G. (1974)*	F	Adrenal cortex	N.S.	N.S.	N.S.	Alive 6 years
(12) Bowden (1974)*	F	"Sarcoma"	N.S.	N.S.	N.S.	DWD 5 + years
(13) 1974 L.T.S. (case 140)**	69 M	Leiomyosarcoma	Synchronous	Solitary	Wedge	DWD 105 months
(14) 1974 L.T.S. (case 172)**	36 F	Fibrosarcoma	132 months	Solitary	RL	DWD 105 months

*In discussion of Longmire, et al.[24]
**Appendix VIII-B.

and Table 8–12 documents the reported and collected cases from all sources of five-year survival after liver resection for embolic metastases from primary tumors other than colon and rectum. Notice that there were no long-term survivors after liver resection for metastatic cancer from the more common tumors that originate in breast, lung, pancreas, and stomach. In fact, there was only one patient who was apparently "cured" among those long-term survivors who did not have a Wilms' or endocrine tumor (the case reported by Straus and Scanlon in 1956 in which the patient died 12 years after resection of a metastatic renal carcinoma, and no tumor was found at autopsy).[39, 43]

Nine patients with melanoma were found in the 1974 LTS whose liver metastases were resected after an interval averaging 85 months after resection of their primary tumors. The primary melanoma had originated on the back in one patient, on the head and neck in three, in the eye in two, on the lower extremity in two, and on the upper extremity in one patient. Appendix VIII–B documents that all did very poorly after resection of their metastases. Eight patients are dead, and the ninth had evidence of widespread disease when she was last seen 22 months after liver resection. Two of the melanoma patients presented with ruptured tumors and intraperitoneal hemorrhage.

The only other metastatic tumors in the overall series of 176 patients who developed necrosis, rupture, and intraperitoneal hemorrhage were two patients with large leiomyosarcomas metastatic to the liver. Palliative resection of liver metastasis occasionally may be required to stop hemorrhage even if known disease is left in the abdomen or elsewhere, but rupture is quite rare with metastatic disease.

SUMMARY AND RECOMMENDATIONS FOR THERAPY

The presence of metastatic cancer in the liver can no longer be considered as an absolute criterion of incurability. Careful preoperative studies and operative evaluation can provide information adequate to form the basis for a reasoned judgment about resection of embolic metastatic cancer. Routine liver scanning, perhaps at yearly intervals during the first five years after colon resection for cancer, may be more useful than repeated barium enemas in finding residual disease before it spreads beyond the hope of a cure. Laminography of the chest has been most helpful in finding disease outside of the liver, and should be done routinely before an attempt is made at metachronous resection.

A look at the results achieved by resection suggests that an aggressive approach is indicated for selected patients with liver metastasis from primary tumors of the colon and rectum. However, when other primary tumors reach the liver, the natural history of the disease may play a more important role than the surgeon in long-term survival, and it is difficult to justify elective liver resection for these other tumor deposits at the present time. When a resectable liver metastasis is found at the time of resection of a primary tumor of the colon and rectum, a decision about simultaneous or delayed resection should be based on the patient's general condition and on the technical factors relating to the ease of synchronous excision. If a decision is made to delay resection, biopsy proof of the metastatic nature of the liver disease is desirable. The best way to follow the growth of a known liver metastasis in the asymptomatic patient is with serial liver scans. The absence of systemic symptoms should encourage an aggressive approach toward resection if an early decision has been made to watch and wait for a few months.

No evidence is yet available to support the need for lobar or segmental liver resection for small metastatic lesions. However, resection through lobar planes may increase the safety of operation for larger metastases.

Although noncurative or "palliative" resections of liver metastasis occasionally may be indicated to control hemorrhage or to remove uncomfortable mass lesions, this practice generally should be discouraged. Reduction of the bulk of a tumor has been recommended as a method of increasing the effectiveness of subsequent chemotherapy; however, because this recommendation has yet to be proved and because the chemotherapist has so few drugs that are effective today against secondary liver tumors, life-threatening noncurative liver resections probably are not yet indicated for that purpose.

When should a surgeon resect the asymptomatic liver metastasis from a primary tumor of the colon and rectum when he finds it at operation for another disease, on physical examination, or with liver scans? On the basis of the evidence presented above, a resection can be justified whenever a metastasis is found *if* the following conditions are met.

(1) The metastatic disease is limited to one lobe of a noncirrhotic liver.

(2) Preoperative and operative evaluation suggest that the liver metastasis is the only remaining tumor.

(3) The condition of the patient, the geography of the tumor, and the experience and skill of the surgeon will allow safe resection.

REFERENCES

1. Almersjö, O., et al.: Hepatic artery ligation as pretreatment for liver resection of metastatic cancer. Rev. Surg. 23:377, 1966.

2. Bengmark, S., et al.: Die chirurgische Behandlung von Lebertumoren. Chirurg. 39:320, 1968.
3. Bengmark, S., Domellöf, L., and Hafström, L.: The natural history of primary and secondary malignant tumors of the liver. III. Prognosis for patients with hepatic metastases from pancreatic carcinoma. Digestion 3:56, 1970.
4. Bengmark, S., and Hafström, L.: The natural history of primary and secondary malignant tumors of the liver. I. The prognosis for patients with hepatic metastases from colonic and rectal carcinoma by laparotomy. Cancer 23:198, 1969.
5. Bengmark, S., and Hafström, L.: The natural history of primary and secondary malignant tumors of the liver. II. The prognosis for patients with hepatic metastases from gastric carcinoma. Digestion 2:179, 1969.
6. Bengmark, S., Hafström, L., and Olsson, A.: The natural history of primary and secondary liver tumors. V. The prognosis for conventionally treated patients with liver metastases from breast cancer. Digestion 6:321, 1972.
7. Brasfield, R. D., et al.: Major hepatic resection for malignant neoplasms of the liver. Ann. Surg. 176(2):171, 1972.
8. Brunschwig, A.: Hepatic lobectomy for metastatic cancer. Cancer 16:277, 1963.
9. Cattell, R. B.: Successful removal of liver metastasis from a carcinoma of the rectum. Lahey Clin. Bull. 2:7, 1940.
10. Filler, R. M., et al.: Hepatic lobectomy in childhood: effects of x-ray and chemotherapy. J. Pediatr. Surg. 4:31, 1969.
11. Flanagan, L., Jr., and Foster, J. H.: Hepatic resection for metastatic cancer. Am. J. Surg. 113:551, 1967.
12. Fortner, J. E., et al.: Major hepatic resection using vascular isolation and hypothermic perfusion. Ann. Surg. 180:644, 1974.
13. Foster, J. H.: Survival after liver resection for cancer. Cancer 26:493, 1970.
14. Galante, M., Dunphy, J. E., and Fletcher, W. S.: Cancer of the colon. Ann. Surg. 165:732, 1967.
15. Gans, H., Koh, S-K., and Aust, J. B.: Hepatic resection. Arch. Surg. 93:523, 1966.
16. Garrè, C.: Contribution to surgery of the liver. Bruns Beitr. Klin. Chir. 4:181, 1888.
17. Goligher, J. C.: The operability of carcinoma of the rectum. Br. Med. J. 2:393, 1941.
18. Hivet, M., Lagadec, B., and Guillard, J.: Place de l'hépatectomie dans les métastases des cancers digestifs. Presse Med. 77:1747, 1969.
19. Howat, J. M.,: Major hepatic resections in infancy and childhood. Gut 12:212, 1971.
20. Jaffe, B. M., et al.: Factors influencing survival in patients with untreated hepatic metastases. Surg. Gynecol. Obstet. 127:1, 1968.
21. Kim, D. K., et al.: Tumors of the liver as demonstrated by angiography, scan, and laparotomy. Surg. Gynecol. Obstet. 141:409, 1975.
22. Lannon, J.: Seventeen cases of hepatectomy. S. Afr. J. Surg. 12:227, 1974.
23. Longmire, W. P., Passaro, E. P., and Joseph, W. L.: The surgical treatment of hepatic lesions. Br. J. Surg. 53:852, 1966.
24. Longmire, W. P., et al.: Elective hepatic surgery. Ann. Surg. 179:712, 1974.
25. Macphee, I. W.: The excision of malignant secondary hepatic deposits. Br. J. Surg. 56:831, 1969.
26. Manheimer, L. H.; Metastasis to the liver from a colonic polyp. N. Engl. J. Med. 272:144, 1965.
27. McDermott, W. V., and Ottinger, L. W.: Elective hepatic resection. Am. J. Surg. 112:376, 1966.
28. McKenzie, A. D., and Wilson, J. W.: Hepatic resection for blood-borne metastases from large bowel carcinoma. Can. J. Surg. 13:159, 1970.
29. Möller, W.: Resection of liver on account of metastatic carcinoma; case. Acta Chir. Scand. 78:103, 1936.
30. Ochsner, J. L., Meyers, B. E., and Ochsner, A.: Hepatic lobectomy. Am. J. Surg. 121:273, 1971.
31. Ozarda, A., and Pickren, J.: The topographic distribution of liver metastases, its relation to surgical and isotope diagnosis. J. Nucl. Med. 3:149, 1962.
32. Pack, G. T., and Ariel, I. M.: Cancer. Boston, Little, Brown & Co., 1960.
33. Pack, G. T., and Brasfield, R. D.: Metastatic carcinoma of the liver: clinical problem and its management. Am. J. Surg. 90:704, 1955.
34. Pack, G. T., and Islami, A. A.: Operative treatment of hepatic tumors. Clin. Symp. 16:35, 1964.

35. Peden, J. C., and Blalock, W. N.: Right hepatic lobectomy for metastatic carcinoma of the large bowel; five-year survival. Cancer *16*:1133, 1963.
36. Pestana, C., et al.: The natural history of carcinoma of the colon and rectum. Am. J. Surg. *108*:826, 1964.
37. Quattlebaum, J. K.: Hepatic lobectomy for benign and malignant lesions. Surg. Clin. North Am. *42*:507, 1962.
38. Raven, R. W.: Hepatectomy, XVI. Congres de la Société Internationale de Chirurgie, Copenhagen. Brussels, Imprimerie Medicale et Scientifique, 1955, p. 1099.
39. Scanlon, E. F.: Personal communication.
40. Smith, W. B., et al.: Partial hepatectomy in metastatic Wilms' tumor. J. Pediatr. *84(2)*: 259, 1974.
41. Smrcka, J., et al.: Arteriographic demonstration and successful removal of metastatic islet cell tumors in liver. Diabetes *16*:598, 1967.
42. Stone, P. W., and Saypol, G. M.: Partial hepatectomy. Surg. Gynecol. Obstet. *95*:191, 1952.
43. Straus, F. H., and Scanlon, E. F.: Five-year survival after hepatic lobectomy for metastatic hypernephroma. Arch. Surg. *72*:328, 1956.
44. Swinton, N. W., Samaan, S., and Rosenthal, D.: Cancer of the rectum and sigmoid. Surg. Clin. North Am. *47*:657, 1967.
45. Wangensteen, O. H.: The surgical problem of gastric cancer. Arch. Surg. *46*:879, 1943.
46. Warren, K. W., and Hardy, K. J.: A review of hepatic resection at the Lahey clinic: 1923–1967. Lahey Clin. Bull. *16*:241, 1967.
47. Wedemeyer, P. P., et al.: Resection of metastases in Wilms' tumor: a report of three cases cured of pulmonary and hepatic metastases. Pediatrics *41*:446, 1968.
48. Woodington, G. F., and Waugh, J. M.: Results of resection of metastatic tumors of the liver. Am. J. Surg. *105*:24, 1963.
49. Adson, M. A.: Major hepatic resections: elective operations. Mayo Clin. Proc. *42*:791, 1967.
50. Adson, M. A., and Jones, R. R.: Hepatic lobectomy. Arch. Surg. *92*:631, 1966.
51. Hoerr, S. O.: Hoerr's law. Am. J. Surg. *103*:411, 1962.

Chapter Nine

PALLIATIVE LIVER RESECTION TO RELIEVE SYMPTOMS OF THE MALIGNANT CARCINOID AND OTHER ENDOCRINE SYNDROMES

INTRODUCTION

Primary epithelial tumors of the liver may be associated with endocrine symptoms such as hypoglycemia, hypercalcemia, virilization, or feminization. When the endocrine manifestations cause enough distress in their own right, liver resection occasionally may be indicated, even if all of the tumor cannot be removed safely. These endocrine paraneoplastic syndromes are not associated with any particular histologic type of hepatocellular carcinoma, and the prognosis of the patient with endocrine symptoms from hepatocellular carcinoma resembles that of other patients with liver cancer, rather than that of patients with metastatic liver deposits from cancers primary in endocrine glands.

235

The 1974 Liver Tumor Survey found five patients with endocrine symptoms from primary liver cancer who underwent liver resection (Cases 15, 62, and 88, Appendix IV; Cases 42 and 66, Appendix V). Although their symptoms were relieved, only one patient has done well during a short period of follow-up. These cases are discussed in Chapters Four and Five and will not be considered further here.

Insulinomas, Zollinger-Ellison tumors, and carcinoids are the exceptions to the general rule that most tumors arising in endocrine glands rarely metastasize to the liver. Such hepatic metastases may or may not be functional, but when they do continue to secrete hormones, and when the rate of tumor growth is slow, the hormonal effects may be much more uncomfortable and much more dangerous to a patient than the effects of tumor growth.

The liver has an enormous capacity to harbor such secondary growths without functional failure. Unfortunately, by the time the problem is recognized, most patients will have multiple and diffuse metastatic spread throughout both lobes of the liver. Occasionally, however, endocrine or metabolic symptoms will be associated with minimal liver disease.[18]

Pharmacologic agents have been used to offset or antagonize the effects of hormones, and chemotherapeutic agents have been employed to control tumor growth. Many patients do not respond to either approach, and the question of palliative resection of the bulk of hepatic metastatic disease is then raised. A significant experience has now accumulated with liver resection for palliation of the malignant carcinoid syndrome, but there is remarkably little experience with other endocrine tumors.

MALIGNANT CARCINOID SYNDROME

Malignant carcinoid tumors are unique in at least two respects: (1) they often grow very slowly so that survival with the disease may be measured in decades, rather than months or years; and (2) they produce a variety of hormones or vasoactive substances that may cause metabolic effects that lead to profound disability, and even death, before tumor growth is widespread. Davis, et al., in a comprehensive review,[7] have summarized the clinical manifestations and therapy of patients with this disease. A minority of carcinoid tumors are malignant, and many that do metastasize do not produce metabolic symptoms. Symptoms occur when the products of functional tumors have access to the systemic circulation prior to hepatic circulation. Most patients with the syndrome have liver metastases that drain directly into the hepatic veins and inferior vena cava. The only well-documented cases of the malignant carcinoid syndrome without hepatic metastases have been associated with very large bronchial carcinoids, or with a very rare carcinoid arising in gonadal teratomas whose venous drainage flows directly into the systemic circulation, bypassing the detoxifying action of the liver.[7]

The syndrome is characterized by episodic flushing of the upper trunk and face with telangiectasis (often precipitated by alcohol ingestion), watery diarrhea with abdominal cramps, bronchospasm, and right heart failure associated with endocardial fibrosis that eventually affects the tricuspid and pulmonary valves. As the symptoms increase, generalized weakness becomes profound, and the patients may become bedridden. Methyldopa has been used to control flushing, methysergide or cyproheptadine may slow diarrhea, and chlorpromazine may reduce vasoactive effects. In general, however, pharmacologic control has been ineffective in patients with severe symptoms.

Several chemotherapeutic agents have been used, alone or in combination. Streptozotocin is perhaps the most popular at the moment and has been used in combination with 5-fluorouracil.[7] Hepatic artery ligation and infusion have been employed, and arterial ligation has been combined with portal vein infusion in a few patients.[17, 20, 22, 24, 29] Unfortunately, the results of therapy have been poor, and a flare in symptoms is often seen upon completion of a course of chemotherapy. Measurement of 5-hydroxyindoleacetic acid in the urine provides a unique method of following the response to therapy for patients with the malignant carcinoid syndrome.

Kincaid-Smith and Brossy reported the removal of an apparently solitary liver metastasis from a bronchial carcinoid in September, 1954 (six and one-half years after pulmonary resection). The operation relieved symptoms of diarrhea in a 64-year-old woman.[13] Palliative resection of liver metastases was also reported by Stanford, et al. in 1958[27] and by Wilson and Butterick in 1959.[32]

Twelve patients with a malignant carcinoid syndrome who underwent liver resection to control vasoactive symptoms were found in the 1974 LTS, five of whom have been reported elsewhere. Table 9–1 outlines the clinical details of these 12 cases. Table 9–2 lists the cases not included in the 1974 LTS which have been reported by others, and Figure 9–1 illustrates the multiple wedge technique that may be required to remove bulky and diffuse disease.

What can we learn from this collected experience of 44 cases? First, there were six operative deaths after 49 liver resections (five patients had re-resection of involved liver). Palliation was achieved in all but one of the 36 patients with follow-up information, and this palliation lasted from a few weeks to more than six years. Flushing and diarrhea usually were alleviated, but cardiac symptoms were unaffected.

Table 9-1. Liver Resection for Carcinoid Syndrome – 1974 Liver Tumor Survey

Case	Age/Sex	Location Primary Tumor	Duration Preop. Symptoms	Operation	Outcome
1.	60M*	Ileum	6 months	RL and left wedge	Relief 4 months, re-resection 8 months, DWD 24 months
2.	58F*	Ileum	4 years	Wedge	Relief 3 years, DWD 46 months
3.	65M*	Bronchus	14 months	Bilat. wedge	Relief 9 months, died at reoperation 15 months
4.	45M*	Bronchus	18 months	Mult. enucleation	No palliation, died with perforated ulcer 2 months.
5.	59M*	Ileum	31 months	Left lobectomy	Poor palliation, alive 26 months
6.	53F	Ileum	Few weeks	Left wedge	Alive with relief, 30 months
7.	51M	Ileum	Few weeks	LL and right wedge	Relief 24 months, alive 28 months
8.	50F	Ileum	4 years	Mult. wedge	Relief 32 months then hepatic artery ligation, alive 47 months
9.	67M	Bronchus	2 years	LL and right wedge	Relief 8 months, died at re-resection 9 months
10.	51F	Ileum	2 years	LLS	Poor palliation, DWD 7 months
11.	55M	Ileum	2 years	RL	Relief 1–2 years, DWD 29 months
12.	60M	Ileum	12 months	LLS	Relief 6½ years, re-resection at 6½ years, alive 10½ years

*Reported elsewhere Case 1,[1] Case 2,[1] Case 3,[6] Case 4,[23] Case 5.[7]

The single patient who survived operation and who was not palliated succumbed to a perforated peptic ulcer two months after enucleation of several carcinoid deposits. At autopsy the liver was filled with metastatic tumor (Case 4, Table 9–1).

Seven patients had reoperation from six months to six and one-half years after initial liver resection because of a recurrence of severe symptoms (Cases 1, 3, 8, 9, and 12, Table 9–1, and Cases 3 and 33, Table 9–2). One had hepatic dearterialization followed by six months of moderate palliation. This patient is still alive 47 months after liver resection and 15 months after dearterialization, but she is quite symptomatic. Another had tumor removed from the mediastinum eight months after liver resection, and eventually died 16 months after the second operation. Second attempts to remove liver disease were made in five other patients. Two died on the operating table with similar rapid clinical deterioration—i.e., sudden cardiac arrest, which may have been related to a precipitate release of vasoactive amines, to air embolization, to blood loss, or to some other unrecognized vascular catastrophe. Three other patients had a significant period of palliation following the second liver resection, and were alive 16, 36, and 45 months after this second operation when last reported. Two had recurrent symptoms; the other was free of metabolic consequences.

The 39 patients who survived initial liver resection lived from two months to $10\frac{1}{2}$ years. At least 18 were still alive at the last time information was available, and seven had lived more than three years. Although there was a tendency for those with long histories of symptoms before liver resection to do better, worthwhile palliation of long duration was achieved after liver resection in a few patients with fulminant carcinoid syndromes. When most or all of the grossly evident tumor was removed from the liver, palliation was more complete and longer-lasting.

The opportunity to resect liver metastases to alleviate a malignant carcinoid syndrome will present itself only rarely, but since liver resection provides significantly better palliation than any other form of therapy, this possibility should be considered in any patient with the syndrome. Liver scan and arteriography should be done for all such patients. Resection, when feasible, should conserve as much normal liver as possible.[28] Tumor enucleation may be feasible, but these metastases have a rich arterial supply.[30] The gentlest of blunt techniques should be used in the cleavage plane between tumor and liver, and any and all resistances should be clipped or tied. Hilar control of the hepatic artery, with or without ligation, will be helpful if metastatic disease is bulky or central.

If at least 90 per cent of the tumor tissue can be removed, life-threatening liver resection probably is justified for patients disabled by the metabolic consequences of their disease, and who have been unre-

Table 9–2. Liver Resection for Carcinoid Tumor: Reported Cases not Included in 1974 Liver Tumor Survey

	REFERENCE	YEAR	AGE/SEX	LOCATION PRIMARY TUMOR	DURATION PREOP. SYMPTOMS	OUTCOME AFTER RESECTION LIVER METASTASES
1.	13	1956	64 F	Bronchus	10 weeks	Alive, without symptoms 1/2-year
2.	27	1958	54 F	Bronchus	4 months	Alive, without symptoms, 2 months
3.	32	1959	41 M	Ileum	18 months	Relief 2 years, re-resection 4 1/2 years later, with relief additional 3 years
4.	31	1960	58 F	Bronchus		2 years relief, DWD 38 months
5.	21	1963	54 F	Unknown	1 1/2 years	Alive with relief, 3 years
6.	10	1966*	63 M	Ileum	N.S.	DWD 72 months
7.	10	1966*	57 M	Ileum	N.S.	Operative death
8.	18	1966	60 M	Ileum	11 years	Alive, without symptoms 9 months
9.	11	1967	35 F	Ileum	8 months	4 months relief, DWD 6 months
10.	4	1967	21 M	Ileum	Several months	Alive, without symptoms 6 months
11.	16	1967	49 M	Ileum	2 years	Operative death
12.	33	1969	43 M	Ileum	6 years	Alive 18 months with relief
13.	8	1969	46 F	Ileum	N.S.	Alive 5 1/2 years with relief
14.	2	1969	58 M	Unknown	1/2-year	Alive 10 weeks with relief
15.	2	1969	59 M	Ileum	N.S.	Postoperative death

16.	2	1969	61	M	Ileum	6 months	No follow-up
17.	5	1970	49	M	Bronchus	15 months	No follow-up
18.	28	1972	63	M	N.S.	9 years	Alive 30 months with relief
19.	28	1972	47	M	N.S.	11 years	Alive 2 years with relief
20.	28	1972	56	F	N.S.	7 years	Alive nearly two years with relief
21.	28	1972	59	M	Ileum	7 years	Alive 1½ years with relief
22.	28	1972	51	M	Bronchus	2 years	Alive 1 year with relief
23.	7	1973	N.S.	N.S.	N.S.	N.S.	Relief 8 months, DWD 18 months
24.	7	1973	N.S.	N.S.	N.S.	N.S.	Alive 30 months with relief
25.	9*	1974	64	F	N.S.	N.S.	Operative death
26.	9*	1974	39	F	N.S.	N.S.	Alive, 9 months
27.	12	1974	49	M	Ileum	8 years	Alive 12 months with relief
28.	12	1974	76	M	Ileum	4 months	Alive 4 months with relief
29.	15	1974	40	F	Ileum	Months	Relief 5 months, DWD 8 months
30.	14	1974	48	M	Ileum	1½ years	Relief 6 months, DWD 7 months
31.	19	1974	N.S.	N.S.	N.S.	N.S.	Operative death
32.	3	1974	52		Ileum	10 months	Relief few months, re-resection at 6 months, 9 more months relief, alive 22 months after first liver resection

*Liver resections for metastatic carcinoid, but it is not clear whether there were symptoms of the malignant carcinoid syndrome.

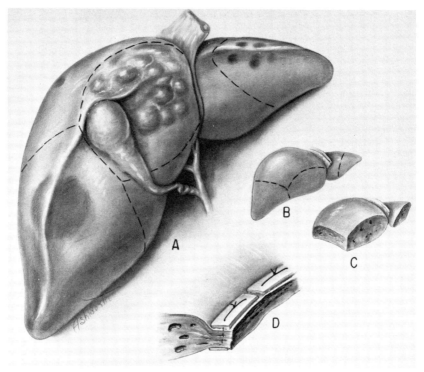

Figure 9–1. Multiple wedge excisions to remove 99 per cent of carcinoid liver metastases in a 65-year-old male with fulminant malignant carcinoid syndrome. (Case 3, Table 9–1). Reprinted courtesy of the Reuben H. Donnelly Corporation, New York, N.Y.

sponsive to medical therapy. However, if a significant volume of tumor tissue is left, little palliation can be expected.

Seven other patients were found in the 1974 LTS who had liver resection for metastatic carcinoid tumors that were not associated with a malignant carcinoid syndrome. In three instances the hospital pathologist had identified these tumors as primary liver tumors, but careful study and special stains have convinced us that they probably were carcinoid tumors. The primary site of these carcinoid tumors was eventually found in four patients and was located in the ileum, the jejunum, a Meckel's diverticulum, and the stomach respectively. One patient died after operation, but five of the six survivors are still alive from 14 to 90 months after liver resection. The last patient died 62 months after liver resection, with disease, but without metabolic symptoms. One of the patients had undergone resection of two separate primary carcinomas of the colon, 20 and eight years prior to the discovery of a mass in the liver that was presumed to be a metastatic lesion when a needle biopsy was reported to show carcinoma. Because of the long interval, liver resection was done, and to everyone's surprise the lesion turned out to be a carcinoid.

Perhaps the most important point to make is that not all liver nodules in patients with a history of other cancers may represent metastatic disease. Biopsy for histologic confirmation should be done before plans for further therapy or thoughts about prognosis are completed.

OTHER ENDOCRINE TUMORS

Although control of hypoglycemic attacks in patients with metastatic insulinomas in the liver would seem an ideal application of liver resection, the opportunity to do so rarely presents itself. In fact, I could

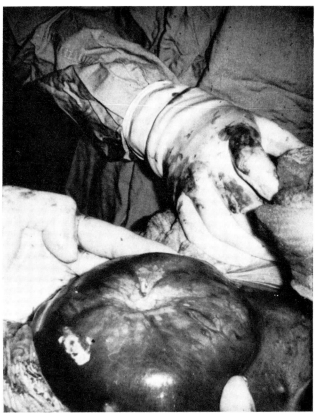

Figure 9–2. Large umbilicated metastasis from a Zollinger–Ellison tumor in left lateral segment of the liver. Wedge excision of most of the segment facilitated total gastrectomy and removed 95 per cent of palpable liver disease.

find only a single report in the literature, and no cases of liver resection for metastatic insulinoma were found in the 1974 LTS. In 1967 Smrcka, et al. reported the story of a young man who had undergone three operations on his pancreas, together with resection of the duodenum and part of the stomach and jejunum, and yet severe hypoglycemic attacks persisted. Finally, arteriography revealed two metastatic lesions in the right lobe of the liver, which were resected. The patient remained symptom-free during the four years of reported follow-up.[25]

Figure 9–2 demonstrates a bilobed metastasis from a Zollinger-Ellison tumor of pancreatic origin. It was found in the left lateral segment of the liver and was resected by the author at the time of total gastrectomy and partial pancreatectomy. Although two tiny nodules of tumor were left in the lateral aspect of the right lobe, left lateral segmentectomy was done to remove the bulk of disease and to provide access to the region of the cardia for esophagojejunal anastomosis. This situation will rarely arise and, since gastrin produces few if any systemic symptoms after total gastrectomy, palliative resection can rarely be justified. However, it is interesting to note that the patient's serum gastrin fell back to normal levels after this resection, and subsequent elevations of serum gastrin were useful in following the course of the disease. Metastatic Zollinger-Ellison tumors usually are very vascular on angiography.[26]

SUMMARY

When the geography of the tumor permits and when metabolic symptoms are disabling, palliative resection of liver metastases should be done for patients with the malignant carcinoid syndrome and for patients with hypoglycemic attacks related to residual disease in the liver.

REFERENCES

1. Adson, M. A.: Major hepatic resections: elective operations. Mayo Clin. Proc. 42:791, 1967.
2. Aronsen, K. F., et al.: Surgical treatment of metastasizing carcinoid tumours. Acta Chir. Scand. 135:177, 1969.
3. Battersby, C., and Egerton, W. S.: A carcinoid saga. Aust. N. Z. J. Surg. 44:32, 1974.
4. Bersohn, I., and Bleloch, J. A.: Right hemi-hepatectomy in secondary carcinoid of the liver—clinical course and liver function tests. S. Afr. Med. J. 44:271, 1967.
5. Blakeney, C. M., and Cullum, P. A.: A single hepatic metastasis from bronchial carcinoid treated by right hepatectomy. Br. J. Surg. 57:237, 1970.

6. Chandler, J. J., and Foster, J. H.: Malignant carcinoid syndrome treated by resection of hepatic metastases. Am. J. Surg. *109*:221, 1965.
7. Davis, Z., Moertel, C. G., and McIlrath, D. C.: The malignant carcinoid syndrome. Surg. Gynecol. Obstet. *137*:637, 1973.
8. Dillard, B. M.: Experience with twenty-six hepatic lobectomies and extensive hepatic resections. Surg. Gynecol. Obstet. *129*:249, 1969.
9. Fortner, J. G., et al.: Vascular problems in upper abdominal cancer surgery. Arch. Surg. *109*:148, 1974.
10. Gans, H., Koh, S-K., and Aust, J. B.: Hepatic resection. Arch. Surg. *93*:523, 1966.
11. Gardner, B., et al.: Studies of the carcinoid syndrome: its relationship to serotonin, bradykinin, and histamine. Surgery *61*:846, 1967.
12. Gillett, D. J., and Smith, R. C.: Treatment of the carcinoid syndrome by hemihepatectomy and radical excision of the primary lesion. Am. J. Surg. *128*:95, 1974.
13. Kincaid-Smith, P., and Brossy, J.: A case of bronchial adenoma with liver metastasis. Thorax *11*:36, 1956.
14. Kune, G. A., and Goldstein, J.: Malignant liver carcinoid: the place of surgery and chemotherapy. Med. J. Aust. 2:777, 1974.
15. Lannon, J.: Seventeen cases of hepatectomy. S. Afr. J. Surg. *12*:227, 1974.
16. Leahy, J., and Moloney, M. A.: The carcinoid syndrome. Ir. J. Med. Sci. *6*:269, 1967.
17. Longmire, W. P., Passaro, E. P., and Joseph, W. L.: The surgical treatment of hepatic lesions. Br. J. Surg. *53*:852, 1966.
18. Ludin, H., Fahrlander, H. J., and Renggli, I.: Zur Darstellung von Karzinoid-lebermetastasen mittels visceraler Arteriographie. Schweiz Med. Wochenschr. *96*:1642, 1966.
19. Martin, R. G.: *In* Discussion of Longmire, et al.: Elective hepatic surgery. Ann. Surg. *179*:712, 1974.
20. Massey, W. H., et al.: Hepatic artery infusion for metastatic malignancy using percutaneously placed catheters. Am. J. Surg. *121*:160, 1971.
21. Mosenthal, W. T.: Resection of massive liver metastases in the malignant carcinoid syndrome. Surg. Clin. North Am. *43*:1253, 1963.
22. Murray-Lyon, I. M.: Treatment of hepatic tumor by ligation of the hepatic artery and infusion of cytotoxic agents. J. R. Coll. Surg. Edin. *17(3)*:156, 1972.
23. Quattlebaum, J. K., and Quattlebaum, J. K., Jr.: Technique of hepatic lobectomy. Ann. Surg. *149*:648, 1959.
24. Rochlin, D. B., and Smart, C. R.: An evaluation of 51 patients with hepatic artery infusion. Surg. Gynecol. Obstet. *123*:535, 1966.
25. Smrcka, J., et al.: Arteriographic demonstration and successful removal of metastatic islet cell tumors in liver. Diabetes *16*:598, 1967.
26. Snyder, H. L., and Klipstein, A. L.: Vascular liver nodules caused by an islet cell tumor. Conn. Med. *40*:312, 1976.
27. Stanford, W. R., et al.: Bronchial adenoma (carcinoid type) with solitary metastasis and associated functioning carcinoid syndrome. South. Med. J. *51*:449, 1958.
28. Stephen, J. L., and Grahame-Smith, D. G.: Treatment of the carcinoid syndrome by local removal of hepatic metastases. Proc. R. Soc. Med. *65*:444, 1972.
29. Watkins, E., Jr., Khazei, A. M., and Nahra, K. S.: Surgical basis for arterial infusion chemotherapy of disseminated carcinoma of the liver. Surg. Gynecol. Obstet. *130*:581, 1970.
30. Watson, R. C., and Baltaxe, H. A.: The angiographic appearance of primary and secondary tumors of the liver. Diagnost. Radiol. *101*:539, 1971.
31. Williams, E. D., and Azzopardi, J. G.: Tumours of the lung and the carcinoid syndrome. Thorax *15*:30, 1960.
32. Wilson, H., and Butterick, O. D.: Massive liver resection for control of severe vasomotor reactions secondary to malignant carcinoid. Ann. Surg. *149*:641, 1959.
33. Zeegen, R., Rothwell-Jackson, R., and Sandler, M.: Massive hepatic resection for the carcinoid syndrome. Gut *10*:617, 1969.

Chapter Ten

LIVER RESECTION TO SATISFY THE "EN BLOC" PRINCIPLE

INTRODUCTION

Carcinoma of the organs adjacent to the liver may grow through their own serosal surface or capsule and become adherent to, or invade into, surrounding organs or structures. When this invasion involves abdominal wall, adjacent bowel, diaphragm, and even pancreas, and when the tumor shows no evidence of distant spread, there still may be hope for cure. Surgeons have long advocated and practiced multivisceral resections for such locally aggressive tumors.

The term "en bloc" is used to describe a technique that avoids any contact with the cancer by cutting only through normal adjacent tissues. When a tumor of the gallbladder, stomach, transverse colon, kidney, or lung has penetrated into the liver, does it make any sense to resect through liver simply to satisfy the en bloc principle?

We will consider this question: (1) by looking at the results achieved by such resections for 92 patients whose data was collected during the 1974 Liver Tumor Survey; and (2) by a brief look at the published reports of others. The literature has not been exhaustively searched in this area, but in the course of seeking information about other liver problems several case reports were encountered. Table 10–1 outlines the 1974 LTS experience, and Appendix X tabulates this information on individual cases. Tumors primary in the gallbladder, stomach, and colon will be discussed separately.

246

Table 10–1.   "En Bloc" Liver Resection for Adjacent Cancers: 1974 Liver Tumor Survey

	Patients	Operative Deaths	Two-Year Survivors	Five-Year Survivors
Gallbladder	35	10	4/32	1/32
Gastric				
Adenocarcinoma	20	3	6/20	3/19
Lymphosarcoma	2	0	0/1	0/1
Leiomyosarcoma	2	0	1/1	—
Colon	15	0	7/11	2/9
Kidney	9	1	3/6	0/3
Adrenal	3	1	0/2	0/2
Esophagus	1	1	—	—
Lung	1	0	0	0
Pericytoma	1	0	1	—
Recurrent cervical cancer	1	0	0	0
TOTAL	90	16	22/74	6/68

LIVER RESECTION FOR GALLBLADDER CARCINOMA

In 1961 Brasfield reported prolonged survival of a woman who at the age of 53 had undergone right hepatic lobectomy for a gallbladder carcinoma that had been an unsuspected finding after routine cholecystectomy.[1] On the basis of that report, many other attempts were made to cure or palliate patients with gallbladder carcinoma by minor or major liver resections, but no one has been able to duplicate Brasfield's success. To the cases previously collected[3] can be added an additional 12, four of which are included in the 1974 LTS (see Appendix X).[2, 6, 8, 10, 11]

Thirty-five patients with gallbladder carcinoma treated by major or minor liver resection were found in the 1974 LTS. All but five had adenocarcinoma. One had an undifferentiated highly anaplastic small cell cancer, and the other four had epidermoid carcinoma, in combination with adenocarcinoma (adenoacanthoma) in three.

In seven cases the carcinoma was found incidentally by a pathologist after the surgeon removed a gallbladder for chronic cholecystitis. Two to eight weeks later a second operation was done, at which time five patients had right lobectomy, and the other two had large wedge resections of the gallbladder bed together with lymphadenectomy of the liver hilum and porta hepatis. In two patients no cancer was found at the time of reoperation; one died postoperatively of septic complications and the other is alive, free of disease, at 18 months (Case 3, Appendix X). The other five patients had residual carcinoma in the gallbladder bed, hilum, or adjacent liver, and the four with adequate follow-up information are all dead.

Twelve patients with a preoperative diagnosis of chronic benign gallbladder disease had enough findings at operation to raise the suspicion of carcinoma. When biopsy proof of cancer was obtained, a synchronous liver resection was combined with cholecystectomy in seven patients—six times by removing a wedge of adjacent liver, and once by right hepatic lobectomy. Three patients had simple cholecystectomy at a first operation and then reoperation one to three months later with wedge resection in one and right lobectomy in two, once combined with Whipple resection. Two patients were transferred to another institution for definitive therapy after initial biopsy without cholecystectomy. Ten of the 12 patients are dead with disease, and the two survivors are alive only five months after their operations, during which tumor was cut across. Both patients have evidence of recurrent disease.

Six patients had evidence more suggestive of cancer than chronic cholecystitis when they first sought medical attention. All had palpable nodular abdominal masses and, when the diagnosis of gallbladder carcinoma was made at laparotomy, wedge resection was done in five patients and right lobectomy in the sixth. Three died after operation, and two more have died with recurrent cancer eight months after liver resection.

Three patients who eventually came to liver resection were followed without reoperation after carcinoma of the gallbladder had been

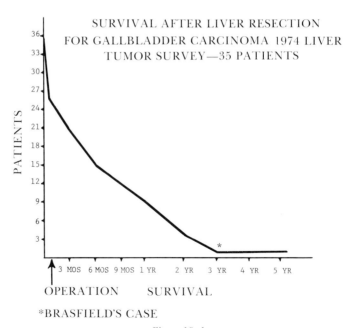

Figure 10–1.

diagnosed at the time of cholecystectomy. When mass recurrences became palpable 14 to 34 months later, they underwent resection of apparently localized recurrent tumor in the liver. Their survival after liver resection was surprisingly long for gallbladder carcinoma (15, 25, and 37 months), but all three patients are dead with metastatic disease.

In six cases the preoperative information was not complete enough to place the patients in one of the categories discussed above, but all six patients are dead after operation or with disease from 0 to 8 months after liver resection (Cases 20–22 and 27–29, Appendix X).

Overall survival after liver resection for gallbladder carcinoma in the 1974 LTS is depicted in Figure 10-1. Of the 22 cases reported in the literature that are not included in the 1974 LTS [3, 6, 7, 8, 10, 11] three are alive at 1½, 3 and 3½ years after liver resection. All the rest are dead with disease from 0 to 36 months after operation. Only Brasfield's case (Case 23, Appendix X) survived five years, and she died 15½ years after liver resection of a recurrent or, more probably, a second primary diffuse cholangiocarcinoma.[2]

RECOMMENDATIONS

The rationale for right hepatic lobectomy for patients with gallbladder carcinoma is obscure, because the gallbladder sits on the central plane between the right and left lobes of the liver. If there is any place for liver resection, it would seem more reasonable to wedge out a suitable portion of the center of the liver anterior to the bifurcation of the major ducts and vessels—an operation that would take parts of both right and left lobes (see Chapter 11).

The suspicion of carcinoma of the gallbladder should be raised whenever the gallbladder is unusually thick, when dissection between the liver and the gallbladder encounters tough white "scar tissue," or when a discrete plaque is seen in the wall of an otherwise normal gallbladder that has been opened in the operating room after excision. Frozen section biopsy will establish the diagnosis and help to determine the depth of invasion. Lymph node biopsy will indicate the extent of disease spread. If the lymph nodes are negative, removal of an appropriate wedge of gallbladder bed with transection by blunt technique without isolation or ligation of the hilar structures is recommended for all but the most superficial of mucosal lesions. If the cancer has obviously spread to regional nodes or is adherent to adjacent organs, little palliation will be achieved by resection.

When an unsuspected diagnosis of carcinoma of the gallbladder is returned by the pathologist several days after routine cholecystectomy, a decision about further therapy may be more difficult. If careful analysis shows only superficial cancer that does not extend to the margin of resection, I would advise waiting for evidence of recurrent disease before offering further therapy. If the tumor does extend to the margin of the resected tissue, and if the patient is in good general health, I would recommend reoperation with wide wedge excision of the gallbladder bed, together with removal of the regional lymph nodes.

When recurrent tumor becomes obvious after a period of observation, re-exploration with liver resection of localized disease will seldom help the patient. If the interval between cholecystectomy and recurrence is long, this may occasionally be justified.

GASTRIC CARCINOMA

Bulky gastric carcinomas sometimes may fix themselves to the undersurface of the left lateral segment of the liver before widespread dissemination has occurred. When the quadrate or caudate lobes of the liver are involved by direct extension, the disease usually is adherent to pancreas and other retroperitoneal structures as well, precluding curative resection.

Twenty-five cases of gastric neoplasms with liver invasion treated by "en bloc" resection were found in the 1974 LTS. Published reports of 30 other cases[3, 5, 7, 8, 9] brings the total to 55. At least six patients have survived more than five years after combined liver-tumor resection without evidence of disease, and are presumed cured. Two of the six patients died at 10 and 18 years after liver resection, and at postmortem examination there was no evidence of persistent carcinoma.

Twenty-one patients in the 1974 LTS had adenocarcinoma, nine with positive regional nodes. Two patients with gastric lymphosarcoma had en bloc liver resections, and the only one who was followed died 11 months later. The two patients who underwent partial resection of the left lateral segment of the liver for adherent gastric leiomyosarcomas are both alive at 16 and 50 months after liver resection.

There were three operative deaths in the 1974 LTS cases (12 per cent), but the deaths were related to pancreatitis, sepsis, and myocardial infarction, rather than to necrosis or hemorrhage from the liver. Fourteen of the 21 operative survivors with adequate follow-up information died of recurrent disease, 11 in the first year and the other three at 21, 22, and 28 months postoperatively. Three are alive without evidence of disease at 16, 36, and 50 months; one died of unrelated causes without evidence of disease at 44 months; and three lived more than five years (3/17 or 18 per cent).

Of the 30 cases reported elsewhere, three lived more than five years, and three are alive without evidence of disease at less than 60 months. Combining this experience with that of the 1974 LTS gives a determinant survival rate (exclusive of operative deaths) of 15 per cent at five years—not very good, but about what could be expected from patients with bulky gastric tumors without liver involvement.

It would seem that wedge resection of adherent liver for gastric malignancies does not affect survival one way or the other. If liver resection is required to satisfy the en bloc principle, it should be done. The fortuitous peripheral location of the portion of liver usually involved allows wedge resection without hilar control. Either the blunt suction technique described in Chapter Eleven, or a row of mattress sutures, will suffice. The crush clamp technique of Lin may be particularly appropriate for these peripheral resections.[4]

COLON CARCINOMA

Fifteen patients in the 1974 LTS had carcinomas of the right side of the colon that had fixed themselves to the free edges of the right lobe of the liver. Wedge resection of small segments of liver was done in each case without hilar dissection or control, and no patient died after operation. Six patients died with recurrent cancer from two to 42 months later; one is alive 52 months after operation with persistent disease in the retroperitoneum proved at the time of elective cholecystectomy for cholelithiasis; and six are alive and free of any evidence of disease at seven, 12, 12, 32, 51, and 216 months after liver resection. The last two patients died of cardiovascular disease at 59 and 137 months after liver resection. Two months after the primary resection the latter had a biopsy-proved pelvic recurrence that was treated with cobalt irradiation, and there was no further evidence of disease in the 11 ensuing years until death. Six patients had metastatic disease in mesenteric lymph nodes at the time of bowel-liver resection, and nine did not. There is no significant difference in the survival between these two small groups of patients with or without positive nodes.

Reports of eight cases of colon-liver "en bloc" resections were found with two operative deaths, four patients dying of disease at less than three years and two who are alive and free of disease at 13 months and nine years after liver resection.[3, 7, 8]

Liver invasion by colon carcinoma is not a sign of unresectability or incurability. Transection of liver substance by blunt technique, leaving a margin of 1 to 2 cm of normal liver, should be done to afford the patient his best chance of cure.

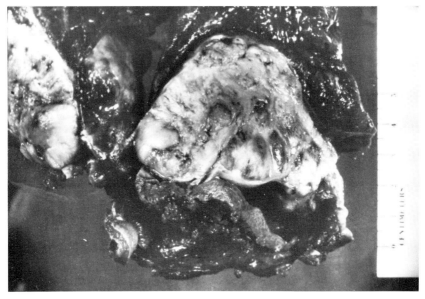

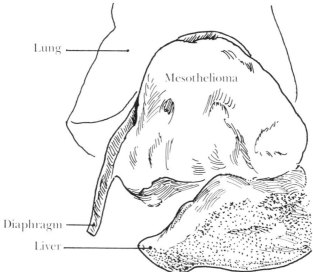

Figure 10–2. Cross section of a nodular mesothelioma of the right diaphragm which had invaded the right lower lobe of the lung and the dome of the right lobe of the liver. A 4 × 8 cm wedge of liver was resected by blunt suction technique together with most of the right diaphragm and the right lower lobe of the lung to satisfy the "en-bloc" principle. The diaphragmatic defect was repaired using Marlex Mesh.

MISCELLANEOUS TUMORS

En bloc resection of liver tumors primary in the kidney and adrenal were done for seven adult patients in the 1974 LTS, and only one short-term survivor remains free of disease at seven months (see Case 76, Appendix X). Four children with Wilms' tumors have done better, but all were treated with postoperative chemotherapy, and two also received radiation therapy.

Every now and then a situation will present itself in which liver resection is required to encompass localized disease that is metastatic from a different primary focus, but has recurred near the liver. One metastatic hemangiopericytoma, and one metastasis from a cervix carcinoma that was causing bowel obstruction, fell into this category in the 1974 LTS.

Figures 10–2 and 10–3 depict a localized mesothelioma of the diaphragm with sarcomatous elements that invaded the diaphragm and liver but had not spread beyond the hope of cure. This tumor was resected recently by the author, and has not been included in the 1974 LTS data. Through a combined thoracoabdominal incision, right lower lobectomy of the lung was performed together with radical excision (with Marlex replacement) of the diaphragm and wedge resection of the dome of the right lobe of the liver. This was done after a frozen

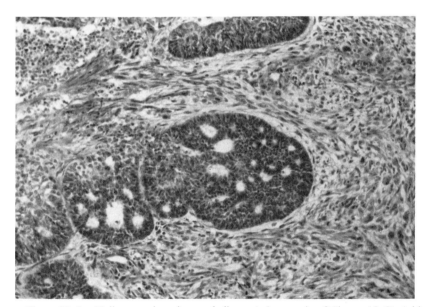

Figure 10–3. Malignant pleural mesothelioma (microscopic of Figure 10–2). A biphasic histologic pattern with adenoid *(left)* and spindle cell *(right)* features.

section diagnosis of malignant mesothelioma was returned by a pathologist. It is too soon after operation to know whether this was worthwhile for this 64-year-old patient.

SUMMARY

Major hepatic lobectomy almost never is indicated when carcinoma or sarcomas of adjacent organs have involved the liver by direct extension. Instead, peripheral wedge excisions to satisfy the "en bloc" principle should be done if the disease appears to be otherwise curable. Although long survival after resection of such invasive tumors is rare, the combination of liver resection should not add to operative risk and may afford the patient at least a chance of cure.

When gallbladder carcinoma is recognized early, wedge resection of the gallbladder bed is recommended. Little evidence is yet available to suggest that this will add significantly to long-term survival, but it seems reasonable to make the attempt if it can be done without unnecessary risk to the patient's life.

REFERENCES

1. Brasfield, R. D.: Right hepatic lobectomy for carcinoma of the gallbladder. Am. Surg. *153*:567, 1961.
2. Brasfield, R. D., Bowden, L., and McPeak, C. J.: Major hepatic resection for malignant neoplasms of the liver. Ann. Surg. *176(2)*:171, 1972.
3. Foster, J. H.: Survival after liver resection for cancer. Cancer *26*:493, 1970.
4. Lin, T. Y.: A simplified technique for hepatic resection. Ann. Surg. *180*:285, 1974.
5. Longmire, W. P., Passaro, E. P., and Joseph, W. L.: The surgical treatment of hepatic lesions. Br. J. Surg. *53*:852, 1966.
6. Longmire, W. P., et al.: Elective hepatic surgery. Ann. Surg. *179*:712, 1974.
7. Martin, R. G.: *In* Discussion of Longmire, W. P., et al.: Elective hepatic surgery. Ann. Surg. *179*:1974.
8. McDermott, W. V., and Ottinger, L. W.: Elective hepatic resection. Am. J. Surg. *112*:376, 1966.
9. Ochsner, J. L., Meyers, B. E., and Ochsner, A.: Hepatic lobectomy. Am. J. Surg. *121*:273, 1971.
10. Schottenfeld, L. W.: Surgery of the liver. Am. J. Dig. Dis. *22*:139, 1955.
11. Warren, K. W., and Hardy, K. J.: A review of hepatic resection at the Lahey Clinic: 1923 to 1967. Lahey Clin. Fed. Bull. *16*:241, 1967.

Chapter Eleven

LIVER RESECTION – OPERATIVE TECHNIQUE

INTRODUCTION

The operation is the critical incident in the care of a patient with a solid liver tumor that will determine whether a cure is possible. By increasing the safety of the operation while extending the possibility of resection, the surgeon can provide his patient with the maximum chance for comfortable and long survival. The choice of whether to resect will depend on a thorough knowledge of the surgical anatomy of the liver and of its physiologic reserve and capacity to regenerate. The distressingly high rates of morbidity and mortality reported after liver resection can be reduced significantly by a skilled surgical team.

In this chapter those factors that might contribute to a safer and more effective operation are discussed. First, the experience of the 1974 Liver Tumor Survey will be reviewed to see if a retrospective look at the records of 621 patients undergoing one or more liver resections will yield any lessons. This will be followed by a discussion of the metabolic consequences of major liver resection, and a brief review of what is known about liver regeneration.

Finally, the details of operative technique will be described, emphasizing the personal opinions of the surgeon-author.

255

MORBIDITY AND MORTALITY – 1974 LIVER TUMOR SURVEY

The reliability of what follows is dependent on the accuracy and thoroughness of the medical records and dictated operative notes of 621 patients with solid liver tumors who were cared for in 98 different hospitals. It would be an understatement to say that there was much variety in the usefulness and length of these records. Several surgeons described in brief and controlled terms the details of what were apparently uneventful liver lobectomies for patients whose anesthesia records, in contrast, document the transfusion of enormous quantities of blood – with several episodes of cardiac arrest and massive resuscitative efforts during the procedure. More often, the prose used to describe major hepatic resection was salted with emotional phrases that reflected the surgeon's monumental concern over what he considered to be an even more monumental task. In spite of these limitations, however, enough information was obtained to allow an objective look at mortality and at some of the major types of postoperative morbidity.

Table 11–1 documents operative mortality after particular operations. A brief return to page 4 will refresh the reader's knowledge of the definition of each of these operations and remind him that wedge resection refers to any type of nonsegmental resection, however large. Eighty-two patients died during or after operation, and Table 11–2 further defines this mortality in the 76 patients in whom the time and cause of death could be determined. It was fairly easy to assign a cause

Table 11–1.   Resection for Solid Liver Tumor – 1974 Liver Tumor Survey: Operative Mortality (Deaths/Patients)

	OPERATION						
TUMORS	*XRL*	*RL*	*LL*	*LLS*	*Wedge*	TOTAL	
Primary, malig., adult	3/13	18/50	2/28	1/13	3/29	27/133	20%
Primary, malig., pediatric	5/15	10/46	2/9	0/8	0/12	17/90	19%
Metastatic, colon and rectum	1/4	4/25	0/10	0/20	3/67	8/126	6%
Metastatic, other primary	0/2	2/11	0/2	3/9	1/27	6/51	12%
Liver cell adenoma	0/3	1/9	0/3	0/3	3/19	4/37	11%
Focal nodular hyperplasia	0/1	0/4	0/1	0/4	0/52	0/62	0
Metastatic carcinoid	1/1	0/4	1/3	0/5	1/8	3/21	14%
Miscellaneous tumors	0/1	0/3	0/1	0/2	1/4	1/11	9%
"En bloc" gallbladder	0/0	8/18	–	–	2/17	10/35	29%
"En bloc" other	0/0	1/3	–	1/5	4/47	6/55	10%
	10/40	44/173	5/57	5/69	18/282	82/621	
	25%	25%	9%	7%	6%	13%	

KEY: XRL – Extended right lobectomy.
        RL – Right lobectomy.
        LL – Left lobectomy.
        LLS – Left lateral segmentectomy.

Table 11–2. Liver Resection for Solid Tumor—1974 Liver
Tumor Survey: Cause—82 Operative Deaths*

	DEATH OCCURRED IN			
PRIMARY CAUSE OF DEATH	Operating Room	First 7 Days	7–30 Days	More Than 30 Days
Failure to control hemorrhage	15	4	4	3
Air embolization (probable)	3			
Liver failure due to technical cause		3	6	4
Cardiopulmonary		3		1
Liver failure in cirrhotic patients		2	6	4
Upper gastrointestinal hemorrhage			4	
Sepsis		1	2	1
Liver failure, cause unknown			3	
Recurrent cancer				2
Judgment error		1	4	
	18	14	29	15

*Death during operation, during first 30 days after operation of any cause, or at any interval due to causes related to the operation.

of death for those patients who died on the operating table. However, the compilation of Table 11–2 required the arbitrary assignment of a single cause of death to each patient, and this was often difficult when death followed weeks of combined organ failure, sepsis, hemorrhage, and malnutrition.

Eighteen patients died in the operating room, 15 because of exsanguinating hemorrhage. In at least 11 instances, the loss of control of bleeding occurred at the time when the junction between the major hepatic veins and the inferior vena cava was approached. Fatal hemorrhage occurred from the inferior vena cava during caudate lobe resection in one patient, and from the whole transected surface of the liver in two other patients: one whose liver substance was being divided with cautery (without previous hilar ligation); the other was undergoing a second emergency operation for control of a ruptured adenoma. The site of bleeding was not specified in the very brief operative note of the 15th patient. Eleven other patients died postoperatively as a direct consequence of enormous blood loss during operation, once again usually related to the dissection of the hepatic vein–inferior vena cava junction. Hemostasis remains the cornerstone of the surgical art, and nowhere else is this demonstrated more clearly than in liver resection.

Three patients died suddenly during operation when blood volume replacement seemed adequate. These sudden cardiac arrests occurred during the enucleation of a huge mesenchymal hamartoma in an 8-month-old infant, and during re-resections of liver tumor in two adult patients for palliation of malignant carcinoid syndromes recurrent after previous liver resection. Air embolization was suspected but not proved in all three patients, but the possibility of a sudden release of vasoactive amines also must exist in the carcinoid patients.

Twelve patients died of liver failure caused primarily by technical factors other than hemostasis. Two infants succumbed eight and 15 days after 90 per cent resections with ascites, anasarca, and liver failure. They represent the only two deaths in this large series that may be attributable to the removal of "too much" liver. Five other patients with noncirrhotic livers went on to fulminant liver failure postoperatively, which was proved at postmortem examination to be related to thrombosed hepatic arteries in two patients, and which was associated in the other three patients with long periods of hilar clamping during bloody resections.

Bile duct injury accounted for three "technical" deaths, and common bile duct stones were left in a fourth patient who eventually succumbed to the consequences of bile leakage, sepsis, and reoperation. A 12th patient had mattress sutures placed in the umbilical fissure during extended right lobectomy. At postmortem examination it was clear that these sutures had compromised the blood supply to the remaining left lateral segment of the liver.

Seventeen cirrhotic patients died after the resection of solid tumors. In 13 cirrhotic patients progressive liver failure seemed related primarily to decreased hepatocellular reserve, but in four it was related to other factors (massive upper gastrointestinal hemorrhage in two, intraoperative hemorrhage in one, and abscess and fistula formation leading to sepsis in the fourth). Deaths followed the incomplete resection of tumor in five patients who had preoperative evidence of liver failure and/or purulent exudate in the liver bed. These resections had no chance to cure the patient and little chance to palliate, and these deaths have been assigned to the category of "judgment error" in Table 11–2.

There were four deaths after 111 liver resections for benign tumors. Two occurred in the operating room (one air embolus and one exsanguinating hemorrhage), and one occurred due to an unrecognized hemorrhage on the first postoperative day. Three operations were done electively, and the fourth was done as a second emergency operation for continued hemorrhage from a ruptured adenoma. The fourth death occurred three and one-half months after resection of a large liver cell adenoma, and was related to continuing sepsis and its complications.

Table 11-3. 1974 Liver Tumor Survey: Operative Mortality Versus Operation

CAUSE OF DEATH	EXTENDED RIGHT LOBEC- TOMY	RIGHT LOBEC- TOMY	WEDGE
During operation	2	10	4
Late consequences of operative hemorrhage	2	6	4
Bile duct problem	—	2	—
Other technical complications	6	4	—
Cardiopulmonary	—	2	2
Liver failure, cirrhotic patient	1	6	2
Liver failure, cause unknown	—	3	—
Upper gastrointestinal hemorrhage	—	1	—
Sepsis	—	4	2
Judgment error	—	1	2
Recurrent cancer	—	—	1
Cause not determined	—	4	1

Seventy-two of the 82 postoperative deaths followed extended right lobectomy, right lobectomy, or wedge resection. Table 11-3 attempts to dissect out the cause of death, and it is clear again that more than one-half of the deaths were related to technical factors at operation.

Eighteen patients died after "wedge" resection, but in all but two instances this "wedge" was a large piece of liver tissue measuring more than 7 cm and/or weighing more than 500 gm. The exceptions occurred in two patients who had removal of small peripheral wedges of tissue. The first was done to include an apparently solitary metastasis in a patient undergoing sigmoid resection for primary adenocarcinoma of the colon. Myocardial infarction on the first postoperative day resulted in rapid death. The other small wedge resection was done to resect a 2 cm liver cell cancer proved by biopsy at an earlier operation for a patient with diffuse cirrhosis of the liver, who died six weeks later of progressive liver failure.

COMPLICATIONS

There were many postoperative complications that did not result in death but which prolonged the hospital stay of the patient. Table

Table 11–4. Liver Resection for Solid Tumor—1974 Liver
Tumor Survey: 621 Operations: Postoperative Complications

| | | AFTER | | | | ALL PATIENTS | CIRRHOTIC PATIENTS |
COMPLICATION	XRL	RL	LL	LLS	W	(DEATHS)	(DEATHS)
Upper GI hemorrhage	1	12	4	1	1	19 (12)	6 (6)
Bile fistula	4	10	5	—	2	21 (7)	1 (1)
Subphrenic abscess	4	15	6	3	11	39 (6)	3 (2)
Postop. intra-abdominal hemorrhage	2	5	2	—	4	13 (7)	2 (2)

11–4 lists the incidence of four of the more important complications, and compares their lethality in the cirrhotic and noncirrhotic patients.

Massive upper gastrointestinal hemorrhage occurred in 19 patients, only two of whom had less than total lobectomy. Gastrointestinal hemorrhage usually occurred in the second or third week after resection, and was preceded or accompanied by sepsis or liver failure in at least eight patients. Sawyer has suggested that the use of T-tube decompression of the common bile duct may result in a higher incidence of gastrointestinal hemorrhage after liver resection. Eight of his 50 patients undergoing major hepatic resection bled from stress ulcer, and six died. Bleeding occurred in eight of the 18 patients with T-tube decompression, and in no patient who did not have a T-tube.[45] Our figures tend to support this relationship. Accurate information about postoperative biliary drainage is available for 13 of the 19 patients who suffered massive upper gastrointestinal hemorrhage, and in nine there was creation of a fistula diverting bile from the duodenum (T-tube: seven patients; Roux-en-Y hepatojejunostomy: one patient; and cholecystostomy: one patient). After the major hepatic lobectomies reviewed in the 1974 LTS, bleeding occurred in 3 per cent of the patients without T-tube biliary decompression and in 12 per cent of the patients with T-tube decompression.

All six cirrhotic patients and six of 13 noncirrhotic patients who suffered massive upper gastrointestinal hemorrhage died. Five patients had a second operation to control gastrointestinal bleeding. Plication of a bleeding vessel was done at the time of pyloroplasty and vagotomy for three patients with duodenal ulcer and for one patient with a gastric ulcer, and one patient had a total gastrectomy for bleeding from multiple "stress" ulcers. Three of these five operated patients died, at least one of recurrent gastrointestinal hemorrhage. Nine noncirrhotic patients with massive upper gastrointestinal hemorrhage were treated with replacement transfusion and antacid therapy, and five survived—one after drainage of a subphrenic abscess. Four other patients with progressive liver failure and abnormalities of coagulation went on to suffer upper gastrointestinal hemorrhage as a late, preterminal complication, and all four died.

Many, if not most, of the patients in this series of liver resections had some postoperative fever. Extensive investigation (including negative laparotomy in a few patients) usually failed to find a localized collection of pus requiring drainage. In a patient otherwise doing well after liver resection, fever alone should not be the basis for reoperation or for the long-term use of antimicrobial medication.

However, subphrenic abscess requiring incision and drainage was seen in 39 of the 621 patients (6 per cent). In at least three additional patients, reoperation was required months and even years after liver resection to remove pieces of Ivalon or Teflon used to "bolster" mattress sutures. Only four of the 36 noncirrhotic patients who had subphrenic abscesses requiring drainage died after adequate drainage of the abscess. In several instances necrotic liver was found in the abscess cavity, suggesting that vascular compromise with eventual slough was an important factor in the etiology of the abscess. The use of mattress sutures and crushing clamps probably is closely related to liver necrosis, and the routine use of external drainage of the subphrenic spaces after major liver resection insures a portal of entry for bacteria to colonize devascularized tissue. Mays suggests subperiosteal 12th rib resection after right lobectomy to provide dependent drainage.[29] However, the relatively low incidence of subphrenic sepsis in this large series and my conviction that careful technique will prevent subsequent necrosis lead me to believe that posterior drainage will not often be necessary.

A persistent bile fistula was found in 21 patients, seven of whom eventually died. Because liver resection rarely involved dissection in the area of the distal common bile duct, the occurrence of a postoperative bile fistula was probably related to operative injury to the intrahepatic or hilar ducts. One of the patients developed a biliary fistula after the anastomosis of the remaining hepatic duct to a Roux-en-Y loop of jejunum. Information about surgical drainage of the biliary tree was incomplete in five patients who went on to fistula formation, but five of the remaining 15 patients had their common bile duct decompressed with a T-tube, and ten did not. Stone makes the point that the distal duct may be obstructed by blood clot, rather than by operative injury or kinking.[45] Distal obstruction should be controlled nicely by a common bile duct T-tube. The occurrence of five fistulas with T-tubes in place suggests the presence of an obstruction proximal to the common bile duct tube, and perhaps related to it. Tube decompression of the proximal ducts through the transected major ducts might be a more dependable way to control pressure in the proximal ducts if biliary decompression is to be used at all (see page 300).

An interesting, but unexplained, association of persistent bile fistula with the delayed appearance of recurrent cancer in the fistula tract was noted in several patients. Does the persistent cancer cause the fistula, or does bile soilage promote the growth of cancer? Cytology or brushings of any persistent fistula tract may lead the clinician to an accurate diagnosis of persistent tumor in time to do something about it.

Severe intra-abdominal hemorrhage occurred in 13 patients during the first 24 hours after liver resection. Four patients, all of whom died, were not returned to the operating room because hemorrhage was unrecognized in one patient; was associated with a severe coagulopathy in another; and continued after unsuccessful attempts to control hemorrhage from ruptured liver cell carcinomas in two patients with diffuse cirrhosis. Nine patients had emergency reoperation as soon as it was apparent that intraperitoneal hemorrhage was severe and continuing, and six eventually survived.

There were many other complications after liver resection, including several instances of dehiscence of the diaphragmatic closure or abdominal wound, bowel fistulas probably related to the prolonged use of hard drains, empyema, wound infection, ascites, pulmonary emboli, and bile peritonitis. Two patients required reoperation to remove metal clamps left in the thorax—an unforgivable complication, but perhaps an understandable one in patients whose thoracic wounds were often made with the patient in a supine position, and whose thoraces were closed by surgeons wearied by several hours of unfamiliar dissection and massive blood loss and replacement.

Four patients suffered an inadvertent injury to, or occlusion of, the remaining bile ducts after lobar resection. Two of the four were reoperated upon one day and one month after liver resection; repair was accomplished, and both of these patients survived. Two other patients were not reoperated upon until liver failure was advanced, and neither survived. If jaundice is persistent or progressive after major liver injury in the noncirrhotic patient, bile duct injury must be suspected and, if found, corrected as early as possible.

Hypothermia was used in 23 instances to support liver resection in seven children and 16 adult patients. In most of these patients, inflow and/or outflow occlusion was never employed during liver transection, although, in a few, total occlusion was necessary for the control of massive hemorrhage from the hepatic vein–inferior vena cava junction. Five patients died after liver resection under hypothermic anesthesia, three of whom did have inflow occlusion. Three patients died of progressive liver failure, a fourth of late surgical complications related to sepsis, and the fifth on the sixth postoperative day of multiple pulmonary emboli. Three other patients recovered after two to three weeks of liver failure and fever. It is not possible to determine whether their problems were related to the use of hypothermia. It is difficult to judge from these figures whether the use of hypothermic anesthesia was beneficial to these patients, but it is possible to state that the crude morbidity and mortality rates are higher in patients with hypothermia than in those in whom hypothermia was not used.

METABOLIC CONSEQUENCES OF LIVER RESECTION

The clinical course of a patient after elective major hepatic resection done in a controlled fashion usually is quite benign – often surprisingly so to the inexperienced surgeon. Mild jaundice may be seen for a few days, but bowel function and appetite return early and the patient's major discomforts are those attendant on any major upper abdominal operation, with or without a thoracic extension of the incision. Even when massive tumors are removed by "90 per cent" resections, most of the bulk of the removed tissue is tumor, and only a minor fraction of functioning liver is lost. If the patient had adequate hepatocellular function preoperatively, he probably will do well postoperatively after resection of up to two-thirds of his liver, provided that the operation does not compromise the blood supply or the bile drainage of the remaining segments.

Stone mentions splanchnic sequestration due to partial obstruction together with diversion of the total portal venous flow through a small remnant of remaining liver, and he associates this with a need for blood replacement in excess of measured losses, and with the development of postoperative ascites after resection of more than 80 per cent of the liver.[56] Certainly the left lobe becomes turgid within minutes of ligation of the right branch of the portal vein, and transient portal hypertension can be demonstrated by direct measurement. But how long does this portal hypertension last after operation? Most of the vascular pathways through the normal liver are open only a fraction of the time, and the liver's potential for adjusting to an increased flow is enormous. Portal hypertension probably does not persist for very long after major hepatic resection, and ascites is more apt to be associated with outflow obstruction (postsinusoidal) than with blockage of the inflow into the hepatic sinusoid.

Several classic papers[22, 31, 42, 56] document some of the biochemical changes that can occur after major liver resection.

Jaundice is very common. Serum bilirubin levels gradually rise to reach peak levels of up to 10 to 15 mg per cent by the seventh day, and usually drop back to normal by the third week. Jaundice may be related to the inability of a "smaller" liver to handle bile pigments until regeneration occurs, but it is related much more commonly to massive transfusion of bank blood, hypotension during operation, sepsis, or anoxia of the remaining hepatocytes due to inflow occlusion during operation. In the noncirrhotic patient a serum bilirubin above 10 mg per cent ten days after liver resection, without other evidence of hepatocellular failure, means mechanical obstruction until proved otherwise. Blockage of a bile duct can be due to kinking, clots, or operative injury, and is easily documented if a T-tube has been placed at operation. The use of endoscopic retrograde cholangiography and/or percutaneous transhepatic cholangiography may be helpful in documenting obstruction in patients without biliary decompression. In any case, an early return to the operating room, before sepsis and hepatic failure occur, is encouraged whenever bile duct injury is proved or strongly suspected.

The serum levels of albumin may fall rapidly after major hepatic resection, probably due to a combination of exudative losses and a decreased synthesis by the compromised liver. Serum albumin concentrations should reach their lowest level about the seventh day, and return quickly toward normal thereafter.[22] Cirrhotic patients may start out with low levels and suffer further postoperative reductions down below 2 gm per cent. A failure to increase endogenous albumin synthesis by the third week is a bad prognostic sign. The transfusion of 25 to 100 gm of salt-poor albumin per day may be required to preserve a serum concentration of 3 gm per cent, but this requirement should decrease rapidly in the second week in uncomplicated cases. Ascites formation will compound the problem of hypoalbuminemia. If ascites does begin to form, all drains, including chest tubes, should be removed early to allow sealing of the abdominal and thoracic walls before ascitic pressure increases.[38] Serum globulin levels may fall slightly for a few days and then rise above normal levels for several weeks.[2] The albumin/globulin ratio may be reversed during the first few weeks after major hepatic resection.

Other liver function tests often are elevated prior to the resection of liver tumors (see Chapter 3). Operative trauma, the stress of anesthesia, multiple transfusions, drug therapy, and surgical complications also can result in abnormal liver function tests after operation, even without liver resection. However, certain biochemical changes that are found after most major liver resections are predictable and bear watching, but require no specific therapy. These changes usually are maximal at the end of the first week, and rapidly return toward normal in the second and third weeks after uncomplicated resection.

Total serum cholesterol and the esterified fraction invariably decrease for a short period after major liver resection. Bromsulphalein excretion is impaired in all patients, and serum glutamic oxalic transaminase and serum glutamic pyruvic transaminase usually are moderately elevated for a few days, although the elevation may not correlate with the type and extent of resection. Transaminase elevation was less in patients with T-tube decompression, and was inversely proportional to operative time in one study.[1] A continued rise in transaminase values after the first week is not expected and, if present, probably reflects continuing liver necrosis, hepatitis, or toxic hepatocellular injury. Serum triglyceride levels may fall rapidly after massive liver resection, and nonesterified fatty acids may rise for a few days.[22, 27]

The prothrombin time often is delayed during the first postoperative week. Deficiencies in other clotting factors may be seen,[2] but probably relate more closely to multiple transfusions, and the consumption of essential factors by continuing hemorrhage, than to specific hepatocellular insufficiency. Zucker, et al. have reported deficiencies in Factors V and VII, fibrinogen, and platelets after major hepatic resection.[53] Our experience with trauma patients suggests that a coagulopathy will be evident by the end of the operation or in the recovery room, if it is ever to be of clinical significance in patients surviving liver resection. Terminal liver failure may be associated with abnormal bleeding, of course, and when it is, survival is very rare and the bleeding usually is not the primary cause of death.

Although blood sugar levels generally are within normal limits after major hepatic resection, they occasionally may drop during the first several days. Large intravenous supplements of up to 250 gm per day usually are given as 10 per cent solutions of glucose in water. The glucose tolerance test may be abnormal for several weeks or months after major liver resection, and its return to normal is proposed as a good test in rabbits and in man for liver regeneration.[19]

The blood urea nitrogen and serum electrolytes usually are within normal limits during an uncomplicated postoperative period. Low serum sodium and potassium values are seen; they probably are not specific sequelae of decreased hepatocellular reserve, but rather are the result of too vigorous hydration or respiratory support, or of the inadequate replacement of electrolytes.

REGENERATION

A patient can survive resection of 80 to 90 per cent of his liver, but 10 to 20 per cent of a normal liver cannot support life. Such a patient will always have a period of relative liver insufficiency, and survival is absolutely dependent on the liver's remarkable ability to regenerate rapidly. It is in that period between resection and restoration of liver cell sufficiency that careful metabolic support is most important.

The unique ability of the liver to regenerate must have been known to the ancients who passed on to us the story of Prometheus, whose liver was devoured by vultures during the day and regrew each night. Modern science has repeated this experiment and proved that the liver can regenerate repeatedly to its original weight after multiple sequential resections in the rat.[9] "Regeneration" may not be the correct term from the biologic point of view for a process consisting first of organ and hepatocellular hypertrophy, and then of intense hyperplasia of all the cellular elements of the liver, but the somewhat mystical connotation of the word "regeneration" seems rather appropriate for this most rapid form of reparative or compensatory tissue growth that occurs in mammals.

The regenerative response is set off by resection of 40 per cent or more of the volume of the normal liver and is proportional to the amount resected,[40] being slightly delayed but most vigorous after subtotal resection. Portal hypertension originally was thought to encourage regeneration, but this has been largely disproved.[6] A humoral factor carried by the portal vein, perhaps of pancreatic origin, has been extensively investigated by Starzl, Price, and others. Some of the data are contradictory, and the effects of insulin, glucagon, and even stress have yet to be fully elucidated. This phenomenon of liver regeneration has been an area of recent intense research interest, and the reader is referred to the scholarly summary of Hays for a general review of the subject.[54]

Pack, et al.[40] Monaco, et al.,[36] and Lin and Chen[22] have studied regeneration in man after major resection. An immediate intraoperative volume increase occurs due to vascular congestion that actually may subside slightly with circulatory readjustment. After a lag period of one to two weeks, the liver begins to gain rapidly in volume, and this gain continues, perhaps intermittently, for months or even years.[22] Most regeneration of the human liver is completed by six months. The regenerated tissue exactly resembles normal liver under the light and electron microscopes, and the standard liver function tests all return to within normal limits, usually well before gain in volume is complete.

Perhaps the most important point for the surgeon to note is the clear demonstration by Lin and Chen that an increase in size does not occur in the cirrhotic liver after resection, nor is there evidence of functional improvement.[22]

TECHNIQUE OF LIVER RESECTION

INTRODUCTION

Most general surgeons with busy surgical practices will be required to perform liver resection several times during a career, on an emergency if not an elective basis. For example, intraperitoneal hemorrhage due to the rupture of a benign or malignant tumor may surprise a surgeon operating for what he thought was a perforated ulcer, a ruptured ectopic pregnancy, or some more common abdominal emergency; during elective resection of carcinomas primary elsewhere in the abdomen, resectable liver metastases may be found that may lend themselves to synchronous resection, or unsuspected liver masses may be discovered as incidental findings at laparotomy for other disease, and excision biopsy may be preferable to incision biopsy and referral. Therefore, it behooves the general surgeon to become familiar with the surgical anatomy of the liver and the techniques of resection.

Too much has been written about special skills, special knowledge, and special tools for liver resection. To many this turgid vascular organ remains a "no man's land." However, an increasing experience with liver trauma has prompted many to learn the essentials, and the experience gained thereby can be usefully applied when the rare necessity for resection of a solid tumor presents itself.

This chapter will express to a greater extent than any other the author's personal biases, based on a moderate experience with both elective and emergency resections of liver tissue. These opinions have been shaded by surveying the results of others and by reading more than 600 operative notes dictated by more than 200 surgeons. However, those notes unfortunately often were deficient in defining the criteria for judgments made and in describing the small but important details of operative technique.

As I read reports of massive blood replacement, of cardiac arrest and resuscitations, and of operative mortality rates as high as 44 per cent,[27] and as I read the recommendations of advocates of hypothermia, aortic clamping, internal shunts, and multiple types of ingenious clamps, I am left both bewildered and bothered. Elective liver resection for tumor can and should be done in a controlled and deliberate fashion in a normotensive and normothermic patient, using techniques familiar to surgeons for many decades. When tumor anatomy requires the resection of portal vein or vena cava, the specialized techniques most recently advocated by Fortner, et al. may have a place,[13] but reported results to date have not convinced me that survival rates achieved by these heroic and gymnastic measures yet justify their common application.

I had an early, limited, and not always happy experience with techniques for liver resection using electrocautery, mattress sutures, sharp dissection, generalized hypothermia, and peritoneal cooling. Because of more recent, more extensive, and more favorable experience with simple techniques, these earlier methods have largely been abandoned. Lin (1954),[21] Tung (1963),[50] and others have re-emphasized the concept of blunt dissection during the last two decades, but we can go back to Keen,[20] who used his thumbnail in 1891 to excise a cystic tumor, for evidence that even the earliest pioneers in liver resection utilized that special quality of liver tissue, the appreciation of which forms the basis for safe liver surgery. That quality is that noncirrhotic liver parenchyma is as soft as cool butter, and once Glisson's capsule has been broached, the only significant resistance to gentle blunt dissection is provided by the blood vessels and major bile ducts. There are no septa and no avascular planes within this solid organ. These facts, plus a knowledge of the gross anatomy of the liver and its vessels, will allow the surgeon to operate safely within this most simple and yet most complicated of the extracranial viscera.

Surgical Anatomy

Figures 11–1, 11–2, and 11–3 depict the essentials of the surgical anatomy of the liver. Thanks to the excellent reviews of Goldsmith and Woodburne,[14] Healey, et al.[15, 16] and Pack and Baker,[39] which simply confirmed what had been pointed out decades before by Cantlie[4] and McIndoe and Counseller,[33] the topographic nomenclature of the liver

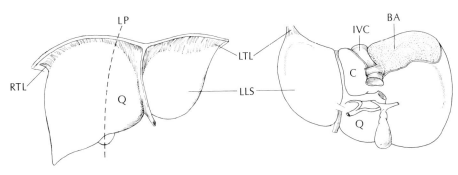

Figure 11–1. Topographic anatomy: anterior, posterior, and superior views.
Code:
  RTL—Right triangular ligament.
  LTL—Left triangular ligament.
  LP —Lobar plane.
  LLS —Left lateral segment.
  IVC —Inferior vena cava.
  BA —Bare area.
  C   —Caudate lobe.
  Q   —Quadrate lobe.
Note:
  (1) The anatomic or interlobar plane is from gallbladder bed to inferior vena cava.
  (2) The inferior vena cava is largely intrahepatic during its short course through the liver.
  (3) The lateral segment of the left lobe is connected to the quadrate lobe behind the round and falciform ligaments—usually by a ligament, but often by a short bridge of liver tissue.
  (4) The bare area is quite posterior.
  (5) The falciform ligament leads the surgeon to the anterior surface of the suprahepatic inferior vena cava through an avascular plane.

has given way to a system based on the divisions of the inflow blood vessels and bile ducts.

Certain points bear emphasis. The "bare area" of the liver, or that nonperitonealized surface contained within the suspensory ligaments, is quite posterior — a fact undoubtedly related to the four-legged posture of our distant ancestors. The exploring hand can pass freely over the dome of the right lobe, and when the surgeon's other hand is placed in Morison's pouch, a careful bimanual evaluation of the thickest (and thus most difficult to assess) part of the liver is quite feasible. Similarly, the left lobe can be evaluated by two sensitive hands in opposition. The caudate lobe hides behind the gastrohepatic ligament (lesser omentum) and its right extreme, the porta hepatis. When tumor affects this most inaccessible lobe, that tumor is very close to the anterior and left surfaces of the inferior vena cava as it lies largely within liver substance.

The bifurcation of the hepatic artery and portal vein into major lobar branches occurs outside of liver substance. Each major branch usually is dissectible for 1 to 3 cm beyond its bifurcations if the surrounding liver is pushed away. The confluence of the right and left hepatic ducts also always occurs outside liver substance, a fact known for many decades to general surgeons handling difficult bile duct problems. The anomalies of biliary drainage are well-known to general surgeons. The portal vein bifurcates at the hilum in three-quarters of patients, but other variations are not uncommon.[44] There are many anomalies of the arterial supply. In as many as 17 to 25 per cent of patients, part or all of the arterial supply of the right lobe of the liver may originate in the superior mesenteric artery; and in perhaps 20 to 25 per cent of patients the left hepatic artery, or at least that part supplying the left lateral segment of the liver, originates from the left gastric artery.[29, 35] The multiple collateral pathways for hepatic arterial blood have been well documented by the surgeons who have used ligation or perfusion of the hepatic artery for the management of patients with trauma or neoplastic disease of the liver.[28, 35]

Portal vein, hepatic artery, and bile duct may reach the hilum of the liver by different routes, but thereafter they travel together into lobe and segment. The caudate lobe receives inflow from both the right and left portal triads, and drains largely through lesser hepatic veins that enter the inferior vena cava below the major right, middle, and left hepatic venous trunks.

Perhaps the key point unknown to, or ignored by, resectionists in the past has been the relation of the falciform-round ligament sulcus (umbilical fissure) to the vascular inflow and bile drainage channels of the medial segment (quadrate lobe) and the lateral segment (classic topographic left lobe) of the left lobe of the liver. These major channels

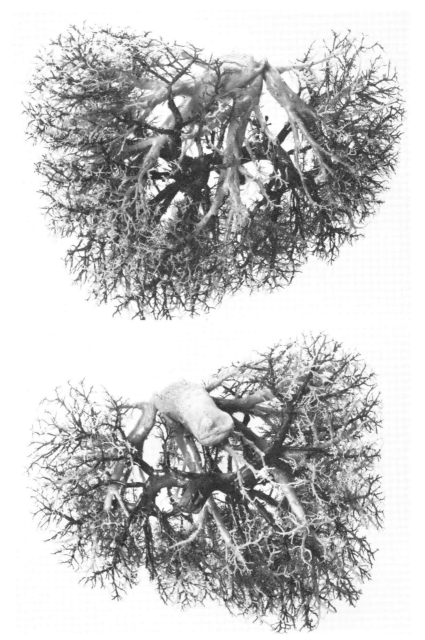

Figure 11–2. Vascular anatomy. Composite picture made up of two photographs and
one line drawing.

Photos are anterior (upper photo) and posterior views of vinyl acetate injection–corrosion casts from which central smaller radicles have been cut away to demonstrate major
vessel anatomy. Inferior vena cava and hepatic veins injected with light-colored plastic.
Portal venous system injected with dark-colored plastic.

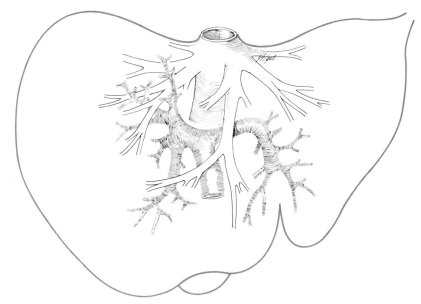

Figure 11–2. Continued.

Note: (1) The left main branch of portal vein is long and curves caudad in the plane of the falciform ligament to supply both the quadrate lobe and the lateral segment of the left lobe.

(2) The right main portal branch is quite short and bifurcates or trifurcates close to junction with main portal vein.

(3) The portal venous branches comes off at right angles from parent trunks.

(4) The right hepatic venous trunk is often as wide as it is long.

(5) The middle hepatic vein drains both the quadrate lobe (medial segment of the left lobe) and the lower anterior segment of the right lobe.

(6) The middle and left hepatic veins join to drain together into the inferior vena cava in most patients.

(7) The hepatic veins branch at less than a right angle.

(8) The most superior branches of the left and right hepatic veins are close to the surface of the liver and are vulnerable during transection of the suspensory ligaments.

(9) The portal and hepatic venous branches interdigitate throughout liver parenchyma, and therefore there are no bloodless planes.

(10) The middle hepatic vein lies in the interlobar plane and is very vulnerable during lobectomy. The line of transection for lobectomy must be kept to the right or left of this major trunk.

lie directly within the plane of the umbilical fissure (Figs. 11–2 and 11–3). Even if transection through this plane does not result in major hemorrhage, it must produce compromise of the afferent blood supply to the remaining segment. The line of resection for tumors of the left lateral segment should keep 1 to 2 cm to the left of the sulcus and its extension beneath the falciform ligament. If a left-sided tumor extends to or beyond the plane of this sulcus, an anatomic left lobectomy will be indicated, with sacrifice of the quadrate lobe as well as the left lateral segment. Some authors have described another potential line of transection 1 to 2 cm to the right of the falciform ligament plane, but this

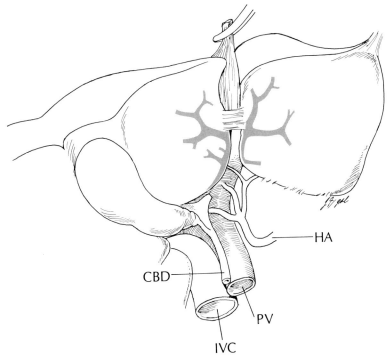

Figure 11–3. Hilum and sulcus of falciform ligament.

Code: CBC—Common bile duct.
         IVC —Inferior vena cava.
         HA —Hepatic artery.
         PV —Portal vein.

Note: (1) The undersurface of the left lobe of the liver reveals that there is a bridge between the medial and lateral segments of the left lobe. This bridge usually is fibrous but may be made of solid liver parenchyma.

(2) Traction on the falciform and round ligaments straightens out the curve of the left portal vein.

(3) Anomalies of the hepatic arterial supply are common. The so-called "middle" hepatic artery is usually a branch of the left hepatic artery, but may come off the main hepatic artery as shown here.

(4) The subhepatic inferior vena cava is readily accessible behind the right border of the gastrohepatic ligament and duodenum. It forms the back wall of the foramen of Winslow.

should be used only for the extension of a right lobectomy, and never for the extension of a left lobectomy.

The middle hepatic vein drains both the quadrate lobe and part of the inferior anterior segment of the right lobe. When tumor anatomy will allow, the middle vein can serve as a most useful guideline for transection during lobectomy (Fig. 11–15).

Because the hepatic veins cross the portal triads at right angles, there can be no truly isolated segments of the liver, nor any avascular

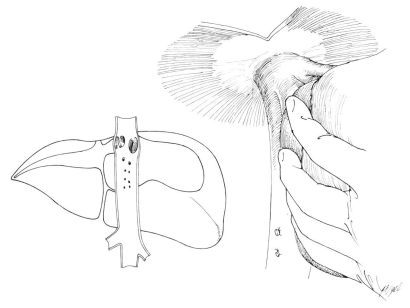

Figure 11–4. The hepatic veins.

Note: (1) With the diaphragm incised and the retroperitoneal attachments of the back of the right lobe of the liver incised, the liver has been rolled to the left to expose the junction of the right hepatic vein and inferior vena cava.

(2) This junction may be outside the liver, but usually its inferior and medial edges are within liver substance. Circumferential dissection therefore may be difficult and dangerous.

. (3) The smaller diagram shows that there may be a few smaller hepatic veins that drain the caudate lobe and the medial portion of the right superior-posterior segment. These enter the inferior cava below the major veins, are variable in number, and rarely are more than 1 cm in diameter. Transection of the most inferior vessels may facilitate right lobectomy, and ligation or clipping should be done in continuity before transection.

planes. In two-thirds of human livers the left hepatic vein joins the middle hepatic vein before entering the inferior vena cava, but this common channel may be quite short (Fig. 11–2). In most cases only the superior aspect of the distal ends of the right and left hepatic veins are accessible outside of liver substance. Circumferential dissection of these trunks, therefore, is very dangerous in most patients (Fig. 11–4). Should hemorrhage occur at this ticklish juncture, no attempt should be made at repair until proximal and distal control of the inferior vena cava is achieved.

Preoperative Preparation

A candidate for elective hepatic resection should come to the operating room well hydrated with an intravenous infusion of glucose running through a large-bore catheter and with a nasogastric tube in place. Unless preoperative studies have indicated a very peripheral and easily accessible location of the tumor, a central venous catheter also should be in place.

Although Pack gave cortisone to patients undergoing right hepatic lobectomy because of experimental evidence that its use enhanced regeneration after subtotal hepatectomy,[42] and although Figueroa, et al. demonstrated that adrenal steroid therapy will prolong the tolerable warm ischemia time of rabbits with hilar clamping,[12] the routine use of preoperative, intraoperative, or postoperative adrenal steroids is not recommended for most patients undergoing elective liver resection. However, antibiotics are used intraoperatively and for a short time after operation, in spite of the lack of any controlled study of their efficacy. Vitamin K_1 oxide is given preoperatively, even to those patients with normal prothrombin levels.

Should an x-ray tunnel be placed beneath the patient on the operating table? Ochsner, et al. have stated that operative cholangiography was the "most valuable method of demonstrating disease deep within the hepatic substance and determining the extent of the lesion,"[37] and Chan feels that "intraoperative portography is the best way to determine spread at laparotomy."[5] However, I prefer not to use the x-ray tunnel because to do so would eliminate the possibility of flexion of the operating table. Preoperative radioisotope scanning and angiography, plus the manual sensitivity of the experienced surgeon, can provide adequate information about the location and extent of disease in most patients. The importance of an ability to flex the operating table overrides the convenience of a radiographic capability that will seldom be used. Proper placement of the patient over a kidney-rest may allow significantly increased exposure of the inferior and posterior

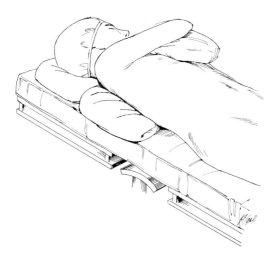

Figure 11–5. Operating table position. For most elective major liver resections, the patient's right shoulder should be raised approximately 30 degrees from the horizontal to allow thoracic extension of a primary abdominal incision. The hips remain flat to facilitate laparotomy. The patient should be positioned so as to allow elevation of the kidney rest, which will increase exposure of the liver hilum.

surfaces of the liver, and thereby may save the patient a thoracotomy wound extension and increase the safety of dissection.

For reasons that will be explained below, I prefer right thoracotomy to median sternotomy extension of an abdominal incision for right lobectomy. Therefore, with hips flat on the table, the patient's right thorax should be rotated about 15 to 30 degrees to the left, with placement of the right arm on an arm rest or ether-screen as diagramed (Fig. 11–5).

THE INCISION

When the patient has a narrow costal margin, a midline incision is probably most suitable for exploration. When the costal margin is flared widely, a subcostal incision can be made on either side and extended or "T-ed" into the right thorax if necessary. In the rare instance when a previous abdominal exploration has revealed a solitary, small, superior, and lateral tumor in either lobe, and when other intraabdominal disease has been carefully ruled out, a thoracotomy incision alone for transdiaphragmatic wedge resection may provide adequate exposure. However, time after time, a nodule carefully described by a referring physician as "solitary" at a previous laparotomy has proved at subsequent operation to have one or more companions in the retroperitoneum or in another area of the liver.

The decision to proceed with resection of an apparently solitary tumor requires thorough exploration of the retroperitoneum and of the posterior regions of the liver at hilum and diaphragm, together with bimanual palpation of the right and left lobes. Thus, unless (1) metastatic disease is obvious; (2) disease is bulky and bilateral; or (3) there is an obvious diffuse cirrhosis of the liver, adequate exploration requires an incision that freely admits two hands.

EXPLORATION

The initial appearance of a liver mass often suggests the correct diagnosis. Hepatocellular carcinomas are soft, often yellow or gray in color, and have prominent surface vascularity. Cholangiocarcinomas and liver metastases from elsewhere in the gastrointestinal tract, breast, or lung usually are quite hard and, in the case of secondary tumors, usually umbilicated. Focal nodular hyperplasia is firm, dark, and often pedunculated. Hepatocellular adenomas are orange–white, quite soft, and often show capsular rupture and hemoperitoneum. Blue and thin-walled cystic lesions usually are benign. Grossly evident calcification suggests echinococcal disease, old trauma, or regressive changes in a hemangioma, but also may be seen occasionally with cystadenoma or cystadenocarcinoma. Abscess and central hematoma may be difficult to differentiate from neoplasm, but the patient's history should have alerted the surgeon to these possibilities prior to operation. Needle aspiration of fluid contents may help with differential diagnosis. Rupture of a cirrhotic liver with hemoperitoneum is due to liver cell carcinoma until proved otherwise.

Fibrous adhesions to the gallbladder, colon, and stomach should be taken down, and the lesser sac should be opened to evaluate the caudate lobe and the lymph node–rich areas along the superior aspect of the pancreas and the roots of the splanchnic arteries. Transection of the round and falciform ligaments will allow a thorough bimanual evaluation of both lobes of the liver and provide an approach to the anterior surface of the inferior vena cava at the diaphragm. However these ligaments are better left uncut if right lobectomy or extended right lobectomy is planned, unless their division is essential for evaluation. The left and right coronary ligaments need not be sectioned until after decision for resection is made in most cases.

Biopsies for frozen section diagnosis should be done early, preferably from a small satellite nodule in the liver or a suspicious extrahepatic lesion. If the tumor is small or pedunculated, excision biopsy may be the safest or most expeditious approach. Simple sharp wedge incision biopsy without suture usually is done safely for the firmer or scirrhous tumors. The softer and more vascular primary hepatocellular carcinomas and hepatocellular adenomas often bleed excessively from biopsy sites. Hemostatic sutures usually are required, but the soft tumor tissue may not hold such sutures well. Needle biopsy may be a less vascular alternative and usually will suffice to establish a frozen section diagnosis. The histologic differentiation between a hepatocellular adenoma and a well-differentiated trabecular hepatocellular carcinoma by frozen section may be difficult, but, since both of these lesions should be resected, this distinction may not have a large clinical significance. Large benign-appearing cystic tumors should be opened if resection is not planned, and their inner lining searched for plaquelike lesions suggesting cystadenoma or cystadenocarcinoma. The liver hilum should be carefully evaluated for evidence of lymph node metastasis and/or portal vein involvement. Primary hepatocellular carcinoma often grows down the portal vein in a retrograde direction, but even when preoperative x-rays have raised this suspicion, the soft tumor in the vein often is difficult to palpate externally. With an index finger in the foramen of Winslow and a thumb anterior to the common bile duct, the portal vein can be ballotted in most patients.

Large tumors of the quadrate lobe and/or the right anterior segment may obscure the hilar structures. Flexion of a patient on the kidney-rest and gentle elevation of these segments will usually allow evaluation up to the major bifurcations.

The critical areas for determining resectability of tumors apparently confined to Glisson's capsule are the portal vein bifurcation, the inferior vena cava, and the umbilical fissure. It may be necessary finally to take down either the left or right triangular ligaments (but not both) to determine whether disease involves the intrahepatic inferior vena cava. The left side of the vena cava can be evaluated with a finger in the lesser sac passing over and under the caudate lobe up to the diaphragm. Opening of the retroperitoneum on the right after section of the right coronary ligament, and rotation of the liver to the left, should give adequate exposure of the right side of the inferior vena cava. Complete division of the falciform ligament will allow careful palpation of the anterior surface of the inferior vena cava at the level of the diaphragm.

After the above steps have been accomplished, a decision should be made about resection. Although others might disagree, at the present time I would not elect resection of a primary malignant tumor of the liver for a patient with one or more of the following findings:

(1) histologic proof of disease outside of the liver;

(2) involvement of the inferior vena cava;

(3) retrograde intraluminal tumor growth in the portal vein to its bifurcation or adventitial involvement of the portal vein at its bifurcation;

(4) discrete tumor nodules in both anatomic lobes; and

(5) involvement of the liver with a diffuse cirrhosis.

Multiple tumor nodules confined to one lobe, or involvement of the medial portion of the opposite lobe by a bulky solitary tumor, are not contraindications to resection of primary tumors. Specific exceptions to these general guidelines are listed in the several chapters discussing particular tumors.

GENERAL PRINCIPLES OF THE TRANSECTION OF LIVER TISSUE

It would take another chapter to describe the multiple techniques that surgeons have advocated for cutting through the liver. A few will be discussed below, but the reader is referred to Chapter Two for a brief outline of some of the historical aspects of hepatic craftsmanship. What is proposed here is a modification of blunt technique that is rapid and that has proved effective in major and minor resections. The anatomic basis and the essential steps for specific lobar and segmental resections will be discussed separately, but in all instances it is necessary to transect liver tissue. The use of clamps, mattress sutures, electrocautery, and sharp instruments is discouraged. Encouraged is the specific control of vessels and ducts under direct vision with hemostatic ties or metal clips of as small size as possible. Vessels should be tied or clipped before they are cut because they will retract into the liver substance following transection, and subsequent control may prove most difficult. For excision of major segments, preliminary hilar ligation should precede, and will greatly simplify, subsequent transection.

The technique proposed is simple, and involves a careful outline of the proposed excision on Glisson's capsule followed by a rapid transection in an anterior-posterior direction.

Step One

After a sharp entry is made with a knife through Glisson's capsule alone, blunt dissection and sharp division of the capsule is continued with a scissors (Fig. 11–6). The capsule dissects readily off normal liver if the right plane is achieved. Capsular division should completely outline the proposed line of resection on the surface of the liver. Spar-

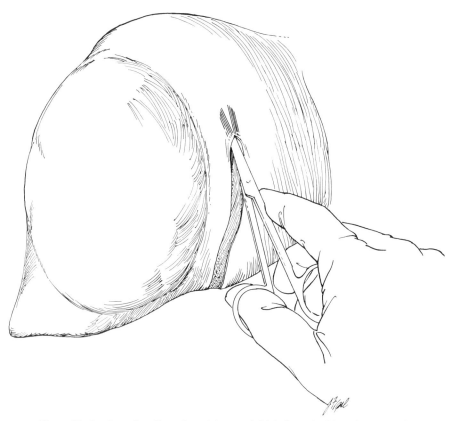

Figure 11–6. Capsular dissection. After an initial sharp incision through Glisson's capsule, the rest of the capsule is dissected bluntly away from the liver parenchyma and then cut so as to completely outline the eventual line of transection. This complete capsular incision will guide the plane for subsequent rapid blunt suction transection.

ing a centimeter or two of capsule on the tumor side of the line of proposed division of liver substance may facilitate eventual treatment of the raw surface.

Step Two

With one hand controlling tumor and the posterior surface of the part to be resected, the surgeon transects liver substance from anterior to posterior with a blunt-nosed metal suction tip held in the dominant hand (Fig. 11–7). Liver tissue is teased away from the vessels by rubbing the suction tip longitudinally along the line of transection. Each

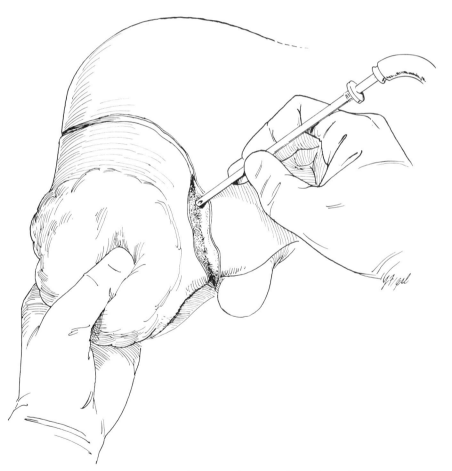

Figure 11–7. Blunt suction technique. After capsular incision, liver substance is teased away from the more resistant vessels, using a blunt-tipped metal suction tip. Small vessels are best treated with clips and/or ties without application of hemostatic clamps. Illustrated is the inner suction tip of an "abdominal" or Poole sucker, which is used after removal of the multi-holed outer sheath.

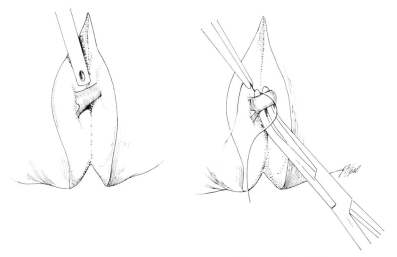

Figure 11–8. Ligation of larger vessels. When blunt suction technique uncovers the anterior surface of a large vessel, circumferential dissection is carefully done with a right-angled clamp. The vessel is then tied on both sides before transection.

and every resistance is clipped and then cut. When larger vessels are encountered by the suction tip, they are carefully encircled with a right-angled clamp and tied before transection (Fig. 11–8). Clips and ties are applied by the first assistant, who also cuts between the ligated vessels. The surgeon maintains direction and control with his non-dominant hand, and with the dominant hand he proceeds rapidly down through liver substance to the posterior capsule in a field kept visible by the suction of the dissecting instrument. With the multiholed metal sheath removed, the inner tip of a Poole abdominal sucker is an ideal size and shape for this technique. Tumor neovascularity is always arterial and often impressive with primary tumors, but if the transection is at some distance from the tumor, each artery will be recognized and specifically tied. Even if major hepatic veins have been tied earlier at their inferior vena cava junction, they should be re-encountered and religated within liver substance if tumor anatomy allows.

An effective team should take no more than five to ten minutes to accomplish transection if the proposed route is carefully defined before the incision of liver substance. The anesthesiologist should be prepared to transfuse blood during transection, but with primary hilar ligation this is not always necessary. Attempts at control of vessels inadvertently transected before ligation should be discouraged until the specimen is removed. Gentle pressure over gauze applied by an assistant will control these bleeding points for a few moments. Remember that the major arteries provide most resistance, and thus usually are found and tied by gentle blunt suction technique. Remember too that the venous compartments are low pressure and readily controlled by surface compression.

Once the transection is complete, a moistened gauze pack should be applied to the raw liver surface for several minutes. This will allow time for inspection of the tissue removed and will provide an opportunity for spontaneous hemostasis by platelet aggregation and clotting in any unligated vessels. Bleeding from small arteries may persist, but this also is best treated initially by pressure and time. Should arterial oozing continue, direct suture control is preferable to clamping and/or clipping. Small bites with a fine suture will usually suffice to surround a point of oozing that often is caused by a side-hole in an intact vessel — a hole that may be enlarged by a clip or torn by a clamp.

Thirty to 50 clips and five to ten ligatures are usually left on the raw surface after lobectomy. Not more than a handful of these clips and ties will be visible after a few minutes of gentle compression, which again illustrates the ability of the transected vessels to withdraw into liver substance.

Speed, teamwork, and attention to details of hemostasis emphasized by Halsted 85 years ago will result in a resection leaving no devitalized or crushed tissue and a minimum of foreign body. Be patient with small oozing vessels and they will stop. Remember that after trauma the normal liver shows a remarkable ability for hemostasis if large vessels are not transected. Delayed hemorrhage from such vessels is very rare unless the problem has been compounded by necrosis caused by massive ligatures, or unless sepsis is encouraged by dead tissue, large foreign bodies, or a "dead space" problem.

The advantages of this blunt suction technique over finger fracture in the elective situation are those of refinement. Most small blood vessels avulsed without ligation by the less discrete finger fracture technique will stop bleeding spontaneously, but small bile ducts thus severed are more liable to leak postoperatively. Meticulous hemostasis will provide meticulous bile stasis.

Most writings on liver resection advise the surgeon to cover the raw surface left after transection by capsule approximation or by attachment of adjacent ligaments or viscera. The only reason to "close" the raw surface exposed by liver transection is to provide hemostasis. Healing of such a surface will take place, as it does for any other abdominal surface denuded of peritoneum, by mesothelial change of wandering peritoneal round cells or underlying connective tissue cells, and of the surface cells of adjacent viscera. This healing is rapidly completed in a few days unless there is infection or necrosis of the underlying liver cells. The other enemy of surface healing is a persistent dead space.

Gentle compression for venous hemostasis sometimes can be secured without vascular compromise by bringing the edges of a concave defect together, using small sutures placed only through liver capsule. Previous blunt capsular dissection facilitates this technique. Closure may encourage hematoma or dead space formation, and a decision will have to be made for each patient based on individual circumstances. I have seldom made any effort to close or cover the raw surface, and have yet to regret this practice. An attempt is always made to fill dead space so that colon, stomach, or omentum are left lying against the transected surface.

The use of electrocautery, specialized clamps, cryosurgery, shunts, hypothermia, surgical adhesives, and other adjuncts to liver resection were dismissed rather summarily in a preceding paragraph. A further explanation is warranted.

Liver resection clamps have been used since Garrè (see Chapter 2).[55] The more modern varieties[3, 10, 11, 48] are temporarily applied to decrease blood loss during transection, and then are removed after ligation of vessels. Their application around central lesions, particularly in the right lobe, is very awkward. Their use may decrease the risk of tumor embolization via the hepatic veins, but to be effective in reducing hemorrhage from central vessels they must also crush and perhaps tear peripheral vessels. Tissue peripheral to the clamp usually is left and may subsequently slough. The newer "crush clamp" technique of Lin avoids this complication.[21]

Large, angled vascular clamps may be used in another fashion without risk of damage to remaining liver, and with at least a theoretic potential for limiting tumor emboli. If tumor anatomy allows, placement of such a clamp around the tumor will provide a convenient "handle" and also limit venous return (Fig. 11–9). Turner used this trick in 1923,[51] and it has proved very useful for peripheral lesions in my experience.

Mattress sutures hold an honored place in the history of the control of hemorrhage from raw liver surface, but currently are esteemed chiefly by those who are unfamiliar with the more discrete methods of vascular control. Mattress sutures tend to cut through soft liver substance if tied tightly enough to control hemorrhage; their placement back from the transected surface risks compromise of vital blood supply and bile drainage to areas of remaining liver, and their size adds an enormous bulk of foreign body, a problem that is only increased if bolsters of Teflon or Ivalon are used to prevent their migration into liver parenchyma. Perhaps the greatest objection to mattress sutures, however, relates to the certain necrosis of liver tissue distal to the ligature. As the use of mattress sutures has decreased, so too has the incidence of postoperative subphrenic sepsis. Tsuzuki, et al. markedly decreased the incidence of abscess formation in dogs by avoiding the use of clamps and mattress sutures, and demonstrated a clear superior-

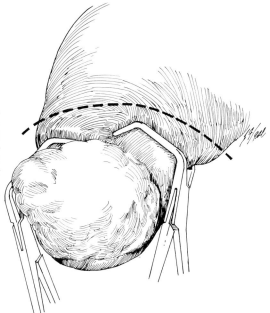

Figure 11-9. Use of clamps as a "handle." Large angled vascular clamps have been placed close to a peripheral tumor to provide a "handle" for traction and to limit venous tumor spread during manipulation. Transection will be done above or central to these clamps.

ity of the finger fracture technique when it was compared with the use of mattress sutures or clamps.[49]

Electrocautery and sharp dissection are decried because both techniques allow withdrawal of transected vessels into liver substance, where subsequent control is most difficult. Cautery is effective in controlling hemorrhage from small vessels, but a trip through a significant thickness of liver tissue will certainly encounter veins 1 cm in diameter or larger, and their transection by cautery will compound rather than solve the hemostatic problem. Blunt technique allows separation of vessels from liver tissue for easier control, whereas cautery and cryosurgical techniques fuse vessels and liver tissue together and make subsequent discrete control more difficult. Cryosurgical transection provides temporary hemostasis after liver transection in experimental animals, but late hemorrhage is very common.[17]

Raffucci, et al. and others have shown that hypothermic dogs will tolerate inflow occlusion for up to 57 minutes, whereas 15 minutes is the limit with normothermia.[43] Many have advocated either systemic or local cooling to "protect" the liver and the patient during ischemic or hemorrhagic crises, but crises should be expected no more often during controlled liver resection than during other major abdominal operations. The cold perfusion and vascular isolation techniques recently reintroduced by Fortner, et al. may prove invaluable when resection of the portal vein and/or inferior vena cava is necessary to develop a free margin around tumor.[13, 46] However, McDermott and Longmire (who investigated the use of cold perfusion many years ago)[32] and Balasegaram[3] share my bias that employment of such techniques is unnecessary in the vast majority of liver resections for solid tumor. Their use actually may increase the risk of operative and postoperative complications. One can only admire the courage and talent of those trying to extend the limits of liver resection by the use of techniques developed by cardiac and transplant surgeons, but the reported results, in terms of patient survival, do not yet warrant a widespread acceptance or utilization of such complex procedures; in fact, they militate against such a recommendation.

The reader is referred to the excellent discussions and illustrations of Madding and Kennedy for a more thorough review of liver anatomy, hemostasis, and the use of various clamps and shunts.[25]

THE TECHNIQUE OF SPECIFIC LOBAR AND SEGMENTAL RESECTIONS

Lobar and segmental resections are based on the anatomic divisions of the inflow blood vessels and bile ducts.[8, 16, 44] The anatomists have helped us to define various segments, but their efforts should not lead us to propose "segmental" operations that increase the operative risk to the patient. For example, the hilar trunks branch quickly to define separate anterior and posterior segments of the right lobe, and these have been further subdivided (Fig. 11–10). Practically, however, lesions in the periphery of the lower part of the right lobe are best resected by wedge excision without "segmental" dissection, and lesions at the dome of the right lobe, unless small enough for a simple wedge excision, are treated more safely by total right lobectomy. To "save" segments of the right lobe by complicated, prolonged, and risk-increasing segmental dissections is theoretically a commendable objective, but it ignores the well-proved ability of the noncirrhotic liver to regenerate. There are really, then, only five standard types of liver resection: wedge; right lobectomy; left lobectomy; left lateral segmentectomy; and central hepatectomy. A right and left lobectomy may be "extended" by taking enough of the medial portion of the opposite lobe to encompass tumor. Starzl, et al. have formalized the right extended lobectomy that includes all of the medial segment of the left lobe, and have called this procedure "trisegmentectomy."[47] These operations will be discussed separately after some general comments are made about the control of the hilar vessels and the inferior vena cava.

PROXIMAL AND DISTAL CONTROL

Dissection of the hilum of the liver begins anteriorly and should be developed as close to the liver as possible. The general surgeon will be

parietal aspect

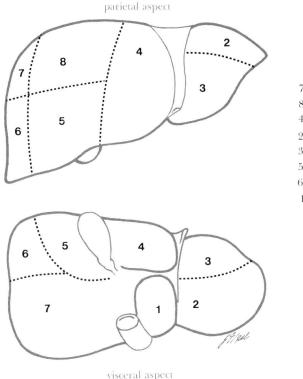

Areas

7: posterior superior
8: anterior superior
4: medial
2: lateral superior
3: lateral inferior
5: anterior inferior
6: posterior inferior
1: caudate

visceral aspect

Figure 11–10. The segments of the liver. Anatomists have emphasized the presence of discrete segments of the liver based on the distribution of the inflow vessels. The segments have been named and numbered as follows:

    (1) Caudate lobe.
    (2) Superior left lateral segment.
    (3) Inferior left lateral segment.
    (4) Medial segment, left lobe.
    (5) Ventrocaudal segment, right lobe.
    (6) Dorsocaudal segment, right lobe.
    (7) Dorsocranial segment, right lobe.
    (8) Ventrocranial segment, right lobe.

The quadrate lobe is the inferior portion of the fourth or medial segment of the left lobe. The distribution of the hepatic venous drainage negates the usefulness to the surgeon of many of these intersegmental "planes."

tempted to isolate the common bile duct beyond the cystic duct junction where he is on familiar ground, so that he can then trace the bile duct proximally to its bifurcation. However, the common hepatic duct is often quite long, and it is possible to have several centimeters of bile duct "hanging in the breeze" after lobectomy, a situation that probably will contribute to the incidence of postoperative bile duct problems. Distal dissection, if done at all, should be limited to the anterior surface of the bile ducts. For either right or left lobectomy, the cystic duct may be isolated and divided early to increase exposure, since the gallbladder eventually will be sacrificed.

Anatomy texts do not often show the extensive network of small blood vessels, lymphatics, and nerves that surround and, to a certain extent, hide the major vessels at liver hilum. The confluence of the right and left hepatic ducts usually is anterior to this network. Circumferential dissection of the bile ducts should be limited to the area of proposed transection. An untied ligature may be placed around the site of proposed ductal ligation, and held for further identification.

Arterial dissection generally is done next, and this should be based on preoperative angiography when possible. Anomalies are common and have been well reviewed by Michels.[35] Gentle elevation of the bile ducts and careful palpation with a finger behind in the foramen of Winslow will allow location of the major arterial trunks, which are always surrounded by dense fibrous, lymphatic, and nervous tissue. The arterial adventitia should be approached early and directly to facilitate further distal dissection and identification of major branches. If positive identification of the arterial branch supplying the segment to be resected is unsure, the injection of a few cubic centimeters of indigo carmine through a fine needle into the suspected trunk will confirm its distal distribution. Once again, an untied ligature will mark the appropriate vessels for subsequent control.

The portal vein usually is approached most easily from the right. It lies posterior to the artery and bile duct. Rotation of the table toward the patient's left side will facilitate its identification. There are no branches on the anterior, right, and posterior surfaces of the portal vein close to the liver. Once the proper plane is achieved, dissection can proceed rapidly up to bifurcation. The inconstant, but dangerous, branches draining into the left or medial side of the portal vein are best left undisturbed. They enter well inferior to the main portal vein bifurcation, and need not be exposed. The major problem with control of the portal vein prior to right lobectomy relates to the length, or rather the lack of length, of the right portal vein. A major posterior segmental trunk that begins immediately at the bifurcation is common, dangerous, and difficult of exposure. This so-called "trifurcation"[52] is best dealt with by delaying the dissection of the right branches until the main portal vein and the left portal vein are encircled for subsequent control. Once this is accomplished, the visible right vein may be encircled distally. Whether this obvious trunk is a common right portal vein or only the anterior segmental branch will become obvious when it is ligated and divided. Should hemorrhage occur, it is easily managed with control of the main and left trunks. Suture ligation is preferred, since a simple tie may be rubbed off during subsequent dissection or retraction.

Control of the inferior vena cava may become necessary for the excision of bulky tumors extending posteriorly, or if accidental injury occurs to major hepatic veins. Formal control is not necessary for most elective resections, and usually can be delayed until needed. If a tear occurs during the dissection of major hepatic veins, gentle pressure will nicely control this low pressure system while the subhepatic and supradiaphragmatic portions of the inferior vena cava are encircled. Attempts to clamp, sew, or tie such lacerations without prior distal and proximal control are fraught with the dangers of exsanguinating hemorrhage and air embolization. After control is obtained, deliberate repair can be done with inflow and outflow occlusion. Heaney recommends subdiaphragmatic aortic clamping during periods of vena cava occlusion,[18] but this is rarely necessary.

One should never attempt to encircle and control the suprahepatic subdiaphragmatic inferior vena cava, since no such possibility exists. The diaphragmatic attachment of the posterior wall of the inferior vena cava usually is inferior to the drainage point of major hepatic veins, so that distal or superior control must always take place in the chest (Fig. 11–11).

Control of the subhepatic inferior vena cava is easily managed after elevation of the duodenum by Kocher's maneuver. The cava

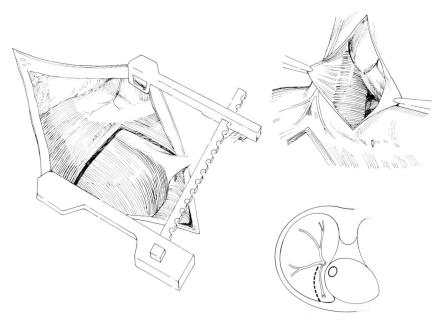

Figure 11–11. Diaphragm incision and vena caval control. After intercostal incision, a radial incision is made in the anterior right diaphragm aiming centrally toward the inferior vena cava. By keeping the branches of the phrenic nerve in sight, the surgeon can preserve all branches by stopping the incision short of the vulnerable anterior branch. The supradiaphragmatic inferior vena cava is approached by incising the pericardium anterior to the phrenic nerve. Blunt dissection below the heart will allow rapid and safe tape encirclement within the pericardium. The phrenic nerve branches are most vulnerable during closure of the diaphragm, and care must be taken to exclude these branches from the large sutures usually used for repair.

should be encircled above the renal veins. The right adrenal vein is occasionally a problem here, and dissection should proceed wherever convenient either above or below this difficult tributary.

Emergency control of the suprahepatic inferior vena cava can be achieved by incision of the diaphragm 2 to 3 cm anterior to the junction of the subdiaphragmatic cava and diaphragm. This leads the surgeon into the pericardium, where rapid blunt dissection allows circumferential control just below the right atrium. If the right thorax is already opened, a more direct and deliberate approach to the intrapericardial vena cava is facilitated.

RATIONALE AND TECHNIQUES OF SPECIFIC TYPES OF LIVER RESECTION

Wedge Resection

A wedge resection is defined as any type of peripheral resection in which no hilar, segmental, or major hepatic venous trunks are transected. The anatomic basis of wedge resection of even large lesions is that peripheral lesions are served by only the terminal branches of the afferent vessels, and only the beginnings of the efferent systems. Wedge resection is most suitable for pedunculated lesions or tumors at the free or lower edge of the liver. However, it is also suitable for removal of small surface lesions from the accessible anterior and superior surfaces of the liver, and from the quadrate lobe.

Technique. The classic technique of surrounding a small tumor with mattress sutures of absorbable material (Fig. 11–12) probably is not bad enough to be entirely discarded, but for the larger lesions it is more dangerous and less effective than the use of the blunt suction

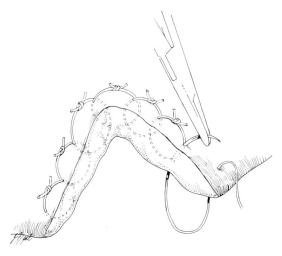

Figure 11–12. Mattress suture wedge excision. Usually, interlocking mattress sutures of heavy absorbable material are placed prior to sharp wedge excision of a peripheral tumor, but they also may be placed after tumor excision if required by hemostasis.

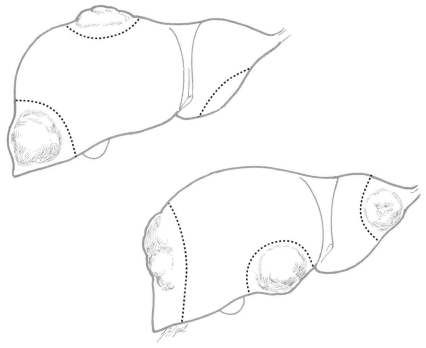

Figure 11–13. Wedge excisions. Although wedge excision is most useful for small tumors along the free edge of the liver, it also may be done for more bulky disease. Typical large wedge excisions are illustrated. Individual circumstances will dictate whether preliminary hilar control is necessary. The upper diagram illustrates the type of peripheral excision of the lower part of the left lateral segment often done to satisfy the "en bloc" principle in removing a large gastric carcinoma that has invaded adjacent liver.

technique described above. Wedge excisions, with or without the use of mattress sutures, can be used for removal of large portions of the right lobe and/or quadrate lobe. Preliminary identification, dissection (but not ligation) of hilar trunks, and careful "mapping" of the line of resection with capsular incision will protect the major vessels and ducts. Figure 11–13 illustrates several common wedge excision sites. The defect created by wedge excision of liver tissue occasionally can be closed by approximation of capsule from either side, but more often is best treated by leaving it alone or by filling the defect with adjacent viscera. These viscera, usually the omentum, may or may not be fixed to the defect with holding sutures. Adequate drainage should be provided when a significant area of liver surface has been transected.

Right Lobectomy

Right lobectomy is defined as the removal of that part of the liver supplied by the right hepatic artery, right portal vein, and right hepatic duct. It includes removal of the area drained by the major right branch of the middle hepatic vein, but it usually is possible to preserve the venous drainage of the quadrate lobe. This operation is the most common type of resection done for large tumor masses, since most types of primary liver tumors have a predilection for the right lobe.

Indications. These are:

(1) any central tumor of the right lobe that requires sacrifice of the right hepatic vein and/or the right inflow vessels; (2) when multiple tumor nodules are in the right lobe, but none are found in the left.

Technique. When a decision for right lobectomy is made for adult patients, the abdominal incision usually should be extended into the thorax. The greater flexibility of a child's rib cage and mobility of the pediatric liver may allow formal right lobectomy without thoracic extension. Thoracic extension can be done by median sternotomy or by right intercostal incision.

Right thoracotomy is preferred for several reasons.

(1) It allows careful palpation of the right lung for evidence of metastatic disease.

(2) It allows supradiaphragmatic evaluation of the back of the liver and the inferior vena cava. On several occasions when the inferior vena cava seemed free of tumor during abdominal exploration, careful transthoracic evaluation has confirmed tumor involvement of this critical area.

(3) Right thoracotomy equalizes abdominal, pleural, and room pressure – thus reducing the danger of air embolization.

(4) When combined with diaphragmatic incision, right thoracotomy allows more direct and deliberate exposure and control of the hepatic vein–inferior vena cava junction from the more accessible lateral and posterior aspect.

(5) The liver can be displaced into the chest to provide wider exposure of the posterior and undersurfaces of the liver. This will facilitate control of the pesky lesser hepatic veins draining the caudate lobe, and will improve exposure of the hilar structures that may be obscured by a large bulky tumor in the right lobe.

However, a right thoracic extension adds to postoperative discomfort and encourages respiratory complications. Also, when ascites forms after liver resection in a patient with thoracic extension, right pleural effusion is a constant finding in spite of a "water-tight" diaphragmatic closure.

The right costal margin is crossed at a point allowing entry into the seventh or eighth intercostal spaces. The skin incision seldom needs to be carried beyond the midaxillary line, and an early entry into the pleural space will allow safe extension laterally. The transected angles of the costal cartilages often seem to fit nicely into the rectangular windows in the blades of the self-retaining thoracotomy retractor, or this retractor may be placed more laterally. The diaphragm is incised radially from costal margin to the anterolateral surface of the pericardium. The phrenic nerve is more likely'to be compromised during suture repair of the transected diaphragm, but also is vulnerable during incision if not carefully watched. (See Figure 11–11).

When thoracic and caval exploration reveals no contraindication to right lobectomy, the liver should be freed of its avascular attachments. Incision of the right suspensory ligaments of the liver and opening of the peritoneum overlying the retrohepatic vena cava are facilitated by: (1) rotation of the table away from the operator; (2) flexion of the patient by elevation of the kidney-rest; and (3) gentle retraction of the right lobe anterior and to the left by the first assistant. Venous return may be compromised by these maneuvers. Usually one or two small phrenic arteries need ligation, as these largely avascular planes are developed from laterally and inferiorly up to the caval junction with the diaphragm.

The liver should then be replaced into its normal position, and hilar ligation should be accomplished by the techniques mentioned above. If there is any doubt about bile duct anatomy, a soft rubber catheter should be inserted into the common hepatic duct or common bile duct to ensure the identification and safety of the left ducts. Once hilar ligation is complete, the table is again rotated away from the surgeon, and the right lobe is retracted to the left. In most patients, a gentle attempt should be made to control the right major hepatic vein at its caval junction, but more often than not the intrahepatic location of this junction will prevent easy circumnavigation of the right hepatic vein, and the effort *should not be pursued.* This vein can be more safely and more easily controlled at the end of transection of liver substance. An attempt to dissect the right hepatic vein at its caval junction should never be made in patients without a thoracic extension of the abdominal incision. In those few instances in which the right hepatic vein is easily encircled, a single, heavy, nonabsorbable ligature should be tied down firmly, but no attempt at clamping, suture ligation, or transection should be made at this point.

With the liver retracted to the left, and with the medial and posterior extent of the tumor appreciated, a decision should be made about ligation of the lesser hepatic veins. Usually not more than one or two of the most inferior veins require ligation. When easy, this is quickly done; when difficult, these short veins are best left alone unless caudate lobe resection is also planned. The line of proposed transection of capsule is identified, and the capsule is cut after blunt dissection away from liver substance. Capsular incision is most difficult and most important around the hilum and near the caudate lobe. It is here that subsequent injury to major *left* inflow trunks is most likely to occur, and these vessels must be kept clearly in sight, as well as mind, when liver substance is transected. The capsular incision is carried superiorly to within 2 or 3 cm of the inferior vena cava, but then veers to the right over the last 3 or 4 cm to allow ligation of a stalk of the right hepatic vein, and to avoid injury to the middle hepatic vein at its junction with the inferior vena cava.

The transection of liver substance is begun on the free edge and anterior surface, and proceeds quickly if the preliminary work described above has been done properly. The only major technical point relates to the right branch of the middle hepatic vein. This is commonly encountered as the first large vessel in the middle of the anterior surface incision. By its direction one can determine whether it drains the quadrate lobe or the anterior segment of the right lobe. The right lobe branches must be taken, but, when tumor anatomy allows, the quadrate lobe branch and middle hepatic trunk provide useful landmarks to limit the medial margin of resection. With one hand behind the right lobe and tumor, and the other hand on the sucker tip, the surgeon controls to the millimeter the appropriate line of resection as his assistant ties, clips, and cuts. This bimanual technique allows accurate appreciation of the direction and depth of transection.

When the posterior capsule is approached, the dissection moves to the right of the inferior vena cava. The major right hepatic trunk or trunks are always impressively large, but ligation should not be difficult since control occurs when this vessel is the last portion of liver to be transected. At this point a clamp may be applied or, preferably, the right hepatic venous stalk should be tied in continuity. Suture ligation superficial to a simple ligature may be added by the cautious surgeon.

With removal of the right lobe and tumor, the large raw surface is treated as described above. If the falciform and left triangular ligaments have been left intact, there is little problem with hilar angulation. The right subphrenic space is drained with soft and suction catheters and filled with adjacent viscera—usually transverse colon and omentum. The bile ducts should be checked carefully, and if there is any doubt about angulation or patency the biliary tree should be decompressed with some sort of tube.

The diaphragm is closed using heavy nonabsorbable sutures placed at least 1 cm back from the cut edge, with care to avoid branches of the phrenic nerve. The cartilages at rib margin are closed with "figure-of-8" wires, often after excision of a wedge of cartilage. No drains should come out through the abdominal wound, which usually is closed with large "buried retention" sutures of wire or plastic, placed well back in the fascia and carried through all layers except skin and subcutaneous tissue.

Extended Right Lobectomy

Extended right lobectomy usually is defined as removal of the right lobe and the medial segment of the left lobe of the liver, but there is confusion here, based partially on terminology and partially on anatomy. First, the caudate lobe may or may not be included. Starzl clearly describes an operation that he calls "trisegmentectomy" in which all liver tissue drained by the middle hepatic vein is removed together with the right lobe of the liver.[47] Certainly this is an extended right lobectomy, but it is rarely done and probably rarely indicated. The term "extended right lobectomy" is more commonly used for any resection that goes beyond the central plane but no farther than the umbilical fissure. Once understood, it is clear that the vascular anatomy allows resection of varying portions of the quadrate lobe and the more superior portion of the medial segment of the left lobe, depending on tumor anatomy. The term "trisegmentectomy" should be reserved for those resections that leave only the left hepatic vein and the liver parenchyma which it drains.

Indications for Extended Right Lobectomy. This operation is indicated for tumors of the right lobe that extend medial to the gallbladder into the quadrate lobe. When such a tumor involves the inferior vena cava junction of the middle and left hepatic vein, resection is contraindicated. Often, pediatric tumors of the right lobe will extend well to the left of the central plane. When this extension is anterior and inferior, the lower one-half of the medial segment of the left lobe can be wedged out in continuity with right lobectomy. The anatomic points essential to an understanding of extended right lobectomy relate to the drainage areas of the middle hepatic vein and to the origin of the afferent supply to the quadrate lobe. If the middle hepatic vein must be taken to encompass tumor and a margin of normal tissue, the quadrate lobe must go, because it will have no venous drainage. Since the arterial and portal venous flow to the lower one-half of the medial segment of the left lobe comes from vessels in the plane of the umbilical fissure, the line of transection must not compromise this common source of afferent supply to both medial and lateral segments. Any plane to the right of the umbilical fissure is suitable for resection as long as venous drainage is preserved.

Technique. The initial steps for extended right lobectomy are the same as those for right lobectomy. After hilar ligation of the main right trunks, the left portal vein, left hepatic duct, and left arterial supply must be traced out toward the umbilical fissure—usually for a distance of not more than 2 to 3 cm.

The key to extended right lobectomy is to clean off the anterior surface of these vessels by discrete ligation of small branches until an adequate rim of normal liver can be palpated to the left of the tumor.

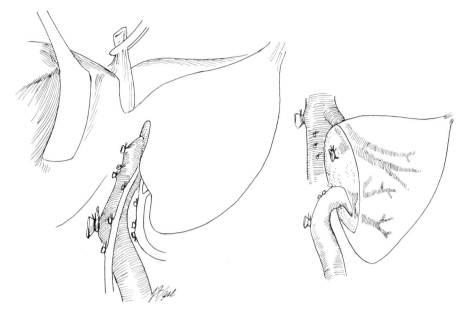

Figure 11–14. Extended right lobectomy. The key to extension of a right lobectomy is the dissection of the undersurface of the left lobe. The left main branch of the portal vein is straightened out by upward traction on the round ligament, and its posterior surface may be visible in the sulcus when fatty areolar tissue is removed. After ligation of the right main trunks at hilum, dissection proceeds to the left along the main trunks with careful ligation of every venous, arterial, or biliary branch going to the portion of the medial segment of the left lobe that is to be resected.

The smaller figure illustrates ligatures on the right hepatic vein, the middle hepatic vein, the right portal vein, and on several smaller hepatic veins that entered the inferior vena cava from the back of a resected caudate lobe.

Tumor involvement of the posterior aspect of the sulcus of the falciform ligament by a bulky right-sided tumor precludes resection.

Once again, it is surprising to the neophyte to find how much can be done without actual transection of liver substance. When portal triad can be safely pushed posteriorly, either blunt suction or mattress suture technique can be used to "wedge" out an appropriate amount of liver tissue by staying *anterior* to the major afferent trunks. Figure 11–14 illustrates the essential anatomy, and the reader is referred to the excellent illustrations in Starzl's paper for a description of the more extensive trisegmentectomy.[47] When it is necessary to come close to the plane of the umbilical fissure, the blunt suction technique is much safer than the use of mattress sutures, and allows close dissection of these major vessels in the umbilical fissure.

Any vertical line of resection between central plane and umbilical fissure is possible, but as transection proceeds down through liver substance toward the right side of the cava, the portal triad must be kept posteriorly and inferiorly. Bleeding will be greater during this transection because neither the inflow nor outflow tracts have been formally controlled.

Transient compression of the hilar structures with a finger or an atraumatic clamp may rarely be necessary. Once again, careful planning and expeditious transection will do more than anything else to limit blood loss. The raw area left after extended right lobectomy may be less than after right lobectomy, and requires no specific treatment. The adequacy of biliary drainage without leakage should be carefully checked, since the greater length of dissection exposes the bile ducts to an increased risk of injury.

Left Lobectomy

Classically, the term "left lobectomy" referred to the excision of the liver to the left of the umbilical fissure. Here, and in all other modern discussions of liver surgery, the term "left lobectomy" is used to describe the excision of all liver tissue served by the branches of the left portal vein, left hepatic duct, and left hepatic artery, with or without the caudate lobe.

Indications. Left lobectomy is indicated for tumors of the left lobe that involve the umbilical fissure or liver tissue to the right of that fissure, but which have not yet involved the left hepatic vein–inferior vena cava junction. When a bulky left-sided tumor pushes to the right of the middle hepatic vein, an anatomic left lobectomy may be "extended" by taking part of the anterior segment of the right lobe. However, this is rarely indicated, since tumors originating in the "thinner" left lobe that are bulging to the right will usually have compromised the inferior vena cava also, and thus be unresectable. Tumors involving the lower part of the quadrate lobe, without involvement of the umbilical fissure or the lateral segment, may be resected by "middle lobectomy," described below.

Technique of Left Lobectomy. A thoracic extension of the incision is rarely, if ever, indicated for left lobectomy. The right suspensory ligaments and the retroperitoneal attachments on the right should not be incised unless caudate lobectomy is planned. A right subcostal incision will usually suffice, but this can be extended far to the left if necessary. Transection of the falciform and left triangular ligaments, when combined with careful bimanual palpation through the opened lesser sac, will allow adequate evaluation of the extent of the tumor.

No attempt should be made at preliminary control of the caval roots of the left or middle hepatic vein. Hilar ligation is done as described above. Preoperative arteriography will have identified left-sided arteries coming off the left gastric or celiac trunks, and these should be ligated separately. Arterial identification is facilitated by opening the lesser sac and searching near the umbilical fissure. Capsule incision to outline the proposed transection is more difficult with left lobectomy because of the caudate lobe. This curious hindquarter of the liver is wrapped around the inferior vena cava, and should be left if tumor anatomy allows. It alone among liver segments has inflow from both the right and left lobar vessels, and its venous drainage is largely through lesser hepatic veins posteriorly. It will survive either right or left lobectomy, therefore, and the surgeon should not be particularly concerned about its nourishment.

Transection beginning inferiorly and anteriorly through the central plane will identify the branches of the middle hepatic vein. When possible, the major right anterior segmental branch or branches, and the middle hepatic venous trunk, should be preserved by keeping to the left of this important landmark. Because most patients will have a common trunk draining both the left and middle hepatic veins into cava, the left hepatic vein should be transected at least 3 cm from the

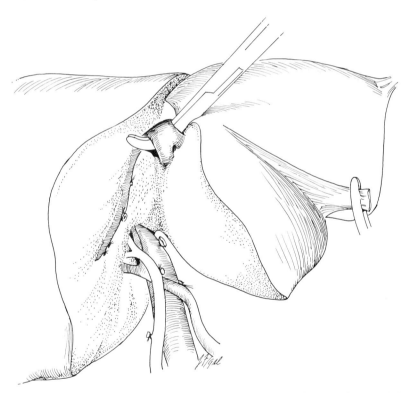

Figure 11–15. Left lobectomy. After ligation of the major left vessels at the hilum, blunt dissection will soon find a branch of the middle hepatic vein as it lies in the central plane. This vein should be preserved after ligation of its branches from the quadrate lobe. Its lateral margin serves as a useful guide for subsequent dissection, and it will lead the surgeon to the major hepatic venous trunk or trunks that drain the lateral segment of the left lobe. At the superior and posterior aspects of this cleavage "plane," dissection should veer to the left to avoid the caudate lobe, the inferior cava, and the risk of compromise to middle hepatic venous drainage.

inferior vena cava within the liver substance, if tumor anatomy allows (Fig. 11–15).

Difficulty with left lobectomy usually arises when tumor anatomy necessitates removal of a part or all of the caudate lobe. In this case, bleeding will be a problem posteriorly, usually coming from small venous branches that join the inferior vena cava below the diaphragm, and which can best be controlled after removal of the left lobe.

The raw surface after transection is compressed, and then hemostasis is secured. The dead space problem is considerably less than that after right lobectomy. However, drainage should be used and, once again, adequate biliary drainage of the right lobe should be ensured before wound closure.

Left Lateral Segmentectomy

Resection of the left lateral segment of the liver by many surgeons has been followed by disaster, because the umbilical fissure has tempted the unwary into using this "obvious" plane for placement of mattress sutures or a cautery excision. For reasons already thoroughly expounded above, the plane of resection for left lateral segmentectomy must be kept at least 1 to 2 cm to the left of the umbilical fissure. No thoracic extension of the incision is used, and primary hilar dissection and/or ligation is not necessary. Isolated left hepatic arterial branches of the left gastric or celiac trunks should be ligated outside of the liver prior to transection.

The operation is actually a wedge excision of enough tissue to encompass the tumor and an adequate margin of normal liver. It should be tailored to tumor anatomy, and need not include all of the segment. After lysis of the falciform and left triangular ligaments, a peripheral tumor often can be grasped with a large-angled vascular clamp and brought up into the wound. Careful capsular marking, dissection, and transection precedes simple transection by blunt suction technique. If major hemorrhage is encountered near the umbilical fissure from the left portal vein, the surgeon should veer quickly to the left and delay attempts at repair until the specimen is removed.

The left hepatic vein is impressively large when it is encountered near the diaphragm and inferior vena cava. Perhaps the most dangerous part of left lateral segmental excision is when transection of the left triangular ligament is carried too vigorously to the right. If this should occur, it is safer to pack this area and proceed with transection of liver substance than to attempt local control by clamping or further dissection. After removal of the lateral segment, direct control of a lacerated left hepatic vein usually is possible. If not, proximal and distal control of the inferior vena cava can be obtained as described above.

Middle Lobectomy

"Central" or "middle" lobectomy is the only major liver resection that utilizes the hepatic venous drainage, rather than the portal inflow, as the anatomic basis for segmental excision. Pack and Miller first used the term and applied it to segmental excision of the medial portion of the left lobe—i.e., the liver between the central plane and the umbilical fissure.[41] Their illustrations clearly show that some of the anterior segment of the right lobe was also taken in some cases. McBride and Wallace have described variations.[29] In truth, middle lobectomy is simply a large wedge excision suitable for central tumors located anterior to the hilar structures. When the trunk of the middle hepatic vein must be taken, both the anterior segment of the right lobe and the quadrate lobe must be excised. The gallbladder is always sacrificed during middle lobectomy and, if there is any place for liver resection for gallbladder carcinoma (see Chapter 10), middle lobectomy would be a reasonable choice. Control of the inferior vena cava and a thoracic extension of the incision are unnecessary for middle lobectomy.

The key to middle lobectomy is careful dissection of the anterior surface of the bifurcating hilar vessels, with ligation of all small branches within 2 or 3 cm of the central plane. More often than not, there are few, if any, tributaries to be ligated at the hilum before the major trunks can be "pushed" posteriorly and kept out of the way. Using mattress sutures passed from back to front or, preferably, using blunt suction technique, a wedge can be removed extending as cephalad as the inferior vena cava, as far to the left as within 1 or 2 cm of the umbilical fissure, and as far to the right as tumor anatomy dictates. The

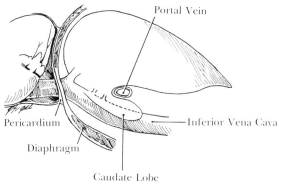

Figure 11–16. Sagittal section, vena caval plane. During middle, right, or left lobectomy the superior and posterior completion of the cleavage of liver parenchyma must come close to the intrahepatic anterior surface of the inferior vena cava. Control of this dissection during right lobectomy is best achieved with the surgeon's left hand placed behind the liver to guide the suction tip toward the palpable right hepatic vein–inferior vena cava junction. Such bimanual control is not possible during middle lobectomy for bulky tumor, and the surgeon must keep the vena cava constantly in *mind,* if not in sight.

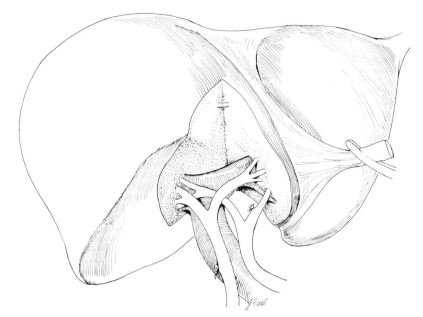

Figure 11–17. Middle lobectomy. Wedge excision of part of the right and left lobes for a tumor close to the gallbladder bed has been accomplished with ligation of the middle hepatic vein. The key to this operation is to maintain the plane of dissection *directly upon* the hilar vessels and ducts until they and their major branches can safely be pushed posteriorly and out of the way.

anterior surface of the inferior vena cava in its intrahepatic portion may be at some risk if the line of transection is carried too far posteriorly above the bifurcation of the portal vein. The plane of transection must be carried parallel to the vertebral column, or sloped anteriorly and superiorly to avoid the slightly anterior course of the intrahepatic vena cava as it traverses the liver below the diaphragm (Fig. 11–16).

After middle lobectomy, the major bifurcations stand widely exposed at the bottom of the wound (Fig. 11–17). This magnificent exposure will be remembered by a surgeon who has seen it, and he may later use central hepatectomy of normal liver to allow safe operation on difficult benign and malignant bile duct problems above the bifurcation.

REFINEMENTS IN TECHNIQUE

Resection in Small Infants

Various authors[7, 23, 26, 56] have discussed differences in technique when major resection is done in small infants. Thoracic extension of an abdominal incision is usually not necessary, even for right lobectomy. Shed blood must be replaced by a superior vena caval route, and Lin recommends direct "hand-push" transfusion of measured losses.[23] Traction on the liver may produce reflex changes or decreased venous return in infants. Stone emphasizes the role of splanchnic sequestration in infants, and advises against drainage after subtotal resection because of the risk of ascites.[56]

Bile Duct Decompression

After Merendino, et al. introduced the concept in 1963,[34] biliary drainage was widely employed in the care of patients with liver trauma or major elective resection. The work of Lucas and Walt[24] casts some doubt on this practice, and the recent comments of Sawyer suggest that postoperative upper gastrointestinal hemorrhage may be increased in patients with biliary decompression.[45]

The deliberate hilar ligation of major ducts, and discrete clipping or ligation of minor ducts, during the division of parenchyma by blunt suction technique should obviate the need for biliary decompression to prevent leakage from raw surfaces after lobar resection. Placement of a T-tube in the common bile or common hepatic duct will allow radiographic demonstration of the remaining bile ducts in the postoperative period, which may be of help in the differential diagnosis of jaundice and/or sepsis. However, T-tube placement in small normal bile ducts, particularly in children, risks injury.

In most patients, a careful evaluation of the remaining bile ducts after removal of the operative specimen and completion of hemostasis will reveal any significant injury or kinking. Immediate repair of any recognized problem is preferable to the establishment of an external fistula by T-tube drainage.

Therefore, the routine biliary drainage of all patients after uncomplicated major liver resection is not recommended. It probably should be used whenever a significant injury to the remaining bile ducts has occurred, or when a biliary suture line needs "protection."

Drainage

Every surgeon has his own rationale and his own technical preferences for providing abdominal drainage. Most articles written about major liver trauma suggest the use of multiple drains, often of several varieties. I do not wish to interfere with cultural and artistic aspects of drainage, and I cannot defend any specific regimen with scientific data. However, a few principles should be stressed.

The primary purpose of any nonsuction drain is to keep open a hole in the abdominal wall long enough to allow the egress of unwelcome fluid collections. Drainage is encouraged by a generous hole in the abdominal wall placed as laterally and as posteriorly as possible. Posterior rib resection, as proposed by McClelland and Shires,[30] for through-and-through drainage after trauma is seldom necessary after elective resection. Drains are used after liver injury (including elective resection) to encourage the exit of blood or bile that may leak from the raw surface, to obliterate dead space (which should require a suction catheter), and to create a track along which the products of late sepsis will find a way to the surface.

Better than any drain or any number of drains is the use of operative technique that will: (1) provide careful hemostasis and bile-stasis; (2) encourage the filling of "dead space" with adjacent viscera; and (3) avoid infection in a clean field by reducing necrosis and limiting the amount of foreign body left in the wound.

Suction drains are hard, and therefore may erode adjacent structures, and they tend to plug with fibrin clots. However, they are more effective when the leakage of blood or bile is great. Use them for a day or two if the field is not "dry" at the end of a major resection, but get them out early. Soft rubber drains will serve for most patients, and should be placed near the transected liver surface and beneath the leaf of the diaphragm exposed by the liver resection. They can be twisted and shortened by the fourth or fifth day, and should be out of most patients in seven days. When drainage is profuse, the hole in the abdominal wall should be kept open until this has subsided, but the long-continued presence of a foreign body deep within the subphrenic spaces will encourage, rather than eliminate, the dangers of sepsis.

Packing

There is little or no place for the use of gauze-packing after elective or emergency liver resection. If there is any role for such packing today (which is doubtful) it may be as a temporary hemostatic measure to control hemorrhage from a ruptured hepatocellular adenoma or carcinoma long enough to allow transfer to another hospital for definitive resection. Such packs should be removed as early as possible.

REFERENCES

1. Almersjo, O., et al.: Enzyme and function changes after extensive liver resection in man. Ann. Surg. *169*:111, 1969.
2. Aronsen, K. F., Ericsson, B., and Pihl, B.: Metabolic changes following major hepatic resection. Ann. Surg. *169*:102, 1969.
3. Balasegaram, M.: Hepatic surgery: a review of a personal series of 95 major resections. Aust. N.Z.J. Surg. *42*:1, 1972.

4. Cantlie, J.: On new arrangement of right and left lobes of liver. *In* Proceedings of the Anatomical Society of Great Britain and Ireland, June, 1897. J. Anat. Physiol. *32*:i-xxiv, 1897–1898, iv-ix.

5. Chan, K. T.: The management of primary liver carcinoma. Ann. R. Coll. Surg. *41*:253, 1967.

6. Clarke, M. A., Thomson, R. Y., and Fraenkel, G. J.: Vascular factors in liver regeneration. Surg. Gynecol. Obstet. *45*:126, 1968.

7. Clatworthy, H. W., Schiller, M., and Grosfeld, J. L.: Primary liver tumors in infancy and childhood. Arch. Surg. *109*:143, 1974.

8. Couinaud, C.: Lobes de segments hépatiques. Nôtes sur l'architecture anatomique et chirurgicale du foie. Presse Med. *62*:709, 1954.

9. Dagradi, A., Galanti, G., and Brearley, R.: Regeneration of the liver following multiple resections. Surgery 55:709, 1964.

10. Doty, D. B., Kugler, H. W., and Moseley, R. V.: Control of the hepatic parenchyma by direct compression; a new instrument. Surgery *67*:720, 1970.

11. Duckett, J. W., and Montgomery, H. G.: Resection of primary liver tumors. Surgery *21*:455, 1947.

12. Figueroa, I., and Santiago-Delpin, E. A.: Steroid protection of the liver, during experimental ischemia. Surg. Gynecol. Obstet. *140*:368, 1975.

13. Fortner, J. G., et al.: Major hepatic resection using vascular isolation and hypothermic perfusion. Ann. Surg. *180*:644, 1974.

14. Goldsmith, N. A., and Woodburne, R. T.: The surgical anatomy pertaining to liver resection. Surg. Gynecol. Obstet. *105*:310, 1957.

15. Healey, J. E., Jr., and Schroy, P. C.: Anatomy of biliary ducts within human liver; analysis of prevailing patterns of branching and major variations of biliary ducts. Arch. Surg. *66*:599, 1953.

16. Healey, J. E., Jr., Schroy, P. C., and Sorenson, R. L.: The intrahepatic distribution of the hepatic artery in man. J. Int. Coll. Surg. *20*:133, 1953.

17. Healey, W. V., et al.: Hepatic cryosurgery. Arch. Surg. *103*:384, 1971.

18. Heaney, J. P.: *In* Adson, M. A., and Sheedy, P. F.: Resection of primary hepatic malignant lesions. Arch. Surg. *108*:599, 1974.

19. Ida, T., Ozawa, K., and Honjo, I.: Glucose intolerance after massive liver resection in man and other mammals. Am. J. Surg. *129*:523, 1975.

20. Keen, W. W.: On resection of the liver, especially for hepatic tumors. Boston Med. Surg. J. *126*:405, 1892.

21. Lin, T. Y.: A simplified technique for hepatic resection. Ann. Surg. *180*:285, 1974.

22. Lin, T. Y., and Chen, C. C.: Metabolic function and regeneration of cirrhotic and non-cirrhotic livers after hepatic lobectomy in man. Ann. Surg. *162*:959, 1965.

23. Lin, T. Y., Chen, C. C., and Liu, W. P.: Primary carcinoma of the liver in infancy and childhood: report of 21 cases, with resection in 6 cases. Surgery *60*:1275, 1966.

24. Lucas, C. E., and Walt, A. J.: Critical decisions in liver trauma. Arch. Surg. *101*:277, 1970.

25. Madding, G. F., and Kennedy, P. A.: Trauma to the Liver. 2nd ed. Philadelphia, W.B. Saunders Co., 1971.

26. Martin, L. W., and Woodman, K. S.: Hepatic lobectomy for hepatoblastoma in infants and children. Arch. Surg. *98*:1, 1969.

27. Mays, E. T.: Hepatic lobectomy. Arch. Surg. *103*:216, 1971.

28. Mays, E. T., and Wheeler, C. S.: Demonstration of collateral arterial flow after interruption of hepatic arteries in man. N. Engl. J. Med. *290*:993, 1974.

29. Mays, E. T.: *In* McBride, C. M., and Wallace, S.: Cancer of the right lobe of the liver. Arch. Surg. *105*:289, 1972.

30. McClelland, R., and Shires, T.: Hepatic resection for massive trauma. J. Trauma *4*:282, 1963.

31. McDermott, W. W., et al.: Major hepatic resection: diagnostic techniques and metabolic problems. Surgery *54*:56, 1963.

32. McDermott, W. W., and Longmire, W. P.: *In* Discussion of Fortner, J. G., et al.: Major hepatic resection using vascular isolation and hypothermic perfusion. Ann. Surg. *180*:644, 1974.

33. McIndoe, A. H., and Counseller, V. S.: Bilaterality of liver. Arch. Surg. *15*:589, 1927.

34. Merendino, K. A., Dillard, D. H., and Cammock, E. E.: The concept of surgical biliary decompression in the management of liver trauma. Surg. Gynecol. Obstet. *117*:285, 1963.
35. Michels, N. A.: Newer anatomy of the liver and its variant blood supply and collateral circulation. Am. J. Surg. *112*:337, 1966.
36. Monaco, A. P., Hallgrimsson, J., and McDermott, W. V.: Multiple adenoma (hamartoma) of the liver treated by subtotal (90 per cent) resection. Ann. Surg. *159*:513, 1964.
37. Ochsner, J. L., Meyers, B. E., and Ochsner, A.: Hepatic lobectomy. Am. J. Surg. *121*:273, 1971.
38. Ong, G. B., and Leong, C. H.: Surgical treatment of primary liver cancer. J. R. Coll. Surg. *14*:42, 1969.
39. Pack, G. T., and Baker, H. W.: Total right hepatic lobectomy: report of a case. Ann. Surg. *138*:253, 1953.
40. Pack, G. T., et al.: Regeneration of human liver after major hepatectomy. Surgery *52*:617, 1962.
41. Pack, G. T., and Miller, T. R.: Middle hepatic lobectomy for cancer. Cancer *14*:1295, 1961.
42. Pack, G. T., and Molander, D. W.: Metabolism before and after hepatic lobectomy for cancer. Arch. Surg. *80*:685, 1960.
43. Raffucci, F. L., and Ramirez-Schon, G.: Management of tumors of the liver. Surg. Gynecol. Obstet. *130*:371, 1970.
44. Ryncki, P. V.: Anatomie chirurgicale du foie. Helv. Chir. Acta *41*:543, 1974.
45. Sawyer, J. L.: *In* Discussion of Stone, H. H., et al.: Physiologic considerations in major hepatic resections. Am. J. Surg. *117*:78, 1969.
46. Shiu, M. H., and Fortner, J. G.: Current management of hepatic tumors. Surg. Gynecol. Obstet. *140*:781, 1975.
47. Starzl, T. E., et al.: Hepatic trisegmentectomy and other liver resections. Surg. Gynecol. Obstet. *141*:429, 1975.
48. Storm, F. K., and Longmire, W. P.: A simplified clamp for hepatic resection. Surg. Gynecol. Obstet. *133*:103, 1971.
49. Tsuzuki, T., et al.: Repair of the resected liver stump: an experimental study. Surgery *2*:395, 1972.
50. Tung, T. T., and Quant, N. D.: A new technique for operating on the liver. Lancet *1*:192, 1963.
51. Turner, G. G.: A case in which an adenoma weighing 2 lb. 3 oz. was successfully removed from the liver; with remarks on the subject of partial hepatectomy. Proc. R. Soc. Med. *16*:43, 1923.
52. Wayson, E. E., and Foster, J. H.: Surgical anatomy of the liver. Surg. Clin. North Am. *44*:1263, 1964.
53. Zucker, M. B., et al.: The effect of hepatic lobectomy on some blood clotting factors and on fibrinolysis. Ann. Surg. *146*:772, 1957.
54. Hays, D. M.: Surgical research aspects of hepatic regeneration. Surg. Gynecol. Obstet. *139*:609, 1974.
55. Garrè, C.: On resection of the liver. Surg. Gynecol. Obstet. *5*:331, 1907.
56. Stone, H. H., et al.: Physiologic considerations in major hepatic resections. Am. J. Surg. *117*:78, 1969.

Chapter Twelve

NONRESECTIONAL THERAPY AND TRANSPLANTATION

INTRODUCTION

More often than not, primary and secondary tumors of the liver, when found, are beyond the bounds of cure by resection. Radiotherapy, systemic chemotherapy, regional infusion of the liver with chemotherapeutic agents through the hepatic artery or the portal vein, and hepatic de-arterialization have all been recommended and tried for these unfortunate patients. When liver involvement by tumor is so extensive as to significantly compromise liver function, any therapy that may cause further injury to the hepatocyte is contraindicated. Total hepatectomy with transplantation would seem to offer the only chance of prolonged survival for this group of patients.

Do any of these methods favorably alter the course of a patient with liver cancer? If so, which method will suit which patient best?

This chapter will briefly summarize the published reports of others in an attempt to answer those questions. The 1974 Liver Tumor Survey did not collect information on patients with liver tumors who did not undergo resection, although resected patients who experienced recurrent disease were often treated with one or more of the methods described below. The author's limited experience with each of these methods is insufficient to form the basis for an independent analysis, but has left him with the impressions that: (1) nonresectional therapy occasionally may be followed by transient improvement that may last weeks, but not months; and (2) prolonged survival probably is more often a manifestation of the natural history of a tumor than an effect of chemotherapy or vascular interruption.

Each of the major categories of nonresectional therapy will be discussed separately here, but they are often used in combination in clinical situations.

RADIATION THERAPY

Radiation therapy was used in combination with chemotherapy for two children in the 1974 LTS, and was used alone in a third child to shrink an unresectable primary tumor so that resection eventually could be done. All three patients seemed to benefit from radiation therapy, although two have subsequently died with recurrent disease. Ten children with resected primary liver cancers had radiotherapy for recurrent disease when it became evident, and two of these children survived at least 17 months (see Chapter 5). At least seven adult patients in the 1974 LTS also had radiotherapy for recurrent primary carcinoma. No patient with biopsy-proved recurrent liver cancer lived more than eight months after radiotherapy was begun. However, one patient, who developed a huge nodular liver and whose scan suggested recurrent cancer, survives without evidence of disease eight years after radiation therapy to the presumed recurrence. The mass was never biopsied but it did shrink following irradiation (case 37, Appendix IV).

The liver is quite radiosensitive, and doses of more than 3000 rads at a rate of 1000 rads per week may produce radiation hepatitis. The primary site of radiation injury is the hepatic venule, and a syndrome much like the Budd-Chiari syndrome, with hepatomegaly and ascites, may be confused with progression of neoplastic disease.[40] The kidneys also may be damaged by adequate doses of liver irradiation, and Filler, et al. have warned of the dangers of combining irradiation with resection and chemotherapy in children.[14]

El-Domeiri, et al. reported poor results with radiotherapy of primary tumors in 31 patients. After a tumor dose of 1000 to 3600 rads, 70 per cent of the patients were dead in less than six months, and only one lived more than a year.[13] Lin reported poor results from radiotherapy in 28 collected cases,[25] but Plengvanit, et al. noted relief of pain in 40 per cent and objective remission (for two months or more) in 35 per cent of 32 patients with primary liver cancer who were treated with a tumor dose of at least 4000 rads. Occasional other long-term survivors have been noted following radiotherapy, but, more often, any beneficial effects have been short-lived. Although most authors report little effect after external irradiation to liver metastases, Turek-Maischeider and Kazem noted some palliation in 10 of 11 patients treated with a radiation dose of less than 3000 rads.[50]

In 1967 Ariel, et al. reported the use of radioactive microspheres containing 90-yttrium injected into the hepatic artery. This technique was used alone in 37 patients with either primary and secondary liver cancers, and was combined with chemotherapy in 59 others. Objective response was achieved in more than one-third of these patients.[5]

SYSTEMIC CHEMOTHERAPY

No attempt will be made to discuss the use of specific chemotherapeutic agents in this section. The fluorinated pyrimidines were used most often, but many other agents also were used—singly, in combination, or serially. The reader is referred to the referenced articles for the details of specific drug protocols.

Only one child in the 1974 LTS survived more than 12 months after chemotherapy was begun for the treatment of recurrent primary liver cancer, and that single exception had resection of all known metastatic disease combined with chemotherapy. At least 16 adult patients with primary liver cancer had systemic chemotherapy when recurrent disease was diagnosed; ten were dead within six months of the start of that therapy, three more were dead by the end of 12 months, and three patients lived two years or more (24, 24, and 31 months). Although it is tempting to attribute the 31-month survival to the effects of methotrexate and Cytoxan systemic chemotherapy, the fact that this longest survivor went 70 months between liver resection and recognition of recurrent disease (before chemotherapy was started) suggests that the natural history of the cancer was in favor of long survival.

Most reports of the results of systemic chemotherapy for a primary or secondary liver cancer are discouraging. For primary liver cancer, Nelson, et al. found no significant difference in the survival of treated or untreated controls,[37] and the evidence of others concurs with this finding.[2, 25, 27] When systemic chemotherapy was combined with radiation therapy, the results were no better in one report.[13] The levels of AFP changed very little in 14 patients receiving chemotherapy in one series,[32] but dropped to below 50 per cent of control values in nine of 26 patients in another series, although the drop was transient.[29] Two long-term survivors with systemic chemotherapy are reported, but the documentation of each case leaves some doubt in my mind about the exact nature of the primary disease.[24, 43] A report from Thailand notes poor results in patients with primary cancer after therapy with 5-fluorouracil, cyclophosphamide, and vinblastine, but claims pain relief in 64 per cent and remission for more than two months in 24 per cent of 109 patients treated with systemic nitrogen mustard.[42]

In the treatment of patients with metastatic liver cancer, Ariel found no increase in survival when systemic fluorouracil was used for metastatic colon cancer.[4] Davis, et al. noted survival of more than one year in five of 24 patients with liver metastases from gastric cancer, and in six of 40 patients with pancreatic cancer metastatic to liver.[11] It is hard to be sure that these results are better than the natural history of patients with liver metastases, since neither series had controls. An occasional reduction in size of secondary liver cancer will be noted on a liver scan after chemotherapy for metastatic cancer,[53] but such reductions usually are short-lived. Schein, et al. have summarized recent studies about the systemic use of various chemotherapeutic agents for metastatic colorectal cancer, and they concluded that little impact has been made on the survival of the over-all population of the patients by the use of current techniques.[45]

HEPATIC ARTERY INFUSION OF CHEMOTHERAPEUTIC AGENTS

Pioneered by Klopp, et al. in 1950, intra-arterial infusion therapy is based on the concept that local tissue binding of chemotherapeutic agents will allow higher local doses with decreased systemic toxicity if the agent is injected into the arterial supply of a tumor.[22] In the early 1960s this technique was applied by Sullivan, et al. and others, in the therapy of patients with primary and secondary liver tumors.[48] Watkins, et al., in an encyclopedic report, advocate placement of the catheter at laparotomy. They describe in great detail the technical steps, the vascular anomalies found, and the complications and results attained in 195 patients so treated.[51] Massey, et al. and Ansfield, et al. prefer a percutaneous route for catheter placement,[3, 29] and Sullivan, et al. recommend prolonged infusion, usually for months, using a small chronometric infusion pump for ambulatory patients.[49]

By whatever technique, the results achieved by arterial infusion are reported by most authors to be superior to those achieved by systemic chemotherapy in terms of objective tumor regression. Unfortunately, benefit usually is short-lived and associated with moderate complications and considerable cost and inconvenience to the patient. Toxic reactions and morbidity in 419 patients are well reviewed by Ansfield, et al.[3]

Many patients have had a trial of systemic chemotherapy before a catheter is placed in the hepatic artery. Experience with these techniques has allowed the development of certain criteria for hepatic artery infusion that are broad enough to include many patients who are too sick to tolerate systemic chemotherapy. However, patients with advanced cachexia, ascites, jaundice, or incipient liver coma, and patients with poor oral intake, elevated blood ammonia levels, or a rising BUN generally are excluded as candidates for hepatic artery infusion. Patients with very advanced disease usually do not benefit, and their demise may be hastened by arterial infusion therapy.

About one-half of a small group of patients with primary liver cancer have had a favorable response to hepatic artery infusion with a variety of chemotherapeutic agents.[3, 11, 25, 27, 32, 42, 44, 51] There is more experience with patients with secondary liver carcinoma, particularly of colon and rectum origin. In this group, improvement for more than three months in six of ten patients was reported by Massey, et al.[29] and in 60 of 108 patients by Watkins, et al.[51] Twelve of 24 patients with colon carcinoma had an objective response in one series,[43] and jaundice cleared in 11 of 36 patients in another.[3] Modest to minimal "increases" in survival have been reported for 50 patients with secondary liver involvement by cancers of the stomach, pancreas, liver, and biliary tracts.[10] Symptoms of the malignant carcinoid syndrome, or hypoglycemic attacks associated with metastatic insulinoma, had been relieved in a few patients.[29, 44, 51]

AFP may drop transiently after arterial infusion of patients with primary hepatoma,[32] and alkaline phosphatase will return toward normal in responders.[29] However, in spite of more than a decade of experience with this technique using any and all of the agents currently available, it is difficult to prove a substantial benefit to the patient. Donegan, et al.[12] and Lange, et al.[23] share my concern that the days of useful and comfortable survival at home may not be increased by these procedures. A recent study of the natural history of patients with metastatic colon and rectum cancer raises some question about the comparison of survival of patients receiving chemotherapy with that of reported untreated patients.[6] An adequately controlled clinical trial seems justified by the marginal success of reported results.

Four patients in the 1974 LTS had infusion of chemotherapeutic agents into the hepatic artery. Three were treated when recurrent disease became obvious two, 15, and 42 months after liver resection. The last survived 20 months after hepatic artery infusion, but the other two died within two months of the start of intra-arterial therapy. The fourth patient was a 49-year-old female who had "prophylactic" hepatic artery infusion with 5-fluorouracil after "curative" excision of a small hepatocellular carcinoma from the right lobe of the liver. She was hospitalized three more times in the two years following liver resection for additional hepatic artery infusions, and she has never shown any sign of recurrent disease in the 55 months that she has survived since liver resection (Case 54, Appendix IV).

HEPATIC ARTERY LIGATION

Although normal liver tissue receives most of its nourishment from the portal vein, Bierman, et al.[8] and Breedis and Young[9] demonstrated that the blood supply to liver tumors came almost completely through the hepatic artery. As early as 1952, Markowitz suggested that ligation of the hepatic artery might be a way to reduce the growth of liver tumors,[28] but at that time most surgeons believed that hepatic artery ligation would usually result in a fatal outcome—a belief based largely on the 1933 report by Graham and Cannell[17] of 60 per cent mortality after hepatic artery ligation. Kim, et al. have nicely summarized more recent evidence that demonstrates clearly, in animals and in man, that most patients with noncirrhotic livers and with adequate preoperative liver function will survive hepatic artery ligation.[21] Healey has clarified some of the vascular patterns of metastatic liver tumors.[18] Michels,[33] and more recently Mays and Wheeler,[31] have demonstrated the remarkable ability of collateral vessels to rearterialize the liver after surgical interruption of the arterial supply at liver hilum. Significant changes in liver function tests will follow hepatic artery ligation in most patients. These changes will be maximal in the first week and then will quickly return to normal in most patients.

Scandinavian and Asian surgeons have pioneered the use of hepatic artery ligation for liver tumors in man. Nillson reported improvement in seven patients with metastatic cancer in 1966,[38] and Plengvanit, et al. described modest benefits achieved by a few patients with primary liver carcinoma after hepatic artery ligation at the liver hilum in 40 patients in 1967.[41] Subsequent experience demonstrated that tumor shrinkage was often remarkable, but always of short duration. Operations to effect more complete dearterialization have been developed and advocated by Balasegaram[7] and Plengvanit, et al.,[42] and arterial ligation has been combined with infusion therapy by several investigators.[16, 34]

Two reports from Scandinavia describe hepatic artery ligation for unresectable secondary and primary liver tumors followed five weeks and four months later by resection of the reduced bulk of tumor.[1, 34] One patient with primary liver cancer died 18 months later, and the other patient who had a secondary liver tumor survives four months after resection.

Ninety patients with primary liver cancer were treated in Bangkok by hilar ligation of the hepatic artery, with nine operative deaths. Pain was relieved in 50 per cent of the patients, and remission lasted more than two months in 35 per cent. Reduction in arterial flow to the tumor tissue was greater than reduction of flow to normal or cirrhotic liver tissue, but in all instances arterial flow returned to preoperative levels within six weeks.[42] Fortner, et al. ligated the hepatic artery in six patients with primary liver cancer and in 17 patients with metastatic disease. Thirteen of these patients also had postoperative infusion of chemotherapeutic agents through the ligated artery. Four postoperative deaths occurred, and nine of the 18 patients evaluated had at least one month of objective remission.[16]

Murray-Lyon treated 11 patients with metastatic disease with hepatic artery ligation combined with arterial infusion chemotherapy. The ten operative survivors had remissions lasting from ten weeks to ten months, and three patients with symptoms of the malignant carcinoid syndrome had some alleviation of disabling attacks of flushing and diarrhea.[36]

Balasegaram performed "complete" hepatic dearterialization in 24 patients with primary liver cancer from Malaysia, and had four operative deaths—three of which occurred in patients with tumor thrombosis of the portal vein. Patients with cirrhosis did poorly with this regimen; none of the five patients who survived more than one year were cirrhotic. Nine patients are still alive at one to 18 months after arterial ligation; some of these have evidence of tumor regrowth after a period of remission. On the basis of this experience, Balasegaram would deny hepatic dearterialization to patients with thrombosis or tumor infiltration of the portal vein, to patients with significant cirrhosis, and to patients with severe liver impairment as manifest by jaundice and/or ascites.[7]

Although the experiences outlined above, and that of others, may demonstrate that hepatic artery ligation can be done safely for selected patients, and that regression of primary and secondary liver tumors will occur in 50 per cent or more of patients, this remission is of short duration and may not long exceed the period of postoperative morbidity. Enough experience has accumulated to indicate that arterial ligation will not significantly prolong the period of useful survival for most patients.

PORTAL VEIN LIGATION

Honjo and associates have suggested that ligation of one of the main branches of the portal vein will reduce the growth of primary and secondary tumors. Reporting on 12 patients with primary liver cancer and eight with metastatic liver disease, these authors describe less morbidity and more effective palliation than they were able to achieve with hepatic artery ligation or palliative resection. They postulate that the gradual atrophy of the liver lobe that follows ligation of a major portal venous branch is accompanied by a reduction in arterial supply, which in turn will affect tumor growth. Noncirrhotic patients and those with hypovascular tumors did better than cirrhotic patients or those with arteriographic evidence of tumor hypervascularity. A remarkable six-year survival has followed portal vein ligation for a patient with metastatic cecal carcinoma, and three other patients have lived for more than two years.[19, 20]

OTHER SUGGESTIONS

Mulcare, et al. have suggested that isolation of the liver with support by an extracorporeal pump-oxygenator system would allow perfusion with high concentrations of cytotoxic agents without systemic toxicity.[35] I have not yet seen reports of a clinical trial of this technique.

Parks, et al. suggest that passive tumor immunotherapy may be possible using antisera developed against specific AFP. Such antisera also might serve as a vehicle for tumoricidal agents.[39] I am not aware of any report of a trial of immunotherapy of any type for human patients with liver cancer, but, with the active present interest in this field, such a report may be expected in the near future.

TRANSPLANTATION

Perhaps the most logical approach to the treatment of patients with massive or diffuse tumors of the liver that remain confined within Glisson's capsule is total hepatectomy. Unfortunately, no extracorporeal replacement for liver function has yet been developed, and liver transplantation for malignant disease using present techniques has met with only limited success.

Starzl in Denver and Calne in Cambridge lead the groups that are most active in liver transplantation during the first half of the 1970s, and the reader is referred to their work and that of others for a more thorough review of this subject.[15, 26, 46, 47, 52]

Dr. John J. Bergan, Director of the Organ Transplant Registry

(Chicago), has been kind enough to provide me with information about liver transplantation for cancer as of January 1, 1976. It is recognized that all transplants are not included in these registry figures, but this service provides more comprehensive and more current information than that from any other source. I am deeply indebted to Dr. Bergan and to the Registry Staff for their assistance.

As of January 1, 1976, 41 transplant teams in 14 countries had done 257 liver transplants in 245 patients for a variety of indications. Seventy-one of these transplants had been done for malignant tumors, the first apparently in 1963. Sixty-five patients underwent total hepatectomy and transplantation for primary carcinoma of the liver, and six others had liver resection with transplantation for metastatic cancer. After an initial burst of activity in the late 1960s, the number of liver transplants for carcinoma has decreased in recent years, probably as a result of the growing appreciation of the unique problems presented by the immunosuppression of patients with malignant disease.

Thirty-nine patients with hepatocellular carcinoma received 36 orthotopic grafts and three heterografts. Twelve survived for more than three months, but nine were dead with recurrent disease within 14 months, and two others died of other causes. The only long-term survivor was a woman who died of biliary obstruction more than five years after orthotopic transplantation. Three patients are alive at one, 22, and 33 months.

Twenty-three patients with cholangiocarcinoma underwent one heterotopic and 22 orthotopic transplants. Nine lived more than three months, one died of tumor recurrence at eight months, and three others died of sepsis at three, five, and eight months. The five remaining patients are alive from three to 23 months after transplantation.

Four patients with metastatic colon carcinoma, and one patient with a metastatic meningioma, died within six months of liver transplantation. The single child with neuroblastoma died of gastrointestinal hemorrhage and hypoglycemic attacks two years after transplantation, but there was no evidence of recurrence. Early death has followed two transplants done for hemangioendothelial sarcomas and one for Kupffer cell sarcoma of the liver.

Overall, then, eight of 71 patients with transplantation for carcinoma have lived as long as one year. Two have survived at least two years, and a solitary patient has lived more than three years. Five of the seven patients who are alive from zero to 33 months after transplantation for primary carcinoma had cholangiocarcinoma.

Although successes with present techniques have been few, future developments may allow total hepatectomy combined with transplantation a chance to provide cure to more patients with primary liver cancer, and to provide a palliation for those with diffuse liver involvement by secondary disease. The difficult problems that accompany transplantation of organs for which prolonged extracorporeal support is not available and the very real effects of immunosuppression on the potential growth of metastatic disease previously "controlled" by intact host defense mechanisms combine to make liver transplantation for malignant tumors an extraordinary challenge.

REFERENCES

1. Almersjo, O., et al.: Hepatic artery ligation as pretreatment for liver resection of metastatic cancer. Rev. Surg. 23:377, 1966.
2. Al-Sarraf, M., Kithier, K., and Vaitkevicius, V. K.: Primary liver cancer. Cancer 33(2):574, 1974.
3. Ansfield, F. J., et al.: Further clinical studies with intrahepatic arterial infusion with 5-fluorouracil. Cancer 36:2413, 1975.
4. Ariel, I. M.: Systemic 5-fluorouracil in hepatic metastases from primary colon or rectal cancer. N.Y. State J. Med. 72:1041, 1972.
5. Ariel, I. M., and Pack, G. T.: Treatment of inoperable cancer of the liver by intra-arterial radioactive isotopes and chemotherapy. Cancer 2:793, 1967.
6. Baden, H., and Andersen, B.: Survival of patients with untreated liver metastases. Scand. J. Gastroenterol. 10:221, 1975.
7. Balasegaram, M.: Complete hepatic dearterialization for primary carcinoma of the liver. Am. J. Surg. 124:340, 1972.
8. Bierman, H. R., et al.: Studies on the blood supply of tumors in man. III. Vascular patterns of the liver by hepatic arteriography in vivo. J. Natl. Cancer Inst. 12:107, 1951.
9. Breedis, C., and Young, G.: The blood supply of neoplasms in the liver. Am. J. Pathol. 30:969, 1954.
10. Davidson, A. R., et al.: The variable course of primary hepatocellular carcinoma. Br. J. Surg. 61:349, 1974.
11. Davis, H. L., Ramirez, G., and Ansfield, F. J.: Adenocarcinomas of the stomach, pancreas, liver and biliary tracts. Cancer 33:193, 1974.
12. Donegan, W. L., Harris, H. S., and Spratt, J. S., Jr.: Prolonged continuous hepatic infusion: results with fluorouracil for primary and metastatic cancer in the liver. Arch. Surg. 99:149, 1969.
13. El-Domeiri, A. A., et al: Primary malignant tumors of the liver. Cancer 27:7, 1971.
14. Filler, R. M., et al.: Hepatic lobectomy in childhood: effects of x-ray and chemotherapy. J. Pediatr. Surg. 4:31, 1969.
15. Fortner, J. G., Kinne, D. W., and Shiu, M. H.: Clinical liver heterotopic (auxiliary) transplantation. Surgery 74:739, 1973.
16. Fortner, J. G., et al.: Treatment of primary and secondary liver cancer by hepatic artery ligation and infusion chemotherapy. Ann. Surg. 178(2):162, 1971.
17. Graham, R. R., and Cannell, D.: Accidental ligation of the hepatic artery: report of one case with a review of cases in the literature. Br. J. Surg. 20:566, 1933.
18. Healey, J. E.: Vascular patterns in human metastatic liver tumors. Surg. Gynecol. Obstet. 120:1187, 1965.
19. Honjo, I., et al.: Ligation of a branch of the portal vein for carcinoma of the liver. Am. J. Surg. 130:296, 1975.
20. Honjo, I., et al.: Evaluation of ligation of a branch of the portal vein for unresectable hepatic tumor. Bull. Soc. Int. Chir. 33:207, 1974.
21. Kim, D. K., Kinne, D. W., and Fortner, J. G.: Occlusion of the hepatic artery in man. Surg. Gynecol. Obstet. 136:966, 1973.
22. Klopp, C. T., et al.: Fractionated intra-arterial cancer chemotherapy with methyl-bis-amine hydrochloride; a preliminary report. Ann. Surg. 132:811, 1950.
23. Lange, M., Falkson, G., and Geddes, E.: Intra-arterial chemotherapy in the treatment of primary liver cancer. S. Afr. J. Surg. 12:245, 1974.

24. Lascari, A. D.: Vincristine therapy in an infant with probable hepatoblastoma. Pediatrics *45*:109, 1970.
25. Lin, T. Y.: Primary cancer of the liver: quadrennial review. Scand. J. Gastroenterol. (Suppl.) *6*:223, 1970.
26. Liver transplantation: Editorial. Lancet *2*:7871, 1974.
27. Longmire, W. P., et al.: Elective hepatic surgery. Ann. Surg. *179*:712, 1974.
28. Markowitz, J.: The hepatic artery. Surg. Gynecol. Obstet. *95*:644, 1952.
29. Massey, W. H., et al.: Hepatic artery infusion for metastatic malignancy using percutaneously placed catheters. Am. J. Surg. *121*:160, 1971.
30. Matsumoto, Y., et al.: Response of alpha-fetoprotein to chemotherapy in patients with hepatoma. Cancer *34*:1602, 1974.
31. Mays, E. T., and Wheeler, C. S.: Demonstration of collateral arterial flow after interruption of hepatic arteries in man. N. Engl. J. Med. *290*:993, 1974.
32. McIntire, K. R., et al.: Effect of surgical and chemotherapeutic treatment on alpha-fetoprotein levels in patients with hepatocellular carcinoma. Cancer *37*:677, 1976.
33. Michels, N. A.: Collateral arterial pathways to the liver after ligation of the hepatic artery and removal of the celiac axis. Cancer *6*:708, 1953.
34. Mokka, R. E. M., et al.: Evaluation of the ligation of the hepatic artery and regional chemotherapy in the treatment of primary and secondary cancer of the liver. Ann. Chir. Gynaecol. Fenn. *64*:347, 1975.
35. Mulcare, R. J., Solis, A., and Fortner, J. G.: Isolation and perfusion of the liver for cancer chemotherapy. J. Surg. Res. *15*:87, 1973.
36. Murray-Lyon, I. M.: Treatment of hepatic tumors by ligation of the hepatic artery and infusion of cytotoxic agents. J. R. Coll. Surg. Edin. *17*:156, 1972.
37. Nelson, R. S., deElizalde, R., and Howe, C. D.: Clinical aspects of primary carcinoma of the liver. Cancer *19*:533, 1966.
38. Nillson, L. A. V.: Therapeutic hepatic artery ligation in patients with secondary liver tumors. Rev. Surg. *23*:374, 1966.
39. Parks, L. C., et al.: Alpha-fetoprotein; an index of progression or regression of hepatoma and a target for immunotherapy. Ann. Surg. *180*:599, 1974.
40. Peckham, M. J.: Therapeutic irradiation of the liver: Br. J. Radiol. *45*:790, 1972.
41. Plengvanit, V., et al.: Treatment of primary carcinoma of the liver by hepatic artery ligation. Tijdschr. Gastroenterol. *106*:491, 1967.
42. Plengvanit, V., Viranuvatti, V., and Chearanai, O.: Treatment of primary liver carcinoma. Med. Chir. Dig. *3*:301, 1974.
43. Ramirez, G., Ansfield, F. J., and Curreri, A. R.: Hepatoma: long-term survival with disseminated tumor treated with 5-fluorouracil. Am. J. Surg. *120*:400, 1970.
44. Rochlin, D. B., and Smart, C. R.: An evaluation of 51 patients with hepatic artery infusion. Surg. Gynecol. Obstet. *123*:535, 1966.
45. Schein, P. S., Kisner, D., and Macdonald, J. S.: Chemotherapy of large intestinal carcinoma. Cancer *36*:2408, 1975.
46. Starzl, T. E., et al.: Progress in and deterrents to orthotopic liver transplantation, with special reference to survival, resistance to hyperacute rejection and biliary duct reconstruction. Transplant. Proc. *6*:129, 1974.
47. Starzl, T. E., et al.: Orthotopic liver transplantation in ninety-three patients. Surg. Gynecol. Obstet. *142*:487, 1976.
48. Sullivan, R. D., et al.: Continuous arterial infusion chemotherapy of human liver cancer using 5-fluoro-2-deoxyuridine. Proc. Am. Assoc. Cancer Res. *4*:66, 1963.
49. Sullivan, R. D., and Zurek, W. Z.: Chemotherapy for liver cancer by protracted ambulatory infusion. J.A.M.A. *194*:481, 1965.
50. Turek-Maischeider, M., and Kazem, I.: Palliative irradiation for liver metastasis. J.A.M.A. *232*:625, 1975.
51. Watkins, E., Jr., Khazei, A. M., and Nahra, K. S.: Surgical basis for arterial infusion chemotherapy of disseminated carcinoma of the liver. Surg. Gynecol. Obstet. *130*:581, 1970.
52. Williams, R., Smith, M., and Shilkin, K. B.: Liver transplantation in man: the frequency of rejection, biliary tract complications, and recurrence of malignancy based on an analysis of 26 cases. Gastroenterology *64*:1026, 1973.
53. Witek, J. T., and Spencer, R. P.: Scan evidence of decrease in size of intrahepatic tumors after chemotherapy. Gastroenterology *67*:516, 1974.

APPENDICES

APPENDIX I: INSTITUTIONS PARTICIPATING IN 1974 LIVER TUMOR SURVEY

STATE/CITY	INSTITUTION	PRIMARY SPONSOR
ALABAMA		
Birmingham	University of Alabama Hospitals	Henry L. Laws, M.D.
	Birmingham V.A. Hospital	Joaquin Aldrete, M.D.
CALIFORNIA		
San Diego	University Hospital	Marshall J. Orloff, M.D.
	Harbor General Hospital	Marshall J. Orloff, M.D.
	Mercy Hospital	Max D. Trummer, M.D.
San Francisco	University of California, Moffit	J. Englebert Dunphy, M.D.
	San Francisco V.A. Hospital	Lawrence W. Way, M.D.
	San Francisco General Hospital	Robert C. Lim, M.D.
COLORADO		
Denver	University of Colorado Hospital	Thomas E. Starzl, M.D.
	Denver General Hospital	Ben Eiseman, M.D.
	Denver V.A. Hospital	Thomas E. Starzl, M.D.
CONNECTICUT		
Hartford	Hartford Hospital	
	St. Francis Hospital	Henry Mannix, Jr., M.D.
Manchester	Manchester Memorial Hospital	Melvin Horwitz, M.D.
New Britain	New Britain General Hospital	William Livingston, M.D.
New Haven	Yale-New Haven Hospital	Robert Touloukian, M.D.
	Hospital of St. Raphael	Douglas Farmer, M.D.
New London	Lawrence and Memorial Hospital	Malcolm Ellison, M.D.
Stamford	Stamford Hospital	Gerald O. Strauch, M.D.
	St. Joseph's Hospital	Gerald O. Strauch, M.D.
DISTRICT OF COLUMBIA		
Washington	George Washington University Medical Center	Paul E. Shorb, Jr., M.D.
FLORIDA		
Miami	Jackson Memorial Hospital	Robert Zeppa, M.D.
	Miami V.A. Hospital	Robert Zeppa, M.D.
GEORGIA		
Atlanta	Grady Memorial Hospital	H. Harlan Stone, M.D.
ILLINOIS		
Chicago	Loyola University Medical Center	Robert J. Freeark, M.D.
	University of Chicago-Billings Hospital	David B. Skinner, M.D.
	University of Illinois Hospital	Tapas K. Das Gupta, M.D.
	Northwestern Memorial Hospital	John M. Beal, M.D.

Table continued on following page.

315

APPENDIX I: INSTITUTIONS PARTICIPATING IN 1974
LIVER TUMOR SURVEY (*Continued*)

STATE/CITY	INSTITUTION	PRIMARY SPONSOR
INDIANA		
Indianapolis	Indiana University Medical Center	John E. Jesseph, M.D.
KENTUCKY		
Louisville	Louisville Children's Hospital	Hiram Polk, M.D.
	Louisville General Hospital	E. Truman Mays, M.D.
LOUISIANA		
New Orleans	Charity Hospital	Isadore Cohn, Jr., M.D.
		Theodore Drapanas, M.D.
	Ochsner Clinic & Hospital	John L. Ochsner, M.D.
MAINE		
Portland	Maine Medical Center	Richard Britton, M.D.
MASSACHUSETTS		
Boston	Beth Israel Hospital	Edwin W. Salzman, M.D.
	Boston Children's Hospital	Judah Folkman, M.D.
	Lahey Clinic	John W. Braasch, M.D.
	Massachusetts General Hospital	Ronald Malt, M.D.
	New England Deaconness Hospital	William V. McDermott, M.D.
	New England Medical Center	Harry H. Miller, M.D.
	Peter Bent Brigham Hospital	Francis D. Moore, M.D.
	University Hospital	Lester Williams, M.D.
Springfield	Western Massachusetts Medical Center	Paul Friedman, M.D.
Worcester	The St. Vincent's Hospital	H. Brownell Wheeler, M.D.
MARYLAND		
Baltimore	The Johns Hopkins Hospital	George D. Zuidema, M.D.
	University of Maryland Hospital	G. Robert Mason, M.D.
MICHIGAN		
Detroit	Grace Hospital	Alexander Walt, M.D.
	Harper Hospital	Alexander Walt, M.D.
	Henry Ford Hospital	Emerick D. Szilagyi, M.D.
	Michigan Children's Hospital	Jack Hertzler, M.D.
	Wayne County Receiving Hosp.	Alexander Walt, M.D.
MINNESOTA		
Rochester	Mayo Clinic & St. Mary's Hosp.	Martin A. Adson, M.D.
MISSISSIPPI		
Jackson	University of Mississippi Medical Center	George V. Smith, M.D.
MISSOURI		
St. Louis	Barnes Hospital	Walter F. Ballinger, M.D.
	St. Luke's Hospital	C. Alan McAfee, M.D.
NEW YORK		
Albany	Albany Medical Center	Charles Eckert, M.D.
Buffalo	E. J. Meyer Hospital	Gerald P. Burns, M.D.
	Roswell Park Memorial Institute	Harold O. Douglass, Jr., M.D.
New York City	Flower & 5th Ave. Hospitals	Walter L. Mersheimer, M.D.
	George Pack Foundation	Irving Ariel, M.D.
	New York Hospital-Cornell Medical Center	Paul A. Ebert, M.D.
	New York University Medical Center	John H. C. Ranson, M.D.

APPENDIX I: INSTITUTIONS PARTICIPATING IN 1974
LIVER TUMOR SURVEY (*Continued*)

STATE/CITY	INSTITUION	PRIMARY SPONSOR
	The Roosevelt Hospital	Walter A. Wichern, Jr., M.D.
	Presbyterian Hospital	J. B. Price, M.D.
Rochester	Strong Memorial Hospital	Charles Rob, M.D.
Syracuse	Community Hospital	Robert Hall, M.D.
	Crouse-Irving Hospital	Robert Hall, M.D.
	St. Joseph's Hospital	Robert Hall, M.D.
	Syracuse University Hospital	Daniel Burdick, M.D.
	Syracuse V.A. Hospital	Robert Hall, M.D.
NORTH CAROLINA		
Durham	Duke University Hospital	David C. Sabiston, Jr., M.D.
Winston-Salem	North Carolina Baptist Hospital	Richard T. Meyer, M.D.
OHIO		
Cincinnati	Cincinnati Children's Hospital	Lester W. Martin, M.D.
Cleveland	Cleveland Clinic Hospital	Robert E. Hermann, M.D.
Columbus	Columbus Children's Hospital	H. William Clatworthy, Jr., M.D.
	Ohio State University Hospital	John P. Minton, M.D.
OREGON		
Portland	Emanuel Hospital	Guy W. Gorrell, M.D.
	Good Samaritan Hospital	Matthew McKirdie, M.D.
	Multnomah County Hospital	William S. Fletcher, M.D.
	Portland V.A. Hospital	R. Mark Vetto, M.D.
	St. Vincent's Hospital	Joseph W. Nadal, M.D.
	University of Oregon Hospital	William W. Krippaehne, M.D.
PENNSYLVANIA		
Philadelphia	Hahnemann Hospital	Dominic A. Delaurentis, M.D.
	Temple University Hospital	R. Robert Tyson, M.D.
Pittsburgh	Montefiore Hospital	Mark M. Ravitch, M.D.
	Pittsburgh V.A. Hospital	Daniel Elliot, M.D.
	University of Pittsburgh Hospital	Larey C. Carey, M.D.
RHODE ISLAND		
Providence	Rhode Island Hospital	Henry T. Randall, M.D.
TENNESSEE		
Nashville	Vanderbilt University Hospital	John H. Foster, M.D.
TEXAS		
Dallas	Dallas Children's Hospital	Robert F. Jones, M.D.
	Parkland Hospital	Robert F. Jones, M.D.
VIRGINIA		
Charlottesville	University of Virginia Hospitals	Shelton Horsley, M.D.
Richmond	Medical College of Virginia	Walter Lawrence, Jr., M.D.
WASHINGTON		
Seattle	Harborview Hospital	James R. Cantrell, M.D.
	Virginia Mason Clinic	Lucius D. Hill, M.D.
Spokane	Sacred Heart Hospital	Carl P. Schlicke, M.D.
WISCONSIN		
Milwaukee	Milwaukee General Hospital	Joseph C. Darin, M.D.
	Milwaukee V.A. Hospital	Robert Condon, M.D.

APPENDIX IV: PRIMARY EPITHELIAL CANCER IN ADULTS

HEPATOCELLULAR CARCINOMA

A. Trabecular

	Age/Sex	Race	Histology Confirmed	Pathologic Grade	Cirrhosis	Maximum Size of Tumor	Operation	Outcome (Months)
1.	21 F	N	Yes	I	No	10 cm	RL	AFD 56
2.	22 M	W	Yes	I-II	No	11 cm	LL	DWD 13
3.	22 M	W	Yes	III	No	7 cm	RL	AFD 60
4.	25 M	W	Yes	III	No	19 cm	LL	DWD 43
5.	30 F	W	Yes	II	No	15 cm	XRL	DWD 36
6.	34 M	N	Yes	III	No	25 cm	RL	DWD 8
7.	38 M	O	Yes	III	No	15 cm	XRL	AFD 28
8.	41 M	W	Yes	II	No	13.5 cm	RL	DWD 5
9.	41 M	W	Yes	—	No	5 cm	XRL	DWD 3
10.*	42 F	W	Yes	III	No	11 cm	RL	AFD 60
11.*	44 M	O	Yes	III	No	10 cm	Lg. wedge	DWD 64
12.	44 F	W	Yes	III	No	10 cm	LLS + wedge	DWD 26
13.	45 M	O	Yes	II-III	Yes	14 cm	RL	DWD 14
14.	46 M	O	Yes	—	Yes	19 cm	XRL	AWD 15
15.	48 M	W	Yes	III	Yes	11 cm	Pall. RL	OD
16.	50 M	W	Yes	III	Yes	2 cm	Wedge	DWD 31
17.*	52 M	O	Yes	—	No	10 cm	RL	DWD 36
18.	55 M	W	Yes	III	No	10 cm	LLS	AFD 144
19.	55 F	W	Yes	III-IV	Thorotrast	7 cm	RL	DWD 4
20.	55 M	N	Yes	III	Yes	3 cm	Wedge	AFD 22
21.	57 M	W	Yes	I	No	12 cm	RL	OD
22.	57 F	W	Yes	III	No	8 cm	XRL	DWD 34
23.	57 M	W	Yes	—	No	18 cm	XRL	AWD 14
24.	58 M	N	Yes	II	Yes	8 cm	RL	OD
25.	60 M	W	Yes	III	No	10 cm	Wedge	DOD 84
26.	60 F	W	Yes	I-II	No	15 cm	RL	AFD 60

Table continued on following page.

No.	Age	Sex	Race		Grade		Size	Location	Outcome
27.	62	F	W	Yes	II	No	4 cm	RL	OD
28.*	63	M	W	Yes	II	Yes	23 cm	RL	OD
29.*	63	F	W	Yes	I	No	14 cm	Wedge	AFD 128
30.	63	M	O	Yes	II	No	7 cm	LL	AFD 68
31.	63	F	–	Yes	III	No	18 cm	LL	AFD 109
32.*	64	M	N	Yes	III	No	Huge	RL	OD
33.*	66	M	W	Yes	III	No	12 cm	RL	DWD 16
34.	66	M	W	Yes	I	No	10 cm	RL	DWD 17
35.	67	M	W	Yes	II	No	13 cm	RL+ wedge	AWD 32
36.	67	M	W	Yes	I-II	No	15 cm	LL	DOD 2
37.	68	M	W	Yes	III	Yes	21 cm	LW	AFD 94
38.	68	M	N	Yes	III	No	10 cm	LLS	DWD 26
39.	69	M	W	Yes	II	No	8.5 cm	Pall. wedge	DWD 2
40.	70	M	W	Yes	I	No	5 cm	RL	OD
41.	71	M	W	Yes	II	No	14 cm	RL	OD
42.	71	M	W	Yes	I	No	11 cm	LLS	AFD 8
43.	71	F	W	Yes	III	No	15 cm	LLS	DWD 10
44.	71	M	N	Yes	I	No	11 cm	LL	DOD 39
45.	73	F	W	Yes	II	Yes	11 cm	Wedge	DOD 79
46.	74	M	W	Yes	III	No	9.5 cm	RL	OD
47.	78	M	W	Yes	II	No	15 cm	LL	AFD 83
48.	78	M	W	Yes	II	Hemochromatosis	Large	Pall. wedge	DWD 5
49.	82	M	W	Yes	III	No	8 cm	Wedge	DWD 46

B. Adenoid

No.	Age	Sex	Race		Grade		Size	Location	Outcome
50.	22	F	W	Yes	II	No	22 cm	RL	NFU
51.	24	F	N	Yes	–	No	11.5 cm	LLS	DWD 11
52.	46	M	W	Yes	–	No	17 cm	Wedge	A?D 39
53.	49	F	W	Yes	III	No	11 cm	Wedge	NFU
54.	49	F	W	Yes	III	No	7 cm	Wedge	AFD 55
55.	55	M	W	Yes	II	No	8 cm	Wedge	AFD 32
56.	55	M	W	Yes	III	No	18 cm	LL	DWD 10
57.	57	F	W	Yes	–	Yes	15 cm	Pall. RL	DWD 15
58.	57	M	W	Yes	II		9 cm	RL	AFD 15
59.	57	M	W	Yes	II	No	10 cm	LLS	DWD 35
60.*	63	M	Esk	Yes	II	No	17 cm	RL	AFD 24
61.	66	M	N	Yes	I	Yes	10 cm	RL	OD

Table continued on following page.

APPENDIX IV: PRIMARY EPITHELIAL CANCER IN ADULTS (Continued)

	Age/Sex	Race	Histology Confirmed	Pathologic Grade	Cirrhosis	Maximum Size of Tumor	Operation	Outcome (Months)
62.	67 M	W	Yes	III	No	9 cm	RL	OD
63.	67 M	W	Yes	II	No	4 cm	Wedge	DWD 96
64.*	67 F	W	Yes	III	Yes	10+ cm	RL	OD
65.	68 F	W	Yes	III	No	11 cm	LL	AFD 70
66.	69 M	W	Yes	II	Yes	11 cm	LL	OD
67.	72 M	W	Yes	II		2 cm	Wedge	DWD 54
68.	75 M	W	Yes	II	No	5 cm	RL	OD
C. Clear Cell								
69.	16 F	W	Yes	II	No	12 cm	ALL	DWD 6
70.	42 F	W	No	–	–	13 cm	?	DWD 33
71.*	43 F	W	Yes	II	No	8 cm	Wedge	DWD 59
72.	52 M	O	Yes	III	Yes	10 cm	Pall. wedge	OD
73.	53 F	W	Yes	–	No	9 cm	Wedge	AFD 33
74.	66 F	W	Yes	III	No	20+ cm	XRL	AWD 36
75.	67 M	W	Yes	II	Yes	7 cm	LLS	DWD 11
D. Syncytial								
76.	37 F	W	Yes	III	No	12 cm	LLS	AFD 4
77.	67 M	W	Yes	III	No	13 cm	RL+	AFD 73
78.	69 F	W	Yes	III	No	8 cm	Wedge	AFD 30
79.	70 M	N	Yes	III	Yes	12 cm	RL	OD
E. Polygonal Cell with Fibrous Stroma								
80.**	5 F	W	Yes		No	4 cm	Wedge	AFD 18
81.**	14 M	W	Yes		No	18 cm	RL	AFD 112
82.**	14 M	W	Yes		No	12 cm	RL	AFD 9
83.	18 F	W	Yes	II	No	13 cm	LL	AFD 61
84.	18 F	W	Yes	III	No	12 cm	LL	DWD 34
85.	20 F	W	Yes	II	No	14 cm	RL	DWD 16
86.	21 F	W	Yes	II	Yes	20+ cm	LL+	OD

Case	Age	Sex			Stage		Size	Location	Outcome
87.	22	M	W	Yes	II	No	17 cm	LL	A?D 12
88.	27	F	W	Yes	II	No	14 cm	Wedge	AFD 35
89.*	28	F	W	Yes	II	No	12 cm	LLS	AFD 172

F. Peritheliomatous

Case	Age	Sex			Stage		Size	Location	Outcome
90.*	64	F	W	Yes	II	No	20 cm	LL	DWD 44

G. Unclassified

Case	Age	Sex			Stage		Size	Location	Outcome
91.	19	F	W	No	—	—	23 cm	RL	AWD 8
92.	20	M	W	No	—	—	9 cm	LL	AWD 41
93.	23	F	W	Yes	—	No	11.5 cm	LLS	AFD 19
94.*	24	F	W	Yes	IV	No	8 cm	XRL	DWD 3
95.	32	M	W	No	—	No	9 cm	RL	DWD 11
96.*	33	F	W	Yes	—	No	30 cm	RL	DWD 62
97.	35	F	W	Yes	—	No	13 cm	Pall. RL	OD
98.	42	F	W	Yes	—	No	14 cm	XRL	DWD 12
99.	46	M	W	No	—	No	10+ cm	RL	AFD 74+
100.	50	F	N	Yes	II	No	5 cm	RL	AFD 55
101.*	53	F	W	Yes	—	No		LL	DWD 10
102.	56	F	W	Yes	—	Yes	7 cm	RL	DWD 45
103.	59	M	N	No	—	Yes	15+ cm	XRL	OD
104.*	59	M	W	Yes	—	No	15 cm	Wedge	DWD 113
105.	61	F	W	Yes	—	No	21 cm	RL	DWD 5
106.	62	M	N	Yes	—	Yes	5 cm	LL	DWD 8
107.	65	M	W	Yes	III	No	14 cm	RL	DWD 41
108.	66	M	W	Yes	—	—	15 cm	RL	OD
109.	67	M	W	Yes	—	—	14 cm	RL	OD
110.	68	M	W	No	—	No	18 cm	RL	D?D 39
111.	68	M	W	Yes	IV	Yes	6 cm	LL	DWD 8
112.	73	F	W	Yes	—	No	16 cm	XRL	OD

CHOLANGIOCARCINOMA

Case	Age	Sex					Size	Location	Outcome
113.	37	F	W	Yes		No	15 cm	Wedge	AFD 12
114.	37	F	W	Yes		No	6 cm	LLS	AFD 8
115.	44	M	W	No		No	8 cm	RL	DWD 4
116.*	49	F	W	Yes		No	7 cm	RL	DWD 27
117.	52	F	W	Yes		No	8 cm	LL	AFD 4
118.*	58	M	W	Yes		No	10 cm	XRL	DWD 53

Table continued on following page.

APPENDIX IV: PRIMARY EPITHELIAL CANCER IN ADULTS (Continued)

	AGE/SEX	RACE	HISTOLOGY CONFIRMED	PATHOLOGIC GRADE	CIRRHOSIS	MAXIMUM SIZE OF TUMOR	OPERATION	OUTCOME (Months)
119.	59 F	W	Yes		No	4 cm	RL	OD
120.	59 M	W	Yes		Thorotrast	1.5 cm	Wedge	OD
121.	65 F	W	Yes		Thorotrast	10 cm	XRL	OD
122.*	68 F	W	Yes		No	12 cm	LL	DWD 12
123.	68 F	W	Yes		No	9 cm	RL	AFD 2
124.	69 F	W	Yes		No	8 cm	LL	DWD 17
125.	70 F	W	Yes		No	10 cm	RL	AFD 23
MIXED CHOLANGIOCARCINOMA AND HEPATOCELLULAR								
126.	35 F	W	Yes	—	No	15 cm	LL	DWD 36
127.	47 M	W	Yes	—	No	3 cm	Wedge	AWD 9
128.	51 F	W	Yes		No	10 cm	Wedge	AFD 11
129.	71 M	W	Yes	III	Yes	10 cm	Wedge	OD
130.	69 M	W	Yes	—	Hemochromatosis	9 cm	LLS	OD

KEY: Operation: XRL–Extended right lobectomy, RL–Right lobectomy, LL–Left lobectomy, LLS–Left lateral segmentectomy, Wedge–Any sublobar resection, however large.

Outcome: DWD–Dead with disease, AFD–Alive, free of disease, AWD–Alive with disease, OD–Operative death, DOD–Dead without evidence of disease.

Race: W–Caucasian, N–Negroid, O–Oriental, Esk–Eskimo.

*Case reported elsewhere, see below.

**Pediatric cases included in this tabulation, also included in Appendix VII.

REFERENCES: (See bibliography Chap. 4)

Number	Reference	Number	Reference	Number	Reference
10.	24	60.	63, Case 3	96.	78
11.	4, Case 11.	64.	24	101.	78
17.	4, Case 8.	71.	4, Case 9	104.	10
28.	38	89.	63, Case 2, 62	116.	38
29.	4, Case 4, 2, Case 4.	90.	4, Case 3	118.	24
33.	38	94.	2, Case 6	122.	38

APPENDIX V: PRIMARY EPITHELIAL CANCER
IN CHILDREN

CASE	AGE	SEX	RACE	OPERATION	MAXIMUM SIZE OF TUMOR	SOLITARY OR MULTIPLE	OUTCOME (Months)
HEPATOBLASTOMA							
1.	9 days	F	W	RL	—	S	OD
2.*	14 days	F	W	RL	10 cm	M	OD
3.*	1½ months	F	W	RL	8 cm	S	AFD 66
4.*	2 months	F	W	LLS	12 cm	S	AFD 119
5.*	2½ months	M	N	RL	14 cm	S	AFD 143
6.	3 months	M	W	LLS	5 cm	S	AFD 27
7.	3 months	F	N	XRL	13 cm	S	OD
8.	4 months	F	W	LLD	—	S	AFD 41
9.*	4 months	M	W	XRL	14 cm	S	AFD 130
10.*	4 months	F	W	RL	15 cm	S	AFD 62
11.	4 months	F	W	Lg wedge-central	14 cm	S	AFD 14
12.*	4 months	F	W	RL	10 cm	S	AFD 32
13.	5 months	M	W	RL	11 cm	S	AFD 53
14.*	6 months	F	W	LL	"Huge"	S	DWD 2
15.	6 months	M	W	RL	16 cm	S	DWD 11
16.	6 months	M	W	Wedge	9 cm	M	AFD 47
17.*	6 months	M	W	RL	11 cm	S	OD
18.*	6 months	F	W	Wedge LL	10 cm	S	AFD 20
19.	7 months	F	W	RL	7 cm	S	AFD 24
20.	7 months	M	W	RL	10 cm	S	AFD 66
21.*	7 months	M	W	RL	—	S	AFD 58
22.	8 months	F	W	RL	12 cm	S	DWD 18
23.	8 months	F	W	RL	6.5 cm	S	DWD 3
24.	8 months	F	W	RL	13 cm	S	AFD 23
25.	8 months	M	W	RL	12 cm	S	OD
26.	8 months	M	N	LLS	12 cm	S	AFD 14
27.	9 months	M	W	RL	10+ cm	S	OD
28.*	10 months	M	W	RL	13 cm	S	DWD 14
29.	10 months	M	W	RL	13 cm	S	OD
30.	11 months	F	W	RL	15 cm	S	OD
31.	12 months	M	W	RL+	12 cm	S	AFD 25
32.	12 months	M	W	RL	"Huge"	S	AFD 72
33.	15 months	M	W	XRL	17 cm	S	AFD 2
34.	15 months	F	W	XRL	16 cm	S	OD
35.*	18 months	M	N	LL	14 cm	S	DWD 9
36.*	23 months	M	W	XRL	7 cm	S	AFD 87
37.	2 years	F	W	LLS	7 cm	M	DWD 6
38.	2 years	M	W	RL	10 cm	S	AFD 41
39.	2 years	M	W	XRL	12 cm	S	AFD 41
40.	2 years	F	W	RL	9 cm	S	OD
41.	2½ years	M	N	RL+	5 cm	S	DWD 32
42.	2½ years	M	W	Wedge RL	18 cm	S	AWD 10
43.*	3 years	F	W	Wedge RL	"Large"	S	AFD 192
44.	3 years	M	W	RL	8 cm	S	AFD 49
45.	3½ years	F	W	XRL	10 cm	M	DWD 38
46.	4½ years	M	W	XRL + wedge	11 cm	M	NFU
47.	5 years	F	W	Wedge + RL	7 cm	M	DWD 23
HEPATOCELLULAR CARCINOMA							
48.*	5 months	F	W	RL	17 cm	S	DWD 8
49.*	7½ months	F	W	XRL	12 cm	S	OD
50.*	14 months	F	W	XRL	13 cm	S	OD
51.*	17 months	M	W	RL	15 cm	S	DWD 2
52.*	18 months	M	W	LL	13 cm	S	DWD 7
53.	21 months	M	W	RL	8 cm	M	OD
54.	2½ years	M	W	RL	10 cm	S	DWD 13

Table continued on following page.

APPENDIX V: PRIMARY EPITHELIAL CANCER
IN CHILDREN (*Continued*)

CASE	AGE	SEX	RACE	OPERATION	MAXIMUM SIZE OF TUMOR	SOLITARY OR MULTIPLE	OUTCOME (*Months*)
55.	5 years	F	—	LL	8 cm	S	AFD 72
56.	5 years	F	W	Wedge	4 cm	S	AFD 18
57.*	6 years	M	W	Wedge	10 cm	S	DWD 11
58.*	8½ years	M	W	RL	15 cm	M	DWD 6
59.	9 years	M	W	XRL	7.5 cm	S	AFD 8
60.*	10 years	M	W	RL	13 cm	S	AFD 82
61.	11 years	F	W	RL	21 cm	S	DWD 9
62.*	12 years	M	W	RL	12 cm	M	DWD 27
63.	12½ years	F	W	RL	12 cm	M	DWD 36
64.	14 years	M	W	RL	12 cm	S	AFD 124
65.	14 years	M	W	RL	12 cm	S	AFD 9
66.	15 years	F	W	RL	15 cm	S	AFD 11
67.	15 years	F	W	RL	13 cm	S	DWD 12
68.*	15 years	M	W	LL	9 cm	S	AFD 118

"UNCLASSIFIED" EPITHELIAL CARCINOMA

69.	1 year	F	—	RL	11 cm	S	DWD 5
70.	2 years	M	—	XRL	15 cm	S	DWD 3
71.	2½ years	F	W	LLS	13 cm	S	DWD 6
72.	8 years	F	—	LL	14 cm	S	OD

KEY: OD — Operative death.
AFD — Alive, free of disease.
DWD — Dead with disease.
AWD — Alive with disease.
NFU — No follow-up.

*Case reported elsewhere (see bibliography Chap. 5):

Number	Reference	Number	Reference	Number	Reference
2.	71, Case 7	18.	71, Case 5	50.	9, 7, 50, Case 5
3.	9	21.	71, Case 9	51.	9, 7
4.	9, ? 50, Case 8	28.	47, Case 1	52.	7, 50, Case 6
5.	48	35.	11	57.	9, 50, Case 20
9.	47, Case 2	36.	32	58.	47, Case 5
10.	54	43.	49, Case 1	60.	71, 62
12.	71, Case 6	48.	9	62.	47, Case 3
14.	47, Case 4	49.	9, 7	68.	2, Case 5
17.	9, 7				

†N.B. The six cases of hepatocellular carcinoma listed as occurring in children under two years of age (cases 48-53) are probably incorrectly categorized. A recent review from Columbus[9] has categorized cases 48-52 as hepatoblastoma, and the histologic slides for case 53 were not available (probably discarded). The pathologist–author (MB) did not have an opportunity to review any of these six cases, although the surgeon–author (JF) was privileged to review the Columbus experience during his visit.

The various tables and correlations in Chapter V were made using the presumed incorrect classification, but this error was discovered too late to be rectified prior to publication.

APPENDIX VI-A: FOCAL NODULAR HYPERPLASIA: 63 CASES – 1974 LIVER TUMOR SURVEY

CASE	AGE	SEX	RACE	PRESENTING SYMPTOM	SIZE OF TUMOR	SOLITARY OR MULTIPLE	OPERATION	OUTCOME	DRUG HISTORY
1.	10 mos.	M	W	Mass	5 cm	S	Wedge	AFD 2	0
2.	5½ yrs.	F	W	Mass	4 cm	S	RL	AFD 10	0
3.	7	F	W	Mass	Largest 17 cm	2	ML	NFU	0
4.	8	F	W	Mass	9 cm	S	Wedge	NFU	0
5.	9	F	W	Mass	11 cm	S	Wedge	AFD 68	0
6.	10	F	N	Mass	4 cm	S	Wedge	NFU	?
7.	10	F	W	Mass	10 cm	S	XRL	AFD 18	0
8.	10	M	W	Mass	10 cm	S	RL	AFD 118	0
9.	14	M	W	Mass	10 cm	S	Wedge	AFD 5	0
10.	16	F	W	Mass 5 months	7 cm	S	Wedge	AFD 6	0
11.	17	F	W	Abdominal pain	10 cm	S	Biopsy only	AFD 33	0
12.	19	F	W	Mass and pain	10 cm	S	LLS	AFD 31	?
13.	19	F	W	Mass	16 cm	S	Wedge	AFD 25	BCP
14.	20	F	N	Abnormal UGI series	3.2 cm	S	Wedge	AFD 25	0
15.	23	F	N	Mass	13 cm	S	LL	AFD 11	BCP
16.	23	F	W	Abnormal UGI series	2.5 cm	S	Wedge	AFD 5	BCP
17.	23	F	W	Mass	11 cm	S	RL	AFD 18	0
18.	24	F	N	Incidental	2 cm	S	Wedge	AFD 62	0
19.	24	F	W	Incidental	7 cm	S	LLS	AFD 24	0
20.	25	F	N	Incidental	5.5 cm	S	Wedge	AFD 60	0
21.	26	F	W	Incidental	1.3 cm	S	Wedge	AFD 9	0
22.	27	F	W	Incidental at laparotomy for F.U.O.	2, 1.5, 0.1 cm	3	LLS	AFD 68	BCP
23.	27	F	W	Incidental	0.5 cm	S	Wedge	NFU	0
24.	27	F	W	Mass	24 cm	S	LLS	AFD 11	0
25.	28	F	W	Mass, weight loss	8, 5 cm	2	Wedge	AFD 6	0
26.	29	F	W	Incidental	1 cm	S	Wedge	NFU	0
27.	30	F	W	Incidental	3.2 cm	S	Wedge	AFD 11	BCP
28.	30	F	W	Incidental	3.4 cm	S	Wedge	AFD 91	0
29.	31	M	W	Incidental	1.4 cm	S	Wedge	AFD 35	0

Table continued on following page.

APPENDIX VI-A: *Continued.*

Case	Age	Sex	Race	Presenting Symptom	Size of Tumor	Solitary or Multiple	Operation	Outcome	Drug History
30.	32	F	W	Incidental	1.5 cm	S	Wedge	AFD 120	?
31.	32	M	W	Incidental	1.2, 0.8, 0.8 cm	3	Wedge	NFU	0
32.	33	F	W	Mass, weight loss	5 cm	3	Wedge	NFU	0
33.	34	F	W	Incidental	12 cm	S	Wedge	AFD 48	0
34.	34	F	W	Incidental	3 cm	S	Wedge	AFD 1	BCP
35.	35	F	W	Pain	4 cm	S	Wedge	DOD 73	?
36.	35	F	N	Incidental	2 cm	S	Wedge	AFD 13	0
37.	35	F	W	Mass	11, 2.5 cm	2	Wedge	AFD 58	?
38.	35	F	W	Incidental	4.5 cm	S	Wedge	AFD 14	0
39.	36	F	W	Incidental	2 cm	S	Wedge	NFU	0
40.	36	F	N	Incidental	3, 2 cm	2	Wedge	NFU	?
41.	36	F	W	Incidental	3 cm	S	Wedge	AFD 116	?
42.*	36	F	W	Incidental	5 cm	S	Wedge	AFD 256	0
43.	37	F	W	Mass	11 cm	S	Wedge	DOD 39	0
44.*	37	F	W	Incidental	3.5 cm	S	Wedge	NFU	0
45.	37	F	W	Incidental	4 cm	S	Wedge	AFD 41	?
46.	37	F	W	Incidental	1.5 cm	S	Wedge	AFD 81	?
47.	39	F	W	Incidental	Largest 1 cm	2	Wedge	NFU	?
48.	39	F	W	Incidental	1 cm	S	Wedge	AFD 123	?
49.*	41	F	N	Incidental	2.5 cm	S	Wedge	AFD 34	?
50.	42	F	W	Incidental	4 cm	S	Wedge	AFD 83	0
51.	42	F	W	Incidental	5 cm	S	Wedge	NFU	?
52.	42	F	W	Bleeding, pain	3 cm	S	Wedge	NFU	?
53.	43	F	W	Pain	1.5 cm	S	RL	AFD 29	0
54.	45	F	W	Mass	4 cm	S	Wedge	NFU	BCP
55.	47	F	W	Incidental	3 cm	S	Wedge	AFD 113	?
56.	47	F	W	Incidental	2 cm	S	Wedge	AFD 21	0

No.	Age	Sex	Race	Finding	Size		Operation	Outcome	Medication
57.	48	F	W	Incidental	1.5 cm	S	Wedge	DOD 138	Librium
58.	53	F	W	Mass	10 cm	S	Wedge	AFD 27	Premarin
59.	53	F	W	Incidental	4 cm	S	Wedge	AFD 3	?
60.	55	F	W	Incidental	3.5, 3 cm	2	Wedge	NFU	?
61.	55	M	W	Incidental	3 cm	S	Wedge	AFD 42	0
62.	56	F	W	Incidental	6, 1.5, 0.5 cm	3	Wedge	AFD 14	Synthroid and estrogen
63.	70	F	W	Incidental	1.5 cm	S	Wedge	NFU	0

Histologic sections not reviewed for Cases 4, 46, 51, and 52, but pathology reports describe typical lesions.

KEY:

FUO – Fever of undetermined origin.

OPERATION: XRL – Extended right lobectomy.
RL – Right lobectomy.
ML – Middle lobectomy.
LLS – Left lateral segmentectomy.

OUTCOME: AFD – Alive, free of disease.
DOD – Dead without disease.
NFU – No follow-up information.

BCP – Birth control pills.   0 – No hormone medication.   ? – Drug history not known.

*Case reported elsewhere: (see bibliography Chap. 6)
Case 42. ref. 41, Case 1
Case 44. ref. 47, Case 3
Case 49. ref. 47, Case 2
Case 1 age is 10 months all other ages are in years.

APPENDIX VI-B: LIVER CELL ADENOMA: 37 CASES—1974 LIVER TUMOR SURVEY

CASE	AGE	SEX	RACE	PRESENTING SYMPTOM	SIZE OF TUMOR	SOLITARY OR MULTIPLE	OPERATION	OUTCOME	DRUG HISTORY
1.	17	F	W	Abdominal pain due to IPB	Bilobed, 14, 10 cm	S	Wedge	OR death	?
2.	18	F	W	Mass, 4 years	22.5 cm	S	Enucleation	AFD 36	0
3.*	19	F	W	Mass, 3 years, acute IPB	Huge	S	XRL	AFD 20	?
4.*	21	F	W	Mass, 5 months	32 cm	S	XRL	AFD 84	0
5.	21	F	W	3 days IPB	12 cm	S	LL	AFD 5	BCP
6.	22	F	W	Mass	16 cm	S	Wedge	AFD 33	
7.	23	F	W	7 days IPB	6 cm	S	Wedge	AFD 12	
8.*	23	F	W	Mass	15, 12, 8, 4 cm	1 resected, 3 left	Wedge	AFD 5	BCP
9.	25	F	W	Mass found during pregnancy	14 cm	S	RL	AFD 46	0, pregnant
10.*	25	F	W	Mass, 3 months post partum	10 cm	S	Wedge	NFU	BCP, 7 weeks
11.	26	F	W	Mass, acute IPB	9.5 cm	S	Wedge	NFU	BCP
12.	26	F	W	Mass, 7 months	8.5 cm	S	Wedge	AFD 9	BCP
13.	26	F	W	IPB 6 months ago, 1 month post partum, acute 1 day, IPB	12.5 cm	S	RL	AFD 30	BCP
14.	27	F	W	1 day IPB, mass	12 cm	S	Wedge	AFD 43	BCP, 3½ years
15.*	27	F	W	Mass	15 cm	S	LLS	AFD 93	BCP, 6 weeks
16.	29	F	W	Mass, 6 months	7.5 cm	S	Wedge	AFD 101	BCP
17.*	29	M	W	2 days IPB	10 cm	S	Wedge	OR death	0
18.	29	F	W	3 days IPB	11 cm	S	RL	AFD	BCP
19.	29	F	W	IPB 11 months ago	2 cm	2	RL + L wedge	AFD 19	BCP
20.*	29	F	W	1 day IPB	10 cm	S	RL	AFD 18	BCP, 8 years
21.*	29	F	W	Acute IPB	10, 6, 2 cm	3	RL	AFD 3	?
22.	30	F	W	F.U.O. mass. 3 months	12 cm	S	LL	AFD 11	BCP
23.	30	F	W	Pain. scan pos., fever 1 month	9.1 cm	2	RL	AFD 28	BCP 6 years
24.	31	F	W	IPB 3 months ago, mass found now. elective resection	7.5 cm	S	Wedge	AFD 12	?
25.	32	F	W	Mass, 7 months	13 cm	S	Wedge	AFD 38	BCP 7 years
26.	32	F	W	Mass, 13 months, acute IPB	15 cm	S	Wedge	AFD 51	?

	Age	Sex	Race	Presentation	Size	Multiplicity	Operation	Outcome	BCP
27.	34	F	W	Mass, 1 month	9 cm	S	LLS	AFD 52	BCP
28.	34	F	W	Mass	8, 1.5 cm	2	Wedge	AFD 17	BCP
29.	35	F	W	Mass, 4 months	7.5 cm	S	Wedge	NFU	0
30.	36	F	W	Mass, 26 months, acute ITB	12 cm	S	LL	AFD 2	BCP 9–10 years
31.	39	F	W	Mass, 4 months	8 cm	S	Wedge	AFD 10	BCP, 4 years
32.	45	F	W	Mass, 2 months	9 cm	S	RL	OR death	BCP
33.	45	F	N	Mass, 4 months	7 cm	S	LLS	AFD 55	?
34.	54	M	W	Mass	23 cm	S	RL	AFD 54	0
35.	62	M	W	Incidental at cholecystectomy	4 cm	M, only 1 resected	Wedge	AFD 43	?
36.	65	F	W	Mass, 1 year	6 cm	S	Wedge	OR death	0
37.	86	F	W	Mass	11 cm	S	Wedge	DOD 89	0

KEY:

IPB: Intraperitoneal bleed.

FUO: Fever of undetermined origin.

Operation: XRL – Extended right lobectomy.
RL – Right lobectomy.
LL – Left lobectomy.
LLS – Left lateral segmentectomy.

Outcome: AFD – Alive, free of disease.
DOD – Dead without disease.
OR death – Operating Room death.
NFU – No follow-up information.
BCP: Birth control pills.

*Case reported by others: (see bibliography Chap. 6)
3. ref. 68
4. ref. 47, Case 2; also ref. 51
8. ref. 58
10. ref. 69, 4
15. ref. 47, Case 1
17. ref. 47, Case 3
21. ref. 31, Case 1

APPENDIX VIII-A: LIVER RESECTION FOR METASTATIC CANCER (PRIMARY CANCERS OF COLON AND RECTUM)

Case	Age	Sex	Race	Interval	Operation	Multiple or Solitary Tumor	Outcome (months)
A. Primary Cancer of Right Colon or Cecum							
1.	76	F	W	M 101	Wedge	S	AFD 122
2.	55	F	N	S	Wedge	S	AFD 16
3.	36	F	N	S	LL	S	DWD 4
4.	52	M	W	M 42	RL	S	AFD 1
5.	76	M	W	S	Wedge	S	NFU
6.	79	M	W	S	Wedge	S	AFD 4
7.	56	F	W	M 12	Wedge	S	DWD 18
8.	76	F	W	M 66	Pall. RL	S	AWD 26
9.	31	M	W	M 28	Bilat. wedge	S	DWD 16
10.	62	M	W	S	LLS	S	AWD 10
11.	75	F	W	S	Wedge	S	NFU
12.*	29	M	W	S	Pall. RL	M	OD
13.	55	F	W	M 15	Wedge	S	AFD 110
14.	68	F	W	M 20	Wedge	M	DWD 14
15.	73	M		S	Wedge	S	DWD 11
16.		M		S	LLS	S	DWD 14
17.	45	F		S	RL	M	AFD 142
18.	54	F		M 12	LLS	S	AWD 5
19.	37	M		M 24	RL	M	DWD 17
20.*	52	M	W	M 16	XRL	M	AFD 198
21.	41	F	W	M 66	LL	S	DWD 13
22.	76	F	W	S	Wedge	S	DWD 8
23.	67	F	W	S	Pall. wedge	S	DWD 33
24.	57	F	W	M 37	RL	S	DWD 9
B. Transverse Colon							
25.	72	F	W	S	LLS	M	DWD 14(est.)
26.	63	M	W	M 3	RL	M	OD
27.	53	F	W	M 51	LLS	M	AFD 12
28.	50	F	W	M 7	Wedge	S	DWD 11
29.	72	M	W	S	Wedge	S	DWD 16
30.	59	F	W	S	Wedge	S	AFD 30
31.	65	F	W	S	Wedge	S	DWD 42
32.	71	F	W	M 12	Pall. LL	M	DWD 4
33.	76	F	W	S	LLS	S	AWD 80
34.	49	M		S	Wedge	S	AFD 102
35.	61	F		M 70	Pall. LLS	S	AWD 14
C. Left Colon							
36.	58	M	W	S	Wedge	S	AFD 49
37.	39	F	W	M 19	RL	S	DWD 16
38.	58	F	N	M 10	LLS	S	AFD 32
39.	53	M	W	S	Wedge	S	DWD 57
40.	46	M	W	M 20	RL	S	DWD 8
41.	32	F	W	S	Wedge	S	DWD 20
42.	50	M	W	M 35	RL + pall. wedge	M	DWD 19
43.	39	F	W	M 23	Large wedge	M	DWD 24
44.	55	F	W	S	LLS	M	DWD 63
45.	64	M	W	M 12	RL+	M	OD
D. Sigmoid Colon							
46.	76	M	W	S	Wedge	S	DWD 34
47.	53	F	W	M 29	LL	S	DWD 20
48.	56	F	W	S	Wedge	S	DWD 8
49.	71	M	W	M 54	Pall. wedge	S	DWD 22(est.)
50.	66	M	W	M 60	Pall. wedge	M	OD
51.	55	M	W	M 18	RL	S	DWD 10(est.)
52.	47	F	W	S	Wedge	S	DWD 33
53.	61	F	W	M 18	Pall. wedge	S	DWD 18
54.	43	F	W	M 20	LL	S	DWD 14
55.	62	F	W	S	Wedge	S	AFD 100

APPENDIX VIII-A: LIVER RESECTION FOR METASTATIC CANCER (PRIMARY CANCERS OF COLON AND RECTUM) (*Continued*)

Case	Age	Sex	Race	Interval	Operation	Multiple or Solitary Tumor	Outcome (months)
56.	65	M	W	S	Wedge	S	DWD 15
57.	71	F	W	S + M 19	Wedge × 2	S	AFD 62
58.	70	F	W	M 56	LLS	S	DWD 14
59.	71	M	W	S	Wedge	S	AWD 17
60.	72	M	W	M 59	Large wedge	S	DWD 6
61.	61	M	W	M 38	Pall. LLS	M	AWD 11
62.	55	F	W	S	LLS	S	AFD 43
63.	51	F	W	S	Wedge	S	AWD 14
64.	71	M	W	S	Wedge	S	AWD 5
65.	47	F	W	M 28	LLS	M	DWD 14
66.*	46	F	W	M 33	RL	M	DWD 10
67.	68	M	W	S	Wedge	S	DWD 24
68.	75	M	W	S	Wedge	S	DWD 16(est.)
69.	59	F	W	M 11	Wedge	S	AFD 116
70	56	F	W	M 12	Wedge	S	DWD 61
71.	72	F	W	S	Wedge	M	DWD 14
72.*	64	M	W	M 12	RL	M	DWD 16
73.	69	M	W	M 27	LLS	S	DWD 7
74.	39	F	W	M 46	LL	M	DWD 8(est.)
75.	50	F	W	S	LLS	S	DWD 13
76.	47	M	W	S	LLS + wedge	M	DWD 6
77.	42	F		S	Pall. wedge	M	DWD 5
78.	38	F		S	RL	M	DWD 11
79.	55	M		M 27	LLS	M	DWD 21
80.	45	F		S	Wedge	S	DWD 25
81.	49	F		M 78	RL	M	DWD ?
82.	63	M		S	LL	M	DWD ?
83.	78	M		M 86	RL	S	AFD 10
84.	41	F		M 31	RL	S	DWD 10
85.	53	M		M 52	Wedge	M	DWD 9
86.	55	F		M 52	RL	M	DWD 8
87.	63	M		S	RL	M	DWD 26
88.	71	F	W	S	Wedge	S	DWD 8
89.	53	F	W	M 8	RL	S	AFD 10
90.	55	M	O	M 24	XRL	M	DWD 8
91.	48	F	W	S	Wedge	S	DWD 11
92.	65	F	W	S	Wedge	S	OD
93.	48	M	W	M 68	RL	S	DWD 21
94.	64	M	W	S	Wedge	M	AFD 3
95.	36	M	W	S	Wedge	S	DWD 57
96.	67	F	W	S	Wedge	S	DWD 6
97.	53	M		M 3	RL	M	DWD 39
98.	55	F	W	M 17	RL	M	OD
E. Rectum							
99.	60	F	W	S	Wedge	M	AFD 62
100.	62	M	W	S	Wedge	M	DWD 33
101.	52	F	W	S	LLS	S	DWD 93
102.	35	M	W	M 22	XRL	M	OD
103.	64	M	W	M 20	Wedge	M	DWD 73
104.	65	M	W	S	Wedge	M	AFD 16
105.	63	M	W	S	Wedge	M	AWD 80
106.	37	F	W	S	Wedge × 2	M	DWD 8
107.	53	F	W	M 54	LL	S	AFD 5
108.	61	M	W	M 36	Wedge	S	NFU
109.	61	M	W	M 10	LL	S	DWD 5
110.	69	M	W	S	Wedge	S	AFD 12
111.	44	M	W	S	Wedge	S	DWD 23
112.	55	M	W	S	Wedge	S	DWD 35
113.	50	M	W	S	Wedge × 2	M	DWD 32

Table continued on following page.

APPENDIX VIII-A: LIVER RESECTION FOR METASTATIC CANCER (PRIMARY CANCERS OF COLON AND RECTUM) (*Continued*)

CASE	AGE	SEX	RACE	INTERVAL	OPERATION	MULTIPLE OR SOLITARY TUMOR	OUTCOME (MONTHS)
114.	55	M	W	M 47	Wedge	S	DWD 23
115.	57	F	W	M 46	2 Resections	S	DWD 25
				M 54	? Wedge		
116.	39	F		M 49	Pall. wedge × 2	M	OD
117.	52	M		S	LL	M	DWD 7
118.	57	F	W	M 4	Wedge × 4	M	DWD 26
				M 22	LL		
119.	67	F	W	S	Wedge	S	DWD 8
120.	55	F	W	M 16	XRL	M	AFD 3
121.	51	F	W	M 22	Wedge	S	AWD 2
122.	58	M	W	M 17	LLS	S	AFD 6
123.	25	M	W	S	Wedge	S	DWD 38
124.	67	F	W	M 48	Pall. LLS	S	DWD 7
F. Colon Primary: Unspecified Location							
125.	33	F		S	Wedge	S	DWD 19
126.	42	M		M 84	RL+	M	AFD 161

KEY: *Interval:* S—Synchronous, M—Metachronous, number—months interval.

    Operation: Pall.—Palliative, RL—Right lobectomy, LL—Left lobectomy, LLS—Left lateral segmentectomy, XRL—Extended right lobectomy.

    Outcome: OD—Operative death, AFD—Alive, free of disease, DWD—Dead with disease, AWD—Alive with disease.

*Cases reported elsewhere: (see bibliography Chap. 8)

    12. Ref. 50—case 10, ref. 49—case 15.

    20. Ref. 35.

    66. Ref. 50—case 9, ref 49—case 13.

    72. Ref. 50—case 8, ref. 49—case 12.

APPENDIX VIII-B: LIVER RESECTION FOR METASTATIC CANCER (PRIMARY CANCERS *OTHER* THAN COLON AND RECTUM)

CASE	AGE	SEX	RACE	INTERVAL	OPERATION	MULTIPLE OR SOLITARY TUMOR	OUTCOME (MONTHS)
Malignant Melanoma							
127.	58	F	W	M 108	Wedge	S	AWD 22
128.	45	M	W	M 24	XRL	S	DWD 10
129.	35	M	W	M 150	Wedge	S	DWD 4
130.	29	F	W	M 71	RL	M	DWD 8
131.	53	F	W	M 150	RL	S	DWD 2
132.	64	F		M 89	Pall. LLS	S	DWD 9
133.	45	F		M 112	Wedge	S	DWD 17
134.	49	F	W	M 27	Wedge	S	DWD 12
135.	35	F	W	M 36	LLS	S	OD
Leiomyosarcoma							
136.	45	F	W	M 65	Pall. RL	M	DWD 11
137.	87	F	W	S	Wedge	S	AFD 26
138.	44	F	W	S	LLS	S	AFD 11
139.	46	F	W	S	RL	M	OD
140.	69	M	W	S	Wedge	S	DWD 105
141.	63	M	W	M 48	Wedge	S	AFD 8
142.	48	M		M 20	Wedge × 2	M	DWD 13
Breast							
143.	44	F	W	M 9	LLS	S	AWD 3

APPENDIX VIII-B: LIVER RESECTION FOR METASTATIC CANCER (PRIMARY CANCERS *OTHER* THAN COLON AND RECTUM) (*Continued*)

CASE	AGE	SEX	RACE	INTERVAL	OPERATION	MULTIPLE OR SOLITARY TUMOR	OUTCOME (MONTHS)
144.	41	F	W	M 8	Wedge	S	DWD 6
145.	73	F		M 204	LLS	S	OD
146.	52	F		S	RL	M	DWD 8
Renal							
147.	48	F	W	S	Wedge	S	DWD 33
148.	65	M	N	M 7	Wedge	S	DWD 7
149.	49	F	W	M 6	Wedge	S	DWD 2
Wilms' Tumor							
150.	5	M	W	M 10	RL	M	DWD 9
151.	4½	M	N	M 13	Wedge	M	AFD 52
152.	4	F	W	M 4	Wedge	M	DWD 3
Ovary							
153.	18	F	N	M 6	Wedge	S	AFD 16
154.	45	F	W	M 60	RL	S	OD
155.	36	F		Precoc.	RL	M	DWD 12
156.	54	F		M 42	Wedge	M	DWD 21
Cervix							
157.	68	F	N	M 52	LLS	S	D?D 42
158.	39	F	W	M 50	Wedge	S	AWD 7
159.	33	F	W	M 6	Wedge	S	DWD 14
Gastric							
160.	72	F	W	S	Wedge	S	DWD 2
161.	74	M	W	M 60	RL	S	DWD 5
162.	63	M	W	S	Wedge	S	DWD 6
Lung							
163.	67	M	W	Precoc.	Wedge	S	DWD 8
Esophagus							
164.	56	M	N	M 5	Wedge	M	OD
Liposarcoma							
165.	74	M	W	M 240+	Enucleation	S	AWD 15
Neuroblastoma							
166.	3	M	W	S	Pall. LLS	M	DWD 7
Angiosarcoma							
167.	38	F	W	M 168	LL	S	DWD 3
Pancreas							
168.	52	F	W	Precoc.	RL	S	DWD 11
Adrenal							
169.	40	F		S	Wedge	S	AFD 5
Paraganglioma							
170.	43	F	N	M 132	Wedge	S	AWD 31
Pericytoma							
171.	36	F	W	M 60	XRL	M	AWD 32
Fibrosarcoma							
172.	36	F	W	M 132	RL	S	DWD 105
Primary Unknown							
173.	55	F	W	Precoc.	LL	S	DWD 8
174.	62	M	O	Precoc.	LLS	S	OD
175.	59	F	W	Precoc.	LLS	S	DWD 6
176.	65	F	W	Precoc.	Wedge	S	DWD 2

KEY:

Interval: S—Synchronous, M—Metachronous, Precoc.—Precocious, Number—Months' interval.

Operation: Pall.—Palliative, RL—Right lobectomy, LL—Left lobectomy, LLS—Left lateral segmentectomy, XRL—Extended right lobectomy.

Outcome: OD—Operative death, AFD—Alive, free of disease, DWD—Dead with disease, AWD—Alive with disease.

APPENDIX X: 1974 LIVER TUMOR SURVEY—EN BLOC LIVER RESECTIONS

	AGE/SEX		PRIMARY TUMOR	LIVER RESECTION	OUTCOME (MONTHS)
1.	64	F	Gallbladder	RL	OD
2.	58	F	Gallbladder	Wedge	DWD 5
3.	40	F	Gallbladder	RL	AFD 17
4.**	78	F	Gallbladder	Wedge	DWD 22
5.	66	F	Gallbladder	RL	DWD 3
6.	68	F	Gallbladder	Wedge	OD
7.	39	F	Gallbladder	RL	DWD 17
8.	51	F	Gallbladder	RL	OD
9.	46	F	Gallbladder	RL	OD
10.	67	M	Gallbladder	Wedge	DWD 3
11.	71	F	Gallbladder	RL	OD
12.	53	F	Gallbladder	Wedge	A?D 10
13.	72	F	Gallbladder	RL	DWD 6
14.	58	F	Gallbladder	Wedge	DWD 22
15.	68	M	Gallbladder	Wedge	DWD 9
16.	65	F	Gallbladder	Wedge	DWD 6
17.	57	F	Gallbladder	Wedge	AWD 4
18.	74	F	Gallbladder	Wedge	DWD 6
19.	65	F	Gallbladder	Wedge	NFU
20.	60	M	Gallbladder	Wedge	DWD 8
21.	65	M	Gallbladder	RL	OD
22.**	64	F	Gallbladder	RL	DWD 5
23.**	53	F	Gallbladder	RL	DWD 186
24.**	51	F	Gallbladder	RL	DWD 25
25.	68	F	Gallbladder	Wedge	OD
26.		F	Gallbladder	RL	DWD 15
27.		F	Gallbladder	RL	OD
28.	65	F	Gallbladder	RL	OD
29.	72	M	Gallbladder	RL	OD
30.	46	M	Gallbladder	RL	DWD 3
31.	46	F	Gallbladder	RL	DWD 5
32.	56	F	Gallbladder	Wedge	DWD 25
33.	82	F	Gallbladder	Wedge	AWD 8
34.	68	F	Gallbladder	Wedge	DWD 27
35.	58	F	Gallbladder	Wedge	DWD 8
36.	62	M	Stomach	Wedge	DWD 5
37.	62	F	Stomach	LLS	DWD 6
38.	68	M	Stomach	LLS	DWD 6
39.	55	M	Stomach	Wedge	AFD 72
40.	71	M	Stomach	Wedge	DWD 12
41.	69	M	Stomach	Wedge	DOD 126
42.	48	F	Stomach	Wedge	AFD 135
43.	47	M	Stomach	Wedge	NFU
44.	45	F	Stomach	Wedge	DWD 28
45.	53	M	Stomach	Wedge	DOD 44
46.	56	M	Stomach	Wedge	DWD 22
47.	43	F	Stomach	Wedge	D?D 3
48.	77	M	Stomach	LLS	DWD 7
49.	58	F	Stomach	Wedge	DWD 11
50.	?	M	Stomach	Wedge	DWD 4
51.	78	M	Stomach	Wedge	AFD 36
52.	37	M	Stomach	Wedge	DWD 5
53.	45	F	Stomach	Wedge	DWD 9
54.	53	F	Stomach	LLS	OD

APPENDIX X: 1974 LIVER TUMOR SURVEY—EN BLOC LIVER RESECTIONS (*Continued*)

	AGE/SEX	PRIMARY TUMOR	LIVER RESECTION	OUTCOME (MONTHS)
55.	58 F	Stomach	Wedge	DWD 8
56.	41 F	Stomach	LLS	AFD 50
57.	62 F	Stomach	LLS	AFD 16
58.	75 M	Stomach	Wedge	OD
59.	82 F	Stomach	Wedge	OD
60.	76 M	Stomach	Wedge	DWD 21
61.	61 F	Right colon	Wedge	AWD 52
62.	72 M	Right colon	Wedge	DWD 42
63.	75 F	Right colon	Wedge	AFD 22
64.	64 M	Right colon	Wedge	DWD 6
65.	75 F	Right colon	Wedge	DWD 18
66.	58 F	Right colon	Wedge	DWD 35
67.	69 F	Right colon	Wedge	AFD 51
68.	68 M	Right colon	Wedge	DOD 59
69.	69 F	Right colon	Wedge	DOD 137
70.	40 M	Right colon	Wedge	AFD 216
71.	82 F	Right colon	Wedge	DOD 2
72.	58 F	Right colon	Wedge	DWD 15
73.	39 M	Right colon	Wedge	AFD 7
74.	77 F	Right colon	Wedge	AFD 12
75.	33 F	Right colon	Wedge	AFD 12
76.	33 M	Right kidney	Wedge	AWD 7
77.	51 M	Right kidney	RL	DWD 10
78.	44 M	Right kidney	Wedge	DWD 11
79.	67 F	Right kidney	Wedge	AWD 36
80.	58 F	Right kidney	RL	OD
81.	6 F	Wilms' tumor*	Wedge	AFD 28
82.	4 F	Wilms' tumor*	Wedge	NFU
83.	5 M	Wilms' tumor*	Wedge	Alive, 20
84.	3½ M	Wilms' tumor*	Wedge	AFD 40
85.	17 F	Adrenal	RL	AFD 7
86.	68 F	Adrenal	Wedge	OD
87.	34 months F	Adrenal	Right lobe, left wedge	DWD 8
88.	30 F	Pericytoma	Wedge	AWD 52
89.	77 M	Esophagus	Wedge	OD
90.	52 F	Cervix (metastasis)	Wedge	DWD 15
91.	71 M	Lung	Wedge	DWD 17
92.	63 F	Lung	Wedge	AFD 2

KEY:
RL — Right lobectomy.
LLS — Left lateral segmentectomy.
AFD — Alive, free of disease.
DWD — Dead with disease.
DOD — Dead without disease.
AWD — Alive with disease.
NFU — No follow-up information.
OD — Operative death.
*Also had chemotherapy and/or radiation therapy.

**Cases reported by others: (See References, Chapter 10.)
4. May be in Warren and Hardy.[11]
22. Brasfield, et al.[2]
23. Brasfield[1]
24. Brasfield, et al.[2]

Index

Page numbers in *italics* indicate illustrations.
Page numbers followed by (t) indicate tables.